Nursing: Transition to Professional Practice

Nursing: Transition to Professional Practice

Edited by Rob Burton and Graham Ormrod

Series editor Karen Holland

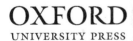
OXFORD
UNIVERSITY PRESS

OXFORD

UNIVERSITY PRESS

Great Clarendon Street, Oxford OX2 6DP

Oxford University Press is a department of the University of Oxford.
It furthers the University's objective of excellence in research, scholarship,
and education by publishing worldwide in

Oxford New York

Auckland Cape Town Dar es Salaam Hong Kong Karachi
Kuala Lumpur Madrid Melbourne Mexico City Nairobi
New Delhi Shanghai Taipei Toronto

With offices in

Argentina Austria Brazil Chile Czech Republic France Greece
Guatemala Hungary Italy Japan Poland Portugal
Singapore South Korea Switzerland Thailand Turkey Ukraine Vietnam

Oxford is a registered trade mark of Oxford University Press
in the UK and in certain other countries

Published in the United States
by Oxford University Press Inc., New York

British Library Cataloguing in Publication Data
Data available

Library of Congress Cataloging in Publication Data
Data available

Typeset by Glyph International, Bangalore
Printed in Great Britain
on acid-free paper by
Ashford Colour Press Ltd, Gosport, Hampshire

ISBN 978-0-19-956843-7

5 7 9 10 8 6

For Lorraine, Tom, and Sarah—
with love, Rob

With special thanks to Pat,
Jake, and Polly—with love, Graham

Series editor preface

Learning to be a nurse requires students to develop a set of skills and a knowledge base that will enable them to make the transition from learner to qualified nurse. As with any transition, this can often seem at times to be a daunting prospect, in the face of which the student may ask: 'How am I ever going to learn all that I need to know to get through this course and become a qualified nurse?'

For student nurses, this experience entails learning in 'two worlds': that of the university and that of the clinical environment. Although there is a physical distinction between the two, it is important that the learning that takes place in one is integrated with the learning in the other. This series of books has set out to do just that.

These 'two worlds' require that a student learns two sets of skills in order to qualify as a nurse and be ready to take on further sets of skills in whatever nursing environment he or she is employed. The skills that will be a core part of this series are numerous, and central to them is the idea of 'coping with the unknown'. Students face a new environment each time they start a new clinical placement, communicating with patients and a large number of health and social care professionals, dealing with difficult and often complex situations, and sometimes stressful clinical experiences. In the university, there are also situations that may be unknown, such as learning new study skills, working and communicating with others, searching and finding information, and managing workloads. It is every student's goal to complete his or her course with the required foundation for the future and it is the essential goal of this series to enable the student to develop skills for a successful learning and nursing experience.

The central ethos of all of the books in this series therefore is to facilitate and enhance the student learning experience and develop his or her skills, through engaging with a variety of reflective accounts, exercises, and web-based resources. We hope that you, as the reader and learner, enjoy reading these books and that the guidance within them supports your goal of successfully completing your course of study.

Karen Holland
Series editor

Preface

As you come towards the end of your nurse training, you will have developed the clinical skills needed to demonstrate your proficiency in your chosen field of practice. You will also have developed a greater awareness of and focus on the complex roles and responsibilities of the qualified nurse. In this book, you will find information, guidance, and exercises that explore the issues that you will experience as you become a qualified nurse. You will need to make decisions concerning both your own practice and the practice of others. Your scope of practice will include the need to make decisions concerning those for whom you are caring, their relatives and carers, the team with which you are working, and the wider interdisciplinary team. All of these areas will generate issues with which you will be expected to deal. The main aim of the book is to provide you with reassurance about these challenges by exploring aspects of practice such as accountability, legal and ethical decision-making, maintaining standards of care, being in charge, teamworking, and teaching others.

Related theories are discussed, deconstructed, and presented to provide a fundamentally practical approach to the types of situation that you will face, no matter what your chosen field of practice. Although this book is primarily designed to assist you in the latter period of your pre-registration course, it will also be invaluable for your initial post-qualification experience, with chapters devoted to areas such as your continuing professional development and getting the job that you want.

Producing the book has involved many people and we would like to thank the following for their kind assistance at various stages: Frank Mitchell for his input in the early stages of development and in shaping the ideas of the book; valued colleagues Nichola Barlow, Graham Thurgood, and Val Ely for their essential contribution; and Sheena Miller, Ruth Elliott, Karen Currell, and Jackie Vasey for the scenarios that they provided as food for thought. Special thanks to Karen Holland for her wise guidance, encouragement, and calming influence, and Geraldine Jeffers again for her patience, advice, and subtle prompts at various stages of writing!

Throughout the book, there are echoes of many people whom we have valued as role models throughout our careers, and students and colleagues too numerous to mention, who have inspired us with their experiences and aspirations. Thanks also to those who continually asked: 'How's the book going?' Thanks to you all for your support!

Lastly, we would like to thank our families for their patience and tolerance while we worked on the book.

Rob Burton and Graham Ormrod

Note: At the time of going to press, all URLs (both within chapters and in the references) were accessed and were working. If you find that this is no longer the case, please undertake a web search using key words from the URL.

Contents

Detailed contents

About the authors

The editors/authors

Dr Rob Burton is a learning disability nurse by background, having mainly worked with people with learning disability and challenging behaviours during his time in practice. He has worked in nurse education for the past 20 years, during which he has contributed in various roles, including course leader, to the development and delivery of the learning disability nursing branch and wider nursing courses, the MSc in Health Professional Education (a teaching course approved by the Nursing and Midwifery Council), and more recently a Professional Doctorate in Human and Health Sciences at the University of Huddersfield. Rob has a keen interest in learning, personal development, and leadership.

Graham Ormrod is currently Divisional Head for Acute Care at the University of Huddersfield, and has extensive experience in both teaching and management in nursing practice. Prior to joining the university, he had a number of roles at the Leeds Teaching Hospitals NHS Trust, including Divisional Nurse and Associate Director of Professional Development. He has a particular interest in enhancing student nurses' experiences and their burgeoning insight into their changing professional roles, ethical decision-making, and recognition of their accountability.

About the contributors

Nichola Barlow works at the University of Huddersfield and has been a nurse for 25 years. The focus of her clinical practice has been acute medicine and acute medicine for the older person. Nichola's areas of special interest within her current role as Senior Lecturer include nursing ethics, professional issues, nursing concepts, and care of the older person. She is also the course leader for a top-up BSc nursing course delivered in Malaysia.

Val Ely works at the University of Huddersfield and has been a nurse for over 30 years. Her early career was spent in surgery and operating theatres, and she was one of the first leaders in day surgery. Since being an educationalist for 20 years, she has specialized in teaching legal and professional issues, and has an MA in Healthcare Law. Her educational role has been exclusively in continuing professional development (CPD). She has taught and published in the non-medical prescribing field and has become recognized for being part of this initiative since its inception. Val's current interest remains in promoting the use of e-learning for CPD. A current project is focusing on the use of e-portfolios in healthcare education.

Dr Graham Thurgood originally qualified as a general adult nurse and subsequently as a district nurse working in nursing roles in both hospital and community settings. He has been a nurse teacher for both pre-registration and post-registration students in a variety of institutions in England and currently works at the University of Huddersfield. He has taught management at both undergraduate and post-graduate levels, developing a specific interest in management skills for nurses. He has an interest in the history of nursing, and has published in this and other areas of nursing. He is currently a Senior Lecturer for Adult Nursing.

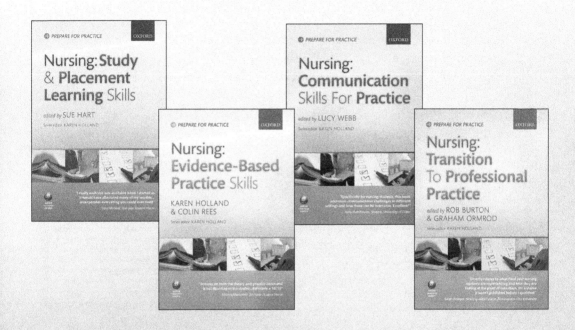

How to use this book

Nursing: Transition to Professional Practice explains the principles of professional practice and outlines the skills required by newly qualified nurses. This brief tour of the book shows you how to get the most out of this textbook and web package.

It's all new to me!

Find what you need fast! The detailed list of contents in the front of the book and the list of aims at the start of each chapter will help you to find what you need quickly.

What does that mean? Each new term is highlighted in colour in the text and explained in the glossary at the back of the book.

> of conduct (NMC, 2008b). This chapter will focus on the various qualified nurse and how this code impacts on them. It outlines nurse in maintaining safety and making ethically sound deci- the concept of ethics will be explored including maintaining a spirit of **beneficence** and **non-maleficence**, and making non-judgemental. Consent, **capacity**, and safeguarding the service users will also be investigated.

Helping you to develop your skills

Theory into action
These activities provide guidance on the underlying theory of professional practice (accountability, leadership, teamwork, etc) and are intended to help you to acquire the practical skills that are required for your academic assignments and your nursing practice.

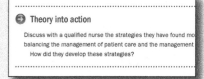

> **Theory into action**
>
> Discuss with a qualified nurse the strategies they have found mo
> balancing the management of patient care and the management
> How did they develop these strategies?

Key points
Essential facts, advice, and tips are highlighted to help you to understand particular issues and to avoid common mistakes.

> **Key points**
>
> If you suspect restraint is being used inappropriately you should
> to your mentor and/or your personal tutor.

Thinking about

Issues relating to professional practice (ethics, law, being in charge, or standards of care, etc) can be complex—these boxes encourage you to develop an awareness of key concepts and practices, and build your knowledge beyond an introductory level.

Thinking about

Imagine an occasion recently where you heard about something t[...] uneasy or worried; that you feel should not have happened. This [...] involves a patient or client who you have cared for or that you hav[...] fellow student or simply something you have heard on a news rep[...]
How did this make you feel? Why do you think you felt this way?[...]

Nursing scenarios

Realistic case studies help you to consider how the theory in the book can be integrated into practice.

Scenario 5.1

On arrival at the stroke ward Mrs Silcox became angry when the s[...] her husband's medications stating:

'This is the fourth time I have had to explain which tablets Bill t[...] me down. I have already told the nurse in casualty and the two d[...] there. Why can't you talk to each other? I'm sure the doctor wrot[...]

Summary mind maps and further information

Every chapter ends with a list of the most important points for readers to take note of and mind maps to aid easy review and revision. You'll then be prompted to visit the Online Resource Centre (where you'll find useful tools) before finding the references to supporting literature.

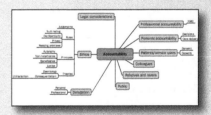

Online Resource Centre

Throughout the final year of the course, students need to make the most of opportunities to prepare for registration and job hunting—this book has a dedicated website to help you to get started. Just bookmark the site in your 'favourites' and go there when instructed to in the book:

www.oxfordtextbooks.co.uk/orc/burton/

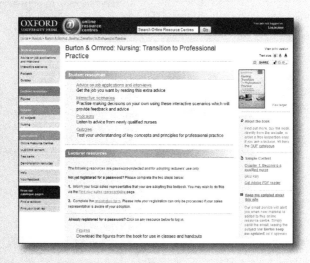

Students can:

- listen to advice from newly qualified nurses who have already made the transition—benefit from their experiences;

- get the jobs they want by reading our extra advice on job applications and interviews;

- practise making decisions on their own using our interactive scenarios, which will provide feedback and advice;

- take some of our quizzes to test their understanding of key concepts and principles for professional practice.

Lecturers can download the figures for the book and use the above resources in their classes.

Becoming a qualified nurse

Rob Burton and Graham Ormrod

The aims of this chapter are to:

- explore the expectations of a newly qualified nurse;
- highlight the experiences of newly qualified nurses;
- discuss the roles of the nurse in different fields of nursing;
- provide an overview of the structure and rationale of the book.

Introduction: how this book can help you to become a qualified nurse

Becoming a qualified nurse is quite an achievement. After three or four years of education involving academic and practice experiences, entering the nursing register of whichever field of nursing you qualify in is something to be proud of. The hard work pays off and you are able to become a professional in your own right. This does bring with it some challenges as well as rewards. You may now find that there are different expectations of you, and a set of roles and responsibilities that are different from those that you experienced as a student under supervision.

The aim of this book is to explore and develop important aspects of the roles and responsibilities of the qualified nurse in order to develop your understanding and to prepare you to successfully make the transition from student nurse to registered professional. It can also be used as a resource for those who may already be qualified and registered, but who are looking for helpful advice and are wishing to continue their professional development. The roles and responsibilities of a qualified nurse include essential professional skills such as:

- leading in care management and care delivery situations;
- maintaining standards of care;

- making ethical and legal decisions;
- being accountable;
- working in teams;
- teaching others.

The focus of the book is not about clinical practice, or the theory of nursing interventions or clinical nursing skills, because in order to become a qualified nurse these aspects should be addressed satisfactorily within the nursing course undertaken to demonstrate **proficiency (Nursing and Midwifery Council**, or NMC, 2010). The intention is to prepare you for the challenges that you will face on being a newly qualified nurse by providing the knowledge and skills required to become effective and accountable practitioners. Clinical decisions will still have to be made in relation to meeting the needs of the people within your care; however, becoming a qualified nurse brings with it wider responsibilities in making and taking decisions related to the nursing team, other staff, and the work environment as a whole. These changes require a large shift from the experience of being a student and a **mentored** supervised learner, so it is essential that you are equipped with all of the skills required to successfully make the transition. There are countless texts available on providing clinical nursing care, but there are few designed specifically to help final-year student nurses to develop the transferable professional skills necessary for the role of the registered nurse, and so this text sets out to assist final-year students by clearly outlining these.

The professional skills that you require as a nurse must be developed in a contemporary context in which nursing careers are changing radically with nurses now working in a wide array of new roles in a variety of healthcare settings. Today, you must be able to demonstrate these skills in job applications and interviews as well as develop employability skills for a career in which continuing professional development will be a key to success. Throughout your career, you may work in a variety of care settings and specialized nursing roles, but you will always require skills in teamworking, management, decision-making, and teaching.

The approach taken throughout the rest of this book will be to provide a discussion of the main theories, concepts, and issues related to the professional skills listed above. We will discuss the meaning of these concepts and their importance for nurses, and provide some practical contextual examples. Throughout the book, you will find exercises designed for you to read and reflect on the material presented and to encourage you to recognize how to use these in your own **field of practice**. Examples from all fields of practice will be used to illustrate the theories, with the inclusion of scenarios to illustrate how to consider and apply these to nursing practice. We also recognize that a pertinent issue in the transition from student to qualified nurse is that of getting a job and building a career, so skills such as preparing for interviews, interview skills, and continuing professional development are also included.

Changing expectations: from student to nurse

Many student nurses will tell you that their three- or four-year nurse education course passed quickly. Within that time, a student would have had a vast range of experiences and been exposed to many theoretical and practical aspects in their educational and practice settings. On qualifying, nurses are required to demonstrate a high level of knowledge, understanding, and application of high-order skills, not only with patients/service users, but also with other team members and those within, entering, and leaving the workplace. These are all skills that they should have developed in their three-year journey to qualifying and are also highlighted as required standards of proficiency (NMC, 2010). The NMC (2007; 2010) provides an account of such skills in its documents related to **Essential Skills Clusters**. These include essential aspects such as care, compassion and communication, organizational aspects of care, meeting needs such as nutrition and fluid management, infection prevention and control, and medicines management.

With registration comes a shift in professional accountability, together with wider clinical, management, and teaching responsibilities. On becoming a qualified nurse, the expectations and dynamics of relationships change, fundamentally. Suddenly, the newly qualified nurse is the one who must 'know the answer', whether it is a query from a patient, a carer, a work colleague or a student. The newly qualified nurse will encounter many challenging situations in which she or he must lead care delivery. This includes dealing with care management within the team, dealing with patients/service users, dealing with other professionals, and dealing with the required needs of the whole workplace environment. The NMC requires a student nurse to demonstrate professional values, communication skills, decision-making, and leadership, and show personal and professional development in order to join the register (NMC, 2010). It is recognized that nurses should be provided with some form of **preceptorship** and supervision in their role for a period of time (four months is suggested by the NMC, 2006) once qualified. Even with this period of preceptorship, there are new expectations and challenges faced by the newly qualified nurse.

Issues and expectations for newly qualifying nurses

Finfgeld-Connett (2008) describes the art of nursing as:

> dynamic and unique to each nursing situation. The art of nursing is shaped by measured risk taking and creativity that is employed in the face of uncertainty. Nursing as an art is actualised through relationship-centred care and is characterised by interpersonal sensitivity and intimacy. Artful nursing results in positive outcomes for both patients and nurses.
>
> FINFGELD-CONNETT (2008: 385)

These are interesting points. They focus on the nurse being able to take risks and show initiative underpinned by the skills of interpersonal communication. These aspects provide the fundamental basis of skills for the nurse in whatever field of practice they belong to. Currently, nurses undertake a three- or four-year programme, which is split 50/50 between theory and practice. In practice, student nurses are supervised throughout by approved mentors, associate mentors, and registrants (NMC, 2008b) to support the application of the theory to practice and to assess the competency and skills of the nurse in clinical health and social care settings. The NMC (2010) explicitly identifies that the qualifying nurse should be competent to practise safely. Therefore the experiences that nurses develop throughout their nursing course should be a vehicle for this. On qualifying, this competence is accepted as a given and highlights that the skills the nurse requires incorporate not only the need for clinical skills and knowledge, but also people and environmental management abilities underpinned by finely tuned interpersonal skills. In this way, the positive outcomes mentioned above for both service users and staff can be ensured. Although the qualifying nurse is given the remit to practise because of the need to meet these standards of proficiency, further and continuing professional development and training is also necessary to ensure that the nurse remains a competent and developing practitioner.

Before going any further, it is appropriate to reflect on one of our own experiences of becoming a newly qualified nurse (many years ago!).

> I had studied and practised hard for three years. Each year I had revised and prepared for my exams and undergone practical examinations. These aimed to demonstrate that the potential qualified nurse was clinically competent, just as the NMC require for those qualifying today. There were some questions and assessments related to managing the clinical area and I had had opportunity to lead shifts in the clinical area under supervision. All of these aspects had gone well. So, on commencing my first job as a qualified nurse, I felt very well prepared for the job with my main fears being related to perhaps being faced with clinical situations that I did not know the answer to.
>
> In my early weeks, I tended to work with more senior nurses and was expected to carry out tasks relevant to the qualified nurse (such as administering and dispensing medications, writing reports, giving handovers and general unit tasks) that had been delegated to me. After a relatively short period of time, the first shift that I was to be solely in charge of came around (these days there is a much more structured approach for preceptorship and support for the newly qualified nurse). The handover was given to me, and the all-important and symbolic 'keys' also handed over. As the previous senior nurse left the area, I was suddenly aware of the eyes of all of the staff on duty being trained towards me. No longer was there any other person for me to turn to for advice and each of these staff were now awaiting instructions in an expectant manner. This was a daunting experience.

I realised that my every move was now being scrutinized and assessed by every member of the team. I had to delegate duties to staff for the coming shift, some of which were less popular than others. This required me having to answer certain questioning staff as to why I had asked them to carry out these tasks (after all, it had been they that had done the same task yesterday!). My answers needed to be good! Over the coming weeks, I realized that it was not to be my clinical knowledge and skills that were put to the test as had been my initial fears; rather it was the tasks related to dealing with staff and aspects such as having to make difficult phone calls to distraught relatives or to other services and professionals where their input was urgently demanded.

I had to quickly develop assertiveness skills. I had to deal with situations such as staff squabbling amongst themselves, refusing to carry out tasks, emergency situations, running out of resources (such basics as there not being enough dinners available for the patients) and much more. I had to account to other professionals and staff why certain things had been carried out in a particular way or not, and defend decisions to others that perhaps I had not even made. I had to defend staff and patients as well as give bad news to patients/clients/service users.

Overall, the first year as qualified nurses was one of adjustment and was very different from our previous expectations. Therefore it might be useful at this juncture for you to reflect on your own expectations on becoming a qualified nurse.

....

➡ Theory into action

What are your expectations, concerns, and anxieties regarding becoming a qualified nurse? Identify positive and negative aspects.

....

A great deal of the literature and policy in place today highlight the fact that the context of health and social care is changing. This is going to require a significant change in values, attitudes, philosophies, and roles of nurses and other health and social care professionals. Nurses are one of the important groups of professionals who will have to respond to these changing roles. Although some years have passed, this quotation from *The NHS Plan* (2000) is still relevant, as it suggested that:

For the first time nurses and other staff, not just in some places but everywhere, will have greater opportunity to extend their roles.

DEPARTMENT OF HEALTH (2000: 6)

Issues such as the above are becoming expectations in today's current nursing roles. These include dealing with the complexity of an increasingly ageing population, and the increase of chronic health conditions such as obesity, and other health and social factors that affect people in being able to live independent lives. The changes are not just related to societal, demographic, and health/illness issues, but also to positive changes such as advances in medical, health, social, and pharmacological interventions, and the rapidly expanding integration of specialized technologies and communication systems and approaches. The Standing Nursing and Midwifery Advisory Committee (SNMAC, 2005) states:

> Advances in biomedical sciences and information technology have created approaches to medical care that extend lifespan, decrease chronic disease, and save the lives of the critically ill.
>
> SNMAC (2005: 2)

Each of these aspects provides nurses with new challenges. They need to be aware of the developments and, with them, the required changes in roles and practices, including the need to take on roles traditionally expected of other health and social care professionals and vice versa.

According to the report *Modernising Nursing Careers*:

> Nurses have taken on new roles, work across boundaries, and are setting up new services to meet patient needs.
>
> DH (2006B: 6)

This is not necessarily a new trend, as these changes in roles, boundaries and services have been slowly gathering pace since the late 1980s and before the inception of 'Project 2000' (United Kingdom Central Council for Nursing, Midwifery and Health Visiting, or UKCC, 1986) and the *Making a Difference* (DH, 1999) types of nurse preparation. The Royal College of Nursing (RCN, 2004) has argued that nurses are crucial in the changing emphasis in health and social care services, which are becoming increasingly person-centred and focused, in order to remove barriers to support for individuals and their families.

> Currently when a nurse qualifies she/he is expected to be competent to work in all environments and situations ... This emerging healthcare system requires a registered Nurse workforce, at all levels post initial registration, capable of critical reflective thinking in order to create this system.
>
> SNMAC (2005: 2–5)

The SNMAC (2005) position paper suggests that developing leadership skills in nurses (and midwives) is important for addressing the complexities of these changes in society and the health and social care systems within it. The Darzi review (Darzi, 2008) suggests that health services need to be fair, personalized, effective, and safe.

Nurses have an important role to play in ensuring that this is the case. They are often seen by the public as the main point of support while receiving care in their own homes or community or during hospital stays. It is therefore important that nurses fulfil their responsibilities and are confident in their roles. The main goal of nurses is to provide holistic health care for their patients/service users and their families while maintaining all aspects of the healthcare environment. This means communicating with, and at times managing, others around them, including other professionals as part of a multi-disciplinary team. The nursing profession is unique because of these characteristics, the interventions that nurses use, their knowledge domains, focus, value base, and commitment to working with others in partnerships (RCN, 2004).

Roles of qualified nurses in differing fields

Longley et al. (2007), on behalf of the NMC, have highlighted the changing provision of health and social care, the main areas in which nurses find themselves operating. Specialist services will become increasingly regionalized, whereas other common health needs will be met in local primary and community care settings. Increasingly, there are moves towards joint working between the National Health Service (NHS) and local government social care providers, as people who require some form of both health and social care support (such as people with mental health issues or people with learning disabilities) are been catered for mainly in community settings. There are currently four branches or fields of nursing in the UK—adult (Ad); children's (CH); mental health (MH); and learning disability (LD)—serving the different patient/client groups.

These fields are all bound by the same code of conduct (NMC, 2008b) and registered with the NMC. They have some very similar underpinning philosophies and some similar knowledge and skills. However, while sharing common nursing goals, each field is also very different, not least because of the client groups they serve, but in identity, environments, and in specific philosophies, attitudes, missions, knowledge, and skills. Just as the armed forces in the main comprise the navy, air force, and army, which have their own strongly defined identities, each with a common purpose (to protect the public and defend the nation) and some shared aspects (uniforms, discipline, and ranking etc.), but each having an entirely different set of values, approaches, and contexts within which they operate and in how they achieve their aims (namely, sea, air, and land), the fields of nursing each have similar but different dimensions too. Therefore there could be seen to be some overlap in the roles and responsibilities of the qualified nurse in the respective fields, although there will be some very specific differences. Below, we provide a brief description of the roles of qualified nurses in each field of nursing. These descriptions are taken from the NMC's 2004 standards of proficiency for pre-registration nursing education, however, they are still pertinent and appropriate today, when students must achieve both generic and field-specific competencies to register as a nurse.

Box 1.1 Adult nurses (NMC, 2004: 23, 24)

This area is concerned with the care of adults, from 18-year-olds to elderly people, in a variety of settings for patients with wide-ranging levels of dependency. The ethos of adult nursing is patient-centred and acknowledges the differing needs, values, and beliefs of people from ethnically diverse communities. Nurses engage in and develop therapeutic relationships that involve patients and their carers in ongoing decision-making that informs nursing care. Adult nurses have skills to meet the physical, psychological, spiritual, and social needs of patients, supporting them through care pathways and working with other health and social care professionals to maximize opportunities for recovery, rehabilitation, adaptation to ongoing disease and disability, health education, and health promotion.

Adult nursing could arguably be seen as the most recognizable field of nursing, particularly in the main public eye. It is the field of nursing with which most of the population has some contact in their experiences with the health services and forms the largest numbers. The Darzi review (2008) states that nurses' roles have changed greatly and that nurses are important in developing the new NHS with responsibilities to provide safe, high-quality, coordinated care. This takes place in acute and other hospital settings and a range of primary care and community settings. As Longley et al. (2007) point out: adult nurses will be involved much more in public health and preventative medicine as well as chronic health conditions. They will need to be responsive to patients' needs and expectations.

Box 1.2 Mental health nurses

Mental health nurses care for people experiencing mental distress, which may have a variety of causative factors. The focus of mental health nursing is the establishment of a relationship with service users and carers to help to bring about an understanding of how they might cope with their experience, thus maximizing their potential for recovery. Users may be cared for in a variety of settings, including the community and their own homes. They may require care for an acute episode or ongoing support for an enduring illness. Mental health nurses work as part of multidisciplinary and multi-agency teams.

According to the DH report *From Values to Action*:

> Mental health nurses (MHNs) are the largest profession working in mental health today. They make a vital contribution to providing care to service users of all age groups and in all settings.
>
> DH (2006A: 3)

Mental health nurses provide a service to those with mental health needs (and conditions affecting their mental stability) in a range of settings. There is a growing emphasis on supporting the service user in the community, although mental health nurses can find themselves in a range of environments, such as acute admission areas and secure environments. The DH (2006b) describes them as the backbone of mental health services, working in every type of service and involved in innovative projects designed to improve care. Longley et al. (2007) suggest that new ways of working in relation to the 'recovery' model is an aspect that will impact on the mental health nurse roles, and they will need to develop skills in responding to the changing approaches to mental health conditions such as Alzheimer's disease and dual diagnosis, while incorporating aspects related to human rights and mental health law into their practice.

Box 1.3 Learning disability nurses

The focus of learning disabilities nursing is influencing behaviours and lifestyles to enable a vulnerable client group to achieve optimum health, and to live in an inclusive society as equal citizens, where their rights are respected. Learning disability nurses work in a variety of residential, day, and outreach service settings, adapting the level of support that they provide according to the complex needs of the individuals, families, and carers with whom they are dealing, and the settings that they are in. Risk assessment and risk management are key components of their work and enable individuals to exercise their individual rights and choices.

Learning disability nurses have had to adapt to changing situations for many years, some of which have challenged or raised questions as to the role of the learning disability nurse. They have long since left institutional settings, as the client group they serve have been increasingly cared for in the community. It could be argued that they are the pioneers in the nursing profession for developing and being involved in interagency, community-based care, and joint working provision. The DH states:

> Learning disability nursing is a person-centred profession with the primary aim of supporting the well-being and social inclusion of people with a learning disability through improving or maintaining physical and mental health.
> DH (2007: 7)

Learning disability nurses are seen as the champions of people with learning disabilities, working in a range of health and social care settings with people with learning disabilities, their families, professions, organizations, and the wider community (DH, 2007). They will need to ensure more user and carer involvement in improving access to mainstream healthcare services and specialist support to increase the client group's involvement in community life (Longley et al., 2007).

Box 1.4 Children's nurses

The philosophy of children's nursing is based on the principle of family-centred care and the belief that children should be cared for by people they know and, wherever possible, within their home environment. Children's nurses understand the complex relationships between personal, socio-economic, and cultural influences on child health and child-rearing practices. Children's nurses work in a variety of settings, across and beyond traditional boundaries, and within a multidisciplinary and multi-agency team. In particular, they contribute to child protection, in collaboration with other key professionals, respecting and promoting the rights of the child.

The role of the children's nurse is to recognize the differences between children/young people and other groups of patients, and subsequently to acquire specialist knowledge and skills in order to care for children and young people. Healthcare professionals caring for children in a variety of settings are encouraged to be proactive in ensuring and advocating that services for children and young people are centred on the child/young person and their family. Longley et al. (2007) indicate that children's and young persons' nurses need to address public health concerns that are being identified in society today: for example, obesity. They will need to adapt their mode of delivery to meet the holistic needs of the child and their family, and assist them through transitions between services.

➡ Theory into action

At this point, take some time to reflect on the roles and responsibilities of the qualified nurse in the different fields. Whichever field you belong to, you may have had experience from placements during your training or by coming into contact with nurses from other fields in your work. Describe the types of patient/service user, the settings/environments in which they worked, and the roles they were undertaking. Identify the similarities and differences between the fields and compare them with your own.

As can be seen above, each field of nursing is a unique speciality. However, within each one there are sub-specialities in which the qualified nurse could choose to work and they can follow specific or broad career paths via their choice of specialization. These specialities recognize that the needs of each client group can be diverse. They can be acute or chronic, health or social-related, involve family members and other members of the multidisciplinary team or a multitude of agencies, and be community or hospital-based. The fundamental transferable skills that all newly qualified nurses require are a high level of communication skills as well as a highly developed awareness of the approaches that can meet the clinical health or social care-related needs of their patients.

Longley et al. (2007) state there will be a need for nurses to be flexible and take in increasing specialist and advanced roles in services in which there is a 'blurring' of boundaries. They will need to be responsive to patient/service user needs and work in teams with other professionals and services in changing contexts. Most of all, they will need to have high levels of knowledge, critical thinking, and **autonomy** at registration. To identify in detail the skills needed by each qualified nurse in their particular field and the requirements is too large a task for this chapter, but they can be found in the NMC's *Standards of Proficiency* (NMC, 2010). These standards set out the generic and field-specific knowledge and skills that nurses must all have and which must be demonstrated in each field before the qualifying nurse can enter the relevant part of the register.

In the final year of the pre-registration course, nursing students are required to demonstrate a high level of knowledge, understanding, and application of high-order skills, not only with the patient/service user, but also with other team members and those entering the workplace. During this period and indeed throughout their pre-registration course, student nurses are still closely supervised and supported in both their academic institution and practice settings. What is evident in scrutinizing the roles and responsibilities of a qualified nurse, to which their nursing education brings them, is that they need to be flexible and able to respond to the needs of their patients/service users in a variety of contexts. There is a need for the ability to work closely with other agencies and disciplines, and there is a need to underpin this with ethical principles and accountability in order to uphold and promote the rights of their patients/service users.

....

➡ Theory into action

Some key words to consider up to this point are: dynamic; unique; measured risk-taking; creativity; relationship-centred care; interpersonal sensitivity and intimacy; positive outcomes; person-centred; community; hospital; safe; effective; multi-professional; ethical principles; clinically competent; flexible; different contexts; rights; values; and specialized.

What do these words mean to you in relation to the role of the nurse?

....

Experiences of newly qualified nurses

With registration and a career as a qualified nurse comes a shift in professional responsibilities. On becoming a qualified nurse, the expectations and dynamics of these relationships change fundamentally. The NMC requires a student nurse to demonstrate professional and ethical practice, be competent in care delivery and care management, and show personal and professional development in order to join the register. This is a large leap from the culture of being a student and a mentored, supervised practitioner, so it is essential that student nurses are equipped with all of the skills required to successfully make the transition. As you can see from our earlier discussion about the differing roles of nurses in different fields, in which we highlighted the similar and different skills and knowledge required by the qualified nurse, the similar broad skills that can be applied to all fields can easily be developed.

Mooney (2007) found that newly qualified nurses were faced with assumptions from others that they should 'know everything'. This was also a high expectation they had of themselves. In meeting the NMC standards of proficiency, the nurse should have demonstrated the relevant knowledge and skills in order to practise in their relevant specialized fields. However, it is important to recognize that not every nurse knows everything about everything in their field, especially if they are practising in highly specialized fields. What they need is to be able to develop and adapt to changing situations. This is similar to the popular metaphor:

> Give someone a fish and they feed for a day, teach them how to fish and they feed for a lifetime!

Therefore, for the nurse, it is impossible to know everything, but they should have developed the skills to find out relevant information, reflect on it, and apply this to their practice. In essence, they should have learned how to learn. There is a great deal to be learned once qualified—especially related to a nurse's 'new' area of work—and a good deal of the development needs to take place 'on the job'. In another study, Lofmark (2006) found that final-year student nurses did find themselves with a good ability to provide care and with a high level of communication skills, teamworking, and a high level of ethical awareness. They stress that the notion of learning how to learn is essential and that staying abreast of developments in the clinical area is critically important.

Whitehead (2001) looked at the experiences of newly qualified children's nurses and found the nurses had concerns in relation to being uncertain about their roles. They also were anxious about taking on the responsibility and accountability. There were some concerns related to their confidence in their own knowledge and skills, and with issues related to management. Another study by Jackson (2005) suggested that a successful transition requires the nurse to develop a self-image relevant to the change in status, that they are be able to 'do the job', and that they meet the expectations of others, with appropriate support.

Mooney (2007) also points out that the duties faced by most newly qualified nurses were not patient contact-centred. There were a lot of duties related to contacting and dealing with other professionals and services. These brought anxieties related to the responsibilities that might be faced as the nurses would become increasingly senior in their roles, with others expecting them to provide the actions and the answers in complex situations. This highlights how the experience of nursing in transition from student to newly qualified nurse can be daunting. In the current environment, there is an expectation that nurses have a preceptor on qualifying to aid in these transitions, but the literature still suggests there is a difficulty in the transition process for such professionals. Gerrish (2000) found that individual accountability, managerial responsibilities (delegating duties without appearing 'bossy'), some challenging clinical situations, such as death and dying, and specialized technological roles were considered to be stressful by qualifying nurses. Issues of the preceptorship of newly qualified nurses become apparent and important in dealing with the transition from supervised student to autonomous practitioner.

⊝ Theory into action

Think of a member of qualified staff with whom you have worked. Describe their qualities in dealing with everyday issues, their clinical knowledge, skills, and abilities to manage people and communicate well with patients/service users and families. What were their attributes, and what were the main aspects of the role that you learned about from working with and observing them?

As already mentioned above, it is apparent that nurses work within different disciplines and fields, specialities, and contexts, and play an important role in health and social services. Change has been a constant in the health and social care services for many years and continues to rapidly develop in response to changing trends in health and societal situations, and the economic and political responses to them. Despite these differences, there are some roles and responsibilities underpinned with relevant theory that are applicable to all nurses and which should always be deemed so, regardless of how services and nursing are reconstructed.

Longley et al. (2007) suggest that healthcare futures, nursing futures, and nurse education futures are inextricably linked. A newly qualified nurse will face challenges in whatever situation they are employed. In analysing the situation in which nurses from all fields find themselves at the current time, one thing is clear is that nursing roles and responsibilities are constantly in a state of flux, having to respond to changing societal and healthcare issues. The newly qualified nurse of the future will not be entering employment into traditional roles. They need to develop skills that transcend the detailed knowledge and skills required to demonstrate that they are fit to enter the NMC register and therefore be eligible to practise as a qualified nurse.

This requires understanding and developing of the professional skills discussed above so that they can be utilized effectively at work by nurses from all fields in a variety of contexts. The following chapters of this book will focus on these aspects in detail, with discussion of the main theoretical underpinnings and practical application.

Professional skills: overview of this book

The focus in this book is related to the professional skills of:

- maintaining standards of care;
- making ethical and legal decisions;
- being accountable;
- teamworking;
- teaching others;
- being in charge.

It is recognized that there is a certain amount of overlap in these professional skills and that some concepts cross all of them, in that there are no clear lines drawn where one skill ends and another starts; however, there is still scope for scrutinizing the particular elements of each. Decisions and actions are taken by nurses in light of the environmental situations that occur in day-to-day practice. You would not usually consider each of the skills or concepts in isolation in relation to particular incidents and environmental situations, but would make a decision based on the factors contributing to the situation. However, when analysing any situation, the decisions made, and the actions taken, some of the individual conceptual principles may be recognized and highlighted. For example, asking a member of staff to complete a task on your behalf is delegating. This fits neatly into leadership theory and also relates to aspects of accountability. Such an approach is something that you may find yourself doing quite often. Completing a health and safety audit in the work environment might relate to management theory. This may be another responsibility you have to take on. Completing a review of an individual's care and setting goals for them in multidisciplinary meetings might relate to teamworking theory. Reporting of poor practices or environments might relate to aspects of accountability and maintaining standards of care. Demonstrating skills related to care needs to junior (or sometimes senior) staff might be considered as teaching and assessing.

However, all of the above aspects could arise from analysing one situation in which the nurse has to make decisions about a certain aspect of care management, consider the human and environmental resources, and report these aspects to their seniors or employers. Therefore all of these aspects are roles and responsibilities of the qualified nurse. The rest of this book will explore each of the following theoretical and practical aspects in more detail.

Chapter 2: Maintaining standards of care

It is important to maintain and develop standards as part of the responsibilities of a qualified nurse. These factors are still important in today's healthcare delivery services.

This chapter will cover the main areas that fall within maintaining standards and the umbrella of **clinical governance**. Aspects such as your responsibilities as a nurse in maintaining standards will be explored. The various bodies and organizations set up to monitor standards in areas in which you might find yourself working as a qualified nurse will be discussed. Relevant policy documents that influence standards of care will be explored so as to identify what they mean in real, practical terms.

Chapter 3: Accountability and ethical decision-making

Nurses abide by a code of conduct (NMC, 2008b). This chapter will focus on the various professional roles of the qualified nurse and how this code impacts on them. It outlines the responsibilities of a nurse in maintaining safety and making ethically sound decisions. Issues relating to the concept of ethics will be explored including maintaining confidentiality, acting in a spirit of **beneficence** and **non-maleficence**, and making decisions while remaining non-judgemental. Consent, **capacity**, and safeguarding the interests of patients and service users will also be investigated.

Chapter 4: Accountability, decision-making, and the law

The legal, professional, and ethical issues, and the decision-making approaches that need to be considered by a qualified nurse, will be discussed in this chapter. The nature of professional employment brings with it many obligations that a nurse must abide by, including aspects related to ensuring anti-discriminatory measures that form the basis of the nurse's practice. The concepts of nurses' responsibilities in relation to civil and criminal law will be discussed. Considerations related to personal and public liabilities will be explored in detail

Chapter 5: Teamwork: working with other people

It is certainly true to say that there are many sorts of team, some of which function better than others. This chapter will look at the ingredients of a good functioning team, how teams differ from simply collections of individuals and what skills are needed in team members. It will also explore how to subsequently lead and manage a team. There will be some discussion related to the formation and structure of teams as well as some exploration of the necessity for **interprofessional teamworking** that is an important factor. Again the established theories in this field will be explored, as will real life management scenarios and experiences both in the NHS and in education. Various roles of other key members of the multidisciplinary team will be highlighted.

Chapter 6: Teaching, mentoring, and assessing

A large part of the responsibilities of a qualified nurse are related to the development of themselves and others around them. This chapter will focus on the personal and professional development issues faced by nurses every day. It will include discussion related to setting outcomes, identifying needs, and taking action to meet them. Theories of learning, managing learning environments and teaching strategies will be discussed, so that the nurse can understand their role in developing themselves and others more clearly. Learning opportunities present themselves in practice every day and it is up to the nurse to seize those opportunities readily when they arise. The NMC has also published a document (NMC, 2008a) on the standards of teaching, mentoring and assessing in practice. The main aspects and requirements of this will be explored in real terms and its application to practice.

Chapter 7: Being in charge: leadership and management

This chapter will look at what it means and what it takes to make that transition from being a student one day to suddenly, the next day, finding out that you are the one who is supposed to be responsible not only for your own welfare, but also for the welfare of the patients/service users, staff, visitors, and anyone else who happens to access the service, whether it is in a hospital or community setting. The focus will be around theories and concepts that you might specifically need to consider when you are leading and managing in a care setting for the first time. It will also address concepts that can be used by the newly qualified nurse instead of having someone to turn to when things get difficult, and you suddenly find that it is others who are turning to you for answers. Leadership and management theories will be discussed to explore how they can help you to carry out one of your most important duties as a nurse.

Chapter 8: Getting the job that you want

The chapter will begin by exploring what interviewing for a job is really about. Success criteria of an interview will be discussed and reframed from the most commonly held misconception that success means 'getting the job' to success means 'getting the *right* job', which might not be the one for which you have just been interviewed. The chapter will next focus on getting the right job, beginning with the filling in of application forms and creating a suitable CV, through to preparing for the interview, dealing with interview 'nerves', and performing well at the interview. We will give some hints and tips for how to answer those awkward questions around the themes of the book. It will also cover how to deal with the 'nightmare' questions.

Chapter 9: Preparation for personal and professional development

Returning to the issues of personal and professional development, this chapter will build from the earlier teaching and facilitating chapter with more of a focus on yourself. Personal development planning and NMC requirements for further education and training will be discussed, including the concept of preceptorship, supervision, and important aspects and requirements related to continuing professional development. We will also touch on **coaching**, regarding how you can use specific goal-setting techniques to enrich your personal and professional life, and how this could then assist you in helping others in your field of practice and work. Future decisions about courses and choices will be explored.

Chapter 10: Preparing for qualification: putting it all together

This concluding chapter has exercises and examples, and will demonstrate how, although we have covered many separate themes, they all come together to form a holistic view of the roles and responsibilities of the newly qualified nurse.

. . . .

➡ Theory into action

Think back to some of the qualified nurses with whom you have worked. Apart from their clinical duties and tasks, in what other aspects have you seen them often involved? Make a list of these other duties and tasks. With regard to the concepts introduced above, which duties and which tasks more readily align with each concept?

. . . .

Starting the journey to becoming a qualified nurse

Successfully completing the nurse preparation course and becoming registered with the NMC may appear to be an end point. However, in reality, it is just the beginning of what could be a long career. An analogy would be that this is the point similar to that at which someone passes their driving test and can take sole control of a car without supervision. In your role as a newly qualified nurse, there may still be some provision of further supervision and support, but in the main, many decisions have to be made by you and you alone. Therefore this book aims to inform you of the considerations needed to make the transition to the role of a newly qualified nurse as smooth as possible. You will, of course, be supported in your transition, but it is not beyond the realms of possibility that you may be called on to demonstrate some of the shift leader and person management aspects within the clinical area in which you begin your career as a qualified nurse sooner rather than later!

The book can be used as a whole to read from beginning to end, or to look at particular sections in which you might be more interested, or you may wish to use it as a reference source. The accompanying exercises are designed to help you to reflect on the information provided and create some dynamic insights for you. Within the book, you will find advice, considerations, or theoretical direction to solve issues that you will come across in your qualified nursing career. Enjoy the journey you are soon to undertake!

Summary

In this chapter, we have looked at:

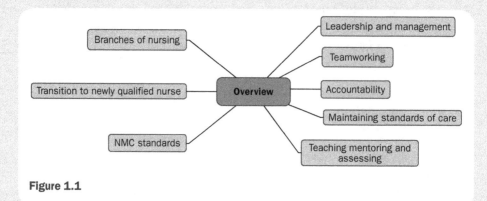

Figure 1.1

Online Resource Centre

 This textbook is accompanied by an Online Resource Centre that provides interactive learning resources and tools to help you to prepare for the transition from student to fully qualified member of staff. After you have completed each chapter and whenever you see this icon, please go to the ORC at your earliest convenience. If you have not done so already, save the ORC web address into your favourites: **http://www.oxfordtextbooks.co.uk/orc/burton**

References

Darzi, Professor, The Lord Of Denham (2008) *High Quality Care For All: NHS Next Stage Review Final Report*. DH, London.

Department of Health (1998) *A First Class Service: Quality in the New NHS*. DH, London.

Department of Health (1999) *Making a Difference: Strengthening the Nursing, Midwifery and Health Visiting Contribution to Health and Health Care*. HMSO, London.

Department of Health (2000) *The NHS Plan: A Plan for Investment, a Plan For Reform*. HMSO, London.

Department of Health (2006a) *From Values to Action: The Chief Nursing Officer's Review of Mental Health Nursing*. DH, London.

Department of Health (2006b) *Modernising Nursing Careers: Setting the Direction*. DH, London.

Department of Health (2007) *Good Practice in Learning Disability Nursing.* DH, London.

Department of Health (2008) *A High Quality Workforce: NHS Next Stage Review.* DH, London.

Finfgeld-Connett D (2008) Concept synthesis of the art of nursing. *Journal of Advanced Nursing,* **62**(3): 381–8.

Gerrish K (2000) Still fumbling along? A comparative study of the newly qualified nurse's perception of the transition from student to qualified nurse. *Journal of Advanced Nursing,* **32**(2): 473–80.

Jackson K (2005) The roles and responsibilities of newly qualified children's nurses. *Paediatric Nursing,* **17**(6): 26–30.

Lofmark A (2006) Competence of newly graduated nurses: a comparison of the perceptions of qualified nurses and students. *Journal of Advanced Nursing,* **53**(6): 721–8.

Longley M, Shaw C & Dolan G (2007) *Nursing: Towards 2015—Alternative Scenarios for Healthcare, Nursing and Nurse Education in the UK in 2015.* NMC, London.

Mooney M (2007) Professional socialization: the key to survival as a newly qualified nurse. *International Journal of Nursing Practice,* **13**: 75–80.

Nursing and Midwifery Council (2004) *Standards for Proficiency for Pre-registration Nursing Education.* NMC, London.

Nursing and Midwifery Council (2006) *Preceptorship Guidelines.* NMC Circular 21/2006. NMC, London.

Nursing and Midwifery Council (2007) *Essential Skills Clusters (ESCs) for Pre-registration Nursing Programmes.* NMC Circular 07/2007. NMC, London.

Nursing and Midwifery Council (2008a) *Standards to Support Learning and Assessment in Practice,* 2nd edn. NMC, London.

Nursing and Midwifery Council (2008b) *The Code: Standards of Conduct, Performance and Ethics for Nurses and Midwives.* NMC, London.

Nursing and Midwifery Council (2010) *Standards for Proficiency for Pre-registration Nursing Education.* NMC, London.

Royal College Of Nursing (2004) *The Future Nurse: The RCN Vision.* RCN, London.

Standard Nursing and Midwifery Advisory Committee (2005). *How to Ensure that Nurse and Midwife Education Keeps Pace with New Models of Care.* Position Paper. SNMAC, London, 1–8.

United Kingdom Central Council For Nursing, Midwifery And Health Visiting. (1986) *Project 2000: A New Preparation for Practice.* UKCC, London.

Whitehead J (2001) Newly qualified staff nurses' perceptions of the role transition. *British Journal Of Nursing,* **10**(5): 330–9.

Maintaining standards of care

Graham Ormrod

The aims of this chapter are to:

- explore your role as a student nurse in maintaining standards and ensuring quality of care;
- explore your subsequent role as a registered nurse in maintaining standards and ensuring quality of care;
- offer practical examples to illustrate key concepts and their application to nursing practice;
- investigate what is meant by 'good quality care'.

While reading this chapter, you will have the opportunity to discover how the experience gained on your placements can help you to contribute to maintaining standards of care. It will help you to develop competence in improving care delivery and management, and explore the mechanisms available to help to develop your authority to deliver and maintain high standards of care confidently.

Standards of care and the nurse's responsibilities

Maintaining and developing quality standards of care is an essential responsibility for all registered nurses. Indeed, the **Nursing and Midwifery Council** *Code: Standards of Conduct, Performance and Ethics for Nurses and Midwives* (NMC, 2008a) reiterates that each nurse must work with colleagues to monitor the *quality* of their work and maintain the safety of those in their care. Similarly, in the document *Framing the Nursing and Midwifery Contribution: Driving Up the Quality of Care* (Department of Health, or DH, 2008b) it is emphasized that nurses should take ownership of the quality of care and be accountable for delivery of the highest standards, while also ensuring that they have the 'authority, skills and mechanisms at their disposal to drive forward continuous quality improvement' (DH, 2008b: 5).

In the White Paper *Equity and Excellence: Liberating the NHS* (DH, 2010), the need to put a stronger emphasis on quality within health care is recognized and it confirms the work led by Lord Darzi in *High Quality Care for All: NHS Next Stage Review* (DH, 2008a)—this document is often referred to as 'the Darzi review'—that high-quality care cannot be delivered in the NHS (or indeed any care environment) without high-quality *nursing* (DH, 2008a: 17).

The coalition government emphasizes in *The Coalition: Our Programme for Government* (HM Goverment, 2010):

> We are committed to the continuous improvement of the quality of services to patients.

This confirms the emphasis and priority articulated by former Prime Minister Gordon Brown in the preface to *High Quality Care for All* (DH, 2008a):

> If the challenge 10 years ago was capacity, the challenge today is to drive improvements in the quality of care.

Similar aspirations are continually voiced by all political parties, as evidenced by the Conservative Party highlighting the plans for the National Health Service (NHS) to deliver some of the 'best healthcare in the world' (Conservative Party Manifesto, 2010: 45, in Lansley, 2010) and the Secretary of State for Health's speech to patients and patients' organizations as he reiterated that it was no longer sufficient to focus 'just on the volume of care but the quality of care, the performance and results' (Lansley, 2010).

It may seem quite odd that statements such as the above need to be made. Is this not obvious? Does it really need confirming that improving quality 'must be the basis of everything we do in the NHS'? (DH, 2008a: 11).

....

⊙ Theory into action

Write down five things that you feel impact positively on the quality and standards of nursing care. Then write down five things that you feel impact negatively on quality and standards.

Think about and write down how you might contribute to addressing these as a newly qualified staff nurse.

Would you expect patients/clients necessarily to have the same opinion on this as nurses?

....

According to Halligan and Donaldson (2001), historically, the NHS seemed to work with an implicit notion of quality—an assumption that if staff were well trained and good facilities and equipment were provided, then high standards of care would inevitably be achieved. Although there is evidence that the NHS has 'greater capacity and infrastructure to deliver good quality care than ever before' (Leatherman & Sutherland, 2008: ix) and evidence would generally indicate improvements in the quality of care for patients or service users (Healthcare Commission, 2008), clearly there are always areas of further improvement. Indeed, as Goodrich and Cornwell (2008) highlight, the defining feature of patients' experiences of care in all kinds of settings was that it was unpredictable and unreliable even hour by hour or shift by shift and ward to ward. Consultations still continue to highlight concerns regarding staff behaviour and attitudes to patients, with 'staff congregating in groups and seemingly ignoring patients' or staff being 'unfriendly and inattentive' (DH, 2008b).

Maben and Griffiths (2008) claim that there are very practical things that all nurses can do to ensure high-quality standards, thereby ensuring a positive experience for those for whom they are caring. They maintain that the essential starting point is always putting the patient/client first because patients want to be 'cared about' as well as 'cared for'. Box 2.1 lists some other fundamental contributions that all nurses can make to maintaining standards and ensuring good-quality nursing care according to Maben and Griffiths (2008).

During your various clinical placements, you will have begun to appreciate the contributions that you can make in many of the areas listed in Box 2.1. Students often spend the most time with patients/service users, assisting in the delivery of the fundamentals of care, and therefore can play an essential part in highlighting the specific requirements

---

Box 2.1 Essential contributions that you could make to ensure good nursing care

- Ensure that you are knowledgeable, skilled, competent, and possess up-to-date and expert knowledge.
- Keep patients informed and involved, encouraging involvement in decision-making.
- Respect privacy, confidentiality, and preserve dignity.
- Have a caring and humane attitude.
- Respect your patients' values and beliefs, and treat them equally.
- **Advocate** for, and listen to, patients.
- Ensure that clinical care is based on sound evidence.
- Identify areas for improvements in patient care and work towards strategies to solve them.
- Ensure effective communication and sharing of good practice across the multidisciplinary teams.
- Contribute to effective leadership where appropriate.
- Recognize that you and every other member of staff have a responsibility for high-quality care and maintaining standards.

and requests of individuals, and consequently ensuring more effective communication and subsequent advocacy. Similarly, you may be aware of the latest research and evidence in a particular aspect of care that you can share with your **mentor** and other staff to help to improve the experience of those for whom you are caring.

So what is high-quality nursing care?

What does it mean to say that a nurse or team of nurses delivered a high standard of care? Interestingly, Goodrich and Cornwell (2008: 22) in their research discovered that nurses and other health professionals struggled with the concept of 'good care' and 'almost universally' respondents said that it was not something they talked about with colleagues.

Key points

According to Maben and Griffiths (2008), there are six core elements to good-quality nursing care:

1. holistic approach to physical, mental, and emotional needs, patient-centred and continuous care;

2. efficiency and effectiveness combined with humanity and compassion;

3. professional, high-quality, **evidence-based practice**;

4. safe, effective, and prompt nursing interventions;

5. patient empowerment, support, and advocacy;

6. seamless care through effective teamwork with other professions. (How this might be achieved will be discussed further in Chapter 5.)

Maben and Griffiths (2008) also highlighted that nurses want many of the same things as patients and the public, the five main aspects being:

- making a difference to patients' lives;
- close contact with patients;
- delivering excellent care;
- working in a team and being a role model;
- continuous development with ongoing learning and improvement.

. . . .

➡ Theory into action

It has been said that some of the enduring qualities of nursing, such as care and compassion, have been lost and are now not demonstrated adequately by nurses. The implication seems to be that the humanity of caring and the more advanced technical tasks and roles that nurses are now undertaking are at polar opposites.

Do you agree with this? Consider and write down why you answered as you did.

. . . .

A brief history of quality in the UK health service

Your experience as a student will probably have helped you to form a perspective and opinion on what makes good-quality nursing care. However, to fully recognize where we currently are and where we might want to be in the future often requires looking back and reflecting on the journey. Think about this as we explore the history of 'the quality agenda' in health care.

It was initially assumed that the UK's National Health Service (NHS), as set up in 1948, with its fundamental welfare principles and aspirations of improving social justice, would *inevitably* result in quality standards of care being delivered. However, as time progressed, it became clear that this was not necessarily so. This realization came due to a number of reasons, not least the changing attitudes and priorities in society. For example, by the 1970s, some of the original aspirations of the welfare state in general and the NHS in particular were being seriously questioned for the first time (Crinson, 2009). This questioning coincided with a steep economic decline in the British economy in that period, leading to shortages and subsequent debates about whether valuable, but limited, resources were being used in the best ways. There was also a dawning realization that the NHS had become far more extensive and complex than originally envisaged and therefore could no longer meet the demands placed on it. The original intention to provide services that met a range of *basic* human needs had changed into a service that was required to cater for the far more complex personalized requirements of the population (Bradshaw & Bradshaw, 2004). Comparable economic pressures in other countries led to similar debates concerning social welfare generally and 'universal' health care in particular.

The election of the Conservative government in the UK under Margaret Thatcher in 1979 indicated a belief that the public services had become **paternalistic** and now had an unhelpful and inappropriate involvement in virtually all aspects of people's personal lives. The 'political' argument was that this created a culture of dependency, resulted in lack of choice in the services that were available, and, fundamentally, constrained individual liberty (Bradshaw & Bradshaw, 2004). Health was seen as an individual's possession and therefore ill health was seen to a large extent to be the fault of the afflicted thereby obscuring any problems arising from socio-economic conditions (Taylor & Hawley, 2010).

Public expectations were also starting to challenge the power of the professionals—in particular, doctors—and this challenge, and what is often called the rise of **consumerism**, resulted in demands for greater choice, more information in any decisions concerning health care, and also a greater accountability of those delivering the service. Harrison and McDonald (2008), however, highlight the possibility of tension between such consumerism and choice, on the one hand, and evidence-based practice, on the other. Simply put, the first suggests that people should have the services that they desire, while the second suggests that they should receive the services that, according to the evidence, are good for them (Harrison & McDonald, 2008: 150).

More and more during this period, health care began to adopt a philosophy that mirrored the world of business (Williamson et al., 2008), resulting in heated discussion of how health care could be run more efficiently, have greater financial accountability, and meet rising expectations. This subsequently led to profound changes in ideas of quality management. The effects of chronic underfunding had led to long waiting times and dilapidated premises, and despite the continued hard work and excellent care being delivered by many, this inevitably resulted in a great deal of hostile commentary in the British media. The shortcomings of the NHS at this time were undeniable, and yet the level of public support for the NHS remained constant (Talbot-Smith & Pollock, 2006).

Following the election of New Labour in 1997, it quickly became clear that one of the new government's priorities would be to attempt to address the concerns that the public had about the quality and standards of healthcare provision. *The New NHS: Modern, Dependable* (DH, 1997: 3.2), for example, promised that the service 'will have quality at its heart' and NHS organizations would have a statutory duty to ensure the quality of their services. Therefore NHS trust chief executives were now made *legally* accountable for clinical standards and each trust had to identify a designated senior clinician to ensure that systems of quality were functioning properly. Similarly, primary care trusts had to nominate a senior health professional to lead on clinical standards and professional development. These 'systems of quality' are often encapsulated under the umbrella term 'clinical governance'.

. . . .

➔ Theory into action

If you are not doing so already, you will probably soon be exploring the job opportunities that are available to you on qualification. If there are jobs available in the organization in which you would like to work, try to find out who is the senior clinician responsible for clinical standards and professional development. Discuss with your mentor what the current initiatives, priorities, and areas of good practice are for the organization.

Is there any information on the organization's website concerning this?

It is very likely that you will be asked questions related to the quality of nursing care at interview and this will be excellent preparation making you 'stand out' at interview. (This is discussed in detail in Chapter 8.)

. . . .

As a student, and soon to be registered nurse, you have a responsibility to recognize the 'systems of quality', reduce risk where possible, and practise in a safe and competent manner (Healy & Spencer, 2007). For example, infection control and reducing the risk of infection is the responsibility of all healthcare workers. Indeed, the Nursing and Midwifery Council (NMC, 2007) **Essential Skills Clusters**, which are designed to ensure safe and effective practice and promote the essential skills in nursing students, include infection prevention and control. Also included within this skills cluster is the expectation that, prior to entry to the NMC register, you will be able to ensure that colleagues are aware of and adhere to local policies concerning infection control procedures.

....

➔ Theory into action

On your final clinical placement, your mentor asks you to consider hypothetically that you are helping to mentor a junior student nurse. They ask you: 'What would you, as a mentor, expect them to know about the immediate remedial action following a needle-stick injury, given that, according to NMC Essential Skills Clusters, each student should have knowledge of this prior to entry to their specific field?'

What considerations would your answer include?

Some points to think about are listed below.

....

Points to consider for the theory into action box: Immediate remedial action following needle-stick injury

Your answer should have included considerations such as (Childs et al., 2009):

- bleed the puncture wound;
- wash the injury with soap and water;
- cover the wound with a waterproof dressing;
- report the injury to your manager;
- complete incident/accident documentation;
- identify the source patient if possible;
- report to occupational health immediately, or accident and emergency department if more appropriate;
- follow up if any testing is required;
- counselling may be advised;
- comply with any given advice.

Clinical governance

It is clear that the history of quality and maintaining high standards in health care is quite a long and complicated one. Let's look in more detail at the current context and explore further the concept of clinical governance.

As previously discussed, quality was initially felt to be an inevitable outcome of healthcare provision in the UK, but it became clear that this assumption was flawed and, by 1970s, for example, UK hospitals began to question and analyse their activity in a more structured way, considering issues such as quality, standards of care, and cost-effectiveness. As time went by, these quality-measuring activities were further supplemented by other ideas. For example, *The Patient's Charter* (DH, 1992) for the first time set out in a very clear way the *rights* that patients had in relation to NHS services and the standards that they could expect in relation to waiting times for operations, ambulance response times, the timely handling of complaints, and so on.

> You have the right to: have any complaint about NHS services (whoever provides them) investigated and to get a quick, full written reply from the relevant chief executive or general manager. The new complaints procedure means this will be within four weeks.
>
> DH (1992)

Also for the first time, each patient in a hospital was required to have an identified nurse to deliver and coordinate their care for the duration of their hospital stay or engagement with health services. Although some criticized many of the rights articulated in *The Patient's Charter* as being too easily achievable (Williamson et al., 2008), if nothing else, it represented a shift in thinking both for the public and also professionals. The historical management of resources and demands by a combination of waiting lists, 'gatekeepng' by general practitioners (GPs) and clinical **autonomy** of physicians was beginning to break down (Harrison & McDonald, 2008). High-quality health care was viewed much more as a *right* and an entitlement rather than a system in which patients were simply passive recipients of care. Not only were such standards introduced, but they were also published, showing how well various organizations were doing in comparison with others. These were presented in the form of 'league tables', highlighting the increasing aspect of 'comparison and competition' in health care and also hinting at the future of patient choice and greater patient and public involvement in healthcare (Bradshaw & Bradshaw, 2004).

Supporters of greater patient and public involvement present the ideal as a shared decision-making model (Crinson, 2009) and highlight certain key characteristics, including that both the patient and the doctor or health professional are involved and share information to build a consensus about the preferred treatment. However, many studies indicate that there is little evidence that this participation in the consultation process occurs (Stevenson et al., 2000; Rogers et al., 2005). Indeed, at best in many cases, patient self-management essentially constituted nothing more than compliance with medical instructions. Similarly, Smith (2001) questioned any developments that might challenge medical autonomy as they inevitably imply distrust of doctors and attempt to replace this trust in the individual with a supposedly more objective trust and confidence in systems: for example, guidelines and performance indicators. This, according to Smith (2001), fractures the therapeutic moral content of the client–practitioner relationship.

However, in theory, not only could patients appropriately expect universal or consistent standards irrespective of where they came in contact with health care, but they could also expect that *all* healthcare practice be supported by sound, current, and robust evidence. According to Hicks (1997), evidence-based practice occurs when decisions that affect the care of patients are taken with regard to all valid, relevant information. This recognizes that research and evidence is only of any real use when it appropriately influences the real world of patient care. It also places an emphasis on 'value for money', clinical effectiveness, and recognizes the importance of **clinical audit** in maintaining and improving practice. While evidence-based practice might be viewed as a common-sense aspiration, not least because the alternative might be random practice or ignorance-based practice and ineffectual practice (Harrison & McDonald, 2008), it is not without its criticisms. Taylor and Hawley (2010), for example, highlight that the guidelines generated by evidence-based practices such as clinical trials, which are subsequently assessed and identified by coordinating bodies such as the National Institute for Health and Clinical Excellence (NICE) as worthy of support by the state healthcare system, can be seen as a way to place limits on what is offered and can therefore be viewed as a form of rationing. Crinson (2009) claims that NICE has actually made very few recommendations to exclude interventions that it had been asked to appraise with regards to patient safety and yet it has frequently recommended the use of cheaper forms of treatment where more expensive ones were judged to provide little or no benefit. However, paradoxically, according to Appleby and Harrison (2006), costs generally under the auspices and advice of NICE are actually increasing and not reducing. Despite these concerns, it is clear that there have been a number of quality initiatives focusing on standards in different aspects of the patient journey. Clinical governance is an amalgamation of all of these initiatives (Ayres, 1999).

Key points

Clinical governance is not a brand new initiative, but a bringing together of several other initiatives under one term.

Definitions of clinical governance

There are many definitions of clinical governance and one of the most famous was included in the 1998 consultation document *A First Class Service: Quality in the New NHS*:

> A framework through which NHS organisations are accountable for continuously improving the quality of their services and safeguarding high standards of care by creating an environment in which excellence in clinical care will flourish.
>
> DH (1998: 33)

According to the Royal College of Nursing (Currie et al., 2003) clinical governance is:

> a framework which helps all clinicians—including nurses to continually safeguard and improve standards of care.

Key points

Unfortunately, there continue to be examples of poor (and worse) practice within some services in the UK. Here are three links to webpages that highlight examples of where the system has 'gone wrong' and the quality of care has been less than patients/clients deserve.

- The Healthcare Commission's report into emergency services at Mid Staffordshire NHS Foundation Trust in March 2009: access **http://www.cqc.org.uk/** and search for 'Mid Staffordshire' to discover the complex aspects of this tragic series of events.

- Issues highlighted by the 2008 Community Mental Health Service Users Survey, which indicate a lack of or limited client involvement in their own care in some areas: access **http://www.cqc.org.uk** and search for 'supporting briefing note'.

- The Ombudsman's (2009) report *Six Lives: the Provision of Public Services to People with Learning Disabilities*: access the Local Government Ombudsman website **http://www.lgo.org.uk/** and search for 'Six Lives'.

Clinical governance is fundamentally about quality of care. It is about making sure that care delivered is safe and patient-centred. Although *all* nurses would probably see this as an important responsibility to aspire to, in many ways, issues of clinical governance can feel very removed from a nurse's daily activity, and therefore it may be quite easy for nurses to feel that clinical governance has nothing to do with them and is simply the responsibility of 'management'—management that is often seen by clinical staff to have different responsibilities and priorities than the day-to-day aspects of patient care. This perception can quite easily be the case for student nurses and newly qualified staff who are unsure of their status and authority, and their role and involvement in clinical governance. Indeed although there was no overt regulation of health professionals inherent in the clinical governance framework, there was an implied demand that encouraged healthcare staff to think in wider strategic terms about resources and efficiency, indicating a belief that they had previously only viewed their roles at the level of individual health professionals treating individual patients (Crinson, 2009).

It is important to recognize that *all* nurses have a significant role to play within clinical governance, as they have a duty to provide individual care of high quality and are expected to practise this wherever they work. In fact, the majority of nurses know and practise clinical governance daily, as it is embedded in their professional values and general concern for others. Something as simple as ensuring that you have communicated information concerning a patient or client fully and appropriately to a more senior colleague is evidence of adhering to the principles of clinical governance. This apparently straightforward activity helps to ensure a high-quality experience for patients by encouraging consistency, reducing risk, and promoting safety.

· ·

⊙ Theory into action

One of the ways in which services and/or care can be improved is by auditing practice. What examples of audits have you seen on your placements?

· ·

Points to consider

Examples of audits regularly used in clinical practice include:

- handwashing audits;
- pressure sore audits;
- nursing documentation audits;
- health and safety audits of various types;
- bed occupancy audits;
- audit/benchmarking utilizing *The Essence of Care: Patient-focused Benchmarking for Health Care Practitioners* (DH, 2003).

Essence of Care

Patient-focused benchmarks for clinical governance (DH, 2001)

The NHS Plan (2000) reinforced the importance of 'getting the basics right' and of improving the patient experience. The 'Essence of Care' (EOC) was introduced to provide a tool to help nurses and other practitioners to take a structured approach to sharing and comparing practice. *Benchmarking* is essentially a means of comparing current practice against a standard. It provides a range of indicators for best practice, and it also encourages the development of plans for addressing poor practice. Nurses work together in a supportive way, auditing and assessing their team's current practice, exploring the evidence of what is best practice and therefore what changes are needed to improve. EOC hopes to thereby thus promote teamwork, networking between different areas, and the sharing, celebration, and learning from good and innovative practice.

The stages involved in benchmarking are as follows (DH, 2001).

- Stage one: Agree best practice
- Stage two: Assess current practice in the clinical area against best practice
- Stage three: Produce and implement an action plan aimed at achieving best practice
- Stage four: Review achievement towards best practice
- Stage five: Disseminate improvements and or review action plan
- Stage six/one: Agree best practice

The areas benchmarked include: principles of self-care; personal and oral hygiene; nutrition; communication; continence and bladder and bowel care; pressure ulcers; safety of clients with mental health needs; record-keeping; privacy and dignity; health promotion; and care environment.

As a student and also a newly qualified staff nurse, it is important that you recognize the significance of the EOC benchmarks and how they not only highlight quality standards of care, but also relate to other essential considerations such as the NMC standards of **proficiency** (NMC, 2004/2010). For example, one of the 'agreed outcomes' of the benchmark for communication, *Benchmarks for Communication between Patients, Carers and Health Care Personnel*, in the EOC is that:

> Patients and carers experience effective communication, sensitive to their individual needs and preferences, that promotes high quality care for the patient.

Similarly, a standard of proficiency for entry to the register insists that students must be able to show that they can communicate safely and effectively with individuals and groups of all ages, using a variety of complex skills and interventions (NMC, 2010). Therefore, knowledge and understanding of initiatives such as the EOC will help you to demonstrate that you have achieved such NMC competencies.

....

⊙ Theory into action

In October 2007, benchmarks were issued covering the care environment. The first benchmark included 'the agreed patient outcome' that 'people are confident that the care environment meets their individual needs and preferences'. The second benchmark rates environment/culture, whereby the atmosphere might range from feeling uncomfortable, afraid, ignored, vulnerable, and abandoned, to feeling comfortable, safe, reassured, confident, and welcome.

Access the *Essence of Care* document (by going to the Department of Health website **http://www.dh.gov.uk** and searching for 'Essence of Care'). There are 13 suggestions for discussion for the second benchmark (see Box 2.2). Discuss with your mentor how these might be implemented in your placement area.

....

Box 2.2 Indicators of best practice: opportunity for communication (DH, 2003)

- Patients and or carers who are physically isolated or unable to communicate directly with significant others are enabled to communicate.
- Patients and or carers have choice about where they exchange information.
- Restrictions to communication are explained.
- Assessment of the needs of patients and or carers identifies where and when communication should take place.
- The inclusion of other people when communication occurs is agreed with the patients and/or carers.
- There is an appropriately furnished, separate and specially designated room.
- The environment is inclusive and adapted to meet differing communication needs in terms of, for example, lighting, acoustic conditions, hearing loops.
- The environment supports communication and audit of the environment, including signage and maps to present information.
- Appointment times are arranged to facilitate communication.
- Mechanisms are in place to ensure necessary follow-up appointments are made.
- Advocacy services are engaged according to the wishes of patients and/or carers.
- Patients and or carers are identified in order to discuss treatment and care when face-to-face communication is not possible, for example by using a password system.
- Communication between patients and/or carers and healthcare personnel is recorded.

The NHS Modernisation Agency, which was established in April 2001 (replaced by the NHS Institute for Improvement and Innovation in 2005) to provide support for modernizing and improving services, claimed that clinical governance was an attempt to create a modern, safe, consistent, patient-led health service. According to Bradshaw and Bradshaw (2004), public confidence had been damaged by incidents such as the investigation and subsequent conviction of the GP and serial killer Dr Harold Shipman, the poor outcomes within paediatric cardiac surgery at Bristol Royal Infirmary (Kennedy, 2001), and the retention of children's organs without consent at Alder Hey Children's Hospital.

Theory into action

For information concerning the above-mentioned high-profile, tragic, and influential events, visit the following.

> http://www.the-shipman-inquiry.org.uk/home.asp
> http://www.bristol-inquiry.org.uk/index.htm
> http://news.bbc.co.uk/1/hi/1136723.stm

Access these resources and discuss their implications with your mentor. What systems and procedures are in place to reduce the likelihood of such things happening again?

As a newly qualified staff nurse, what would you do if you were to become aware of such circumstances happening in *your* practice area?

Such incidents as mentioned above indicated that the NHS was unable to deal effectively with staff who were not performing or undertaking poor practices, and in consequence, patients were left vulnerable and unprotected. Even if this poor practice *was* recognized, these and other incidents seemed to indicate that there was either an inability or a reluctance to do anything about it. Clinical governance was (and is!) an attempt to address this apparent lack of accountability and to reduce the likelihood of future failures (also see Chapters 3 and 4, which cover the issues of accountability in detail). This continues to be essential for all nurses and other health professionals as the delivery of health care continues to change with public expectations, new technologies, policy initiatives, workforce planning, and many other issues contributing to the speed and direction of the change.

Scenario 2.1

The case of nurse Colin Norris, found guilty in March 2008 of murdering four elderly female patients while working in hospitals in Leeds UK, indicates that, despite certain systems being in place, vigilance is still essential. The inquiry report is available at **http://www.yorksandhumber.nhs.uk/document.php?o=4328**

The report is at pains to emphasize that the responsibility for the intentional harming and subsequent deaths of the patients rested with Norris, and that it is always going to be difficult for an organization to design and implement systems and processes that will totally eradicate the risks posed by someone who has such an intent. However, there were also criticisms of the systems in place and subsequent recommendations made. For example, the report recommended an audit of the omission of administration of drugs prescribed, and also raising awareness of the policy for acting on information and concerns expressed by relatives.

The NHS Plan (2000) was the landmark document produced by the Labour government highlighting its vision of this direction of change. This document highlighted a massive ten-year reform of the NHS, with setting and monitoring standards as a central theme. *The Plan* attempted to set in place structures to improve efficiency, effectiveness, access, and quality of services. As Bradshaw and Bradshaw (2004) explain, the strategies chosen by the government concentrated on the formulation of national standards, performance indicators, audit, and inspection. Part of this was to create new structures, bodies, and guidelines to enable the plan to work. These included the setting up of the Commission for Health Improvement (CHI), NICE, the Modernisation Agency, and the introduction of national service frameworks (NSFs) to set minimum standards and expectations for key areas of health.

As we shall see, many of these initiatives have, as you would expect, changed and developed as time has progressed; however, many of the fundamental principles behind their formation—for example, the setting and monitoring of standards—remain at the heart of their purpose. As your career develops, doubtless you will witness further reform of these initiatives in due course, but it is certain that future reform will retain some or all of the central values and aims that you see today. It is important to recognize the significance of initiatives such as these. Not least because the NMC (2008b: 26) highlights in its *Standards to Support Learning and Assessment in Practice*, that students must be able to identify ways in which policy impacts on practice and learn within a context that reflects healthcare policies.

Similarly, the NMC Code (2008a) insists that, as a registered nurse:

> you must take part in appropriate learning and practice [*sic*] activities that maintain and develop your competence and performance.

It also requires that:

> You must act as an advocate for those in your care, helping them to access relevant health and social care, information and support.

Undoubtedly, recognition of the wider healthcare context and knowledge of any changes in national and local policies or procedures is necessary to fulfil these and other aspects of the Code.

....

⊖ Theory into action

How you can ensure that you stay up to date with any new reforms or policies?

....

The key role of the charge nurse in maintaining standards

As discussed throughout this chapter, maintaining standards is the responsibility of all staff; however, in the document *Breaking Down Barriers, Driving up Standards* (RCN, 2009), the Royal College of Nursing recognizes the crucial role of the sister and charge nurse in maintaining standards of patient care. It emphasizes that a strengthening of nurse leadership has a positive impact on quality performance and improved standards of patient care. As the Hay Group (2006) also highlights, however, good and effective leaders require more and different qualities from those that are traditionally perceived as important for a nurse. Kindness, empathy, and a caring attitude are not enough on their own to be successful in a 'management' position. To encourage improvements in standards, sisters/charge nurses or managers need to move away from styles of working with others that aim only to create harmony and a friendly working environment, and by their motivation, influence, and development of team members balance these with being able to deploy styles that provide long-term direction, engagement, and a focus on these standards. This, according to the Hay Group (2006), will ensure that *all* staff are stronger and better able to take decisions and run the ward or unit effectively, even when the charge nurse or manager is not around. The research appeared to find correlations between effective charge nurse leadership, patient outcomes and staff performance such as: lower rates of medication errors; higher levels of patient satisfaction; and lower staff absence, and sickness rates (Hay Group, 2006). However, evidence from the RCN indicated that the pressure placed on charge nurses or sisters from looking after and nursing a group of allocated patients on every working shift, in addition to their leadership responsibilities, has made it very difficult for them to appropriately lead, manage, and *supervise* clinical practice and the ward environment.

According to the RCN (2009), charge nurse/sisters must be supervisory to shifts and therefore be:

- enabled to oversee standards of care delivery and the ward environment;
- more visible to patients, staff, doctors, and other visitors as the nurse leader and the person in charge;
- allowed to set appropriate standards;
- encouraged to know their patients and their healthcare needs;
- able to teach clinical practice and procedures;
- a good role model for good professional practice and behaviours.

....

Thinking about

- What do you think of the RCN guidelines?
- Do you agree that these changes would have a positive impact on patient care?

● In your experience, has the charge nurse/sister played a significant role in maintaining the standards of care in the environment in which you have worked?

● How do you think the ward/department charge nurse/sister can impact on more junior staff's ability to 'run the ward effectively, even when she is not around'?

(This is further discussed in Chapter 7.)

This crucial leadership role is also highlighted in *Front Line Care: The Future of Nursing and Midwifery in England* (Prime Minister's Commission, 2010).

The use of nursing measures or metrics in maintaining standards

Griffiths et al. (2008) discuss how the nursing profession might more consistently provide high-quality standards for all. Their conclusion is that caring and the patient experience needs to be reiterated as the central aspect of nursing. This may be accomplished by the establishment of an agreed set of nursing measures or 'metrics', which can value and measure the nursing contribution to health care. According to Maben and Griffiths (2008), nurses need to act as 'guardians of care quality' and the patient experience, and embrace a new professionalism to re-establish the values, behaviours, and relationships with patients. These changes and values are reiterated in *Framing the Nursing and Midwifery Contribution: Driving up the Quality of Care* (DH, 2008b), which acknowledges the variability in the standards of care throughout the country and challenges nurses to improve the quality of the care as 'guardians' by 'strengthening leadership, developing methods of assessing their contribution, defining accountability and identifying supportive structures' (DH, 2008b: 5). Nurses need to have the authority, skills, and mechanisms to drive forward quality improvements and take lead responsibility for the quality of care.

So what are nursing metrics?

Metrics are an attempt to develop a set of measures to identify and quantify the quality of nursing care. They can involve:

● safety;
● effectiveness;
● compassion.

The metrics are designed to provide information to help to improve nursing care and demonstrate to nurses that nursing care quality can be defined and measured. They are not used in isolation, but in conjunction with other quality initiatives that focus on *outcomes* and encourage the measurement and achievement of the goals of nursing and attempt to encourage flexibility to judge the best way in which to deliver nursing outcomes across different settings and practice areas.

Key points

Metrics may be used to measure practice in relation to areas such as:

- staffing levels;
- medication administration errors;
- pressure ulcers;
- falls;
- healthcare-associated infection—pneumonia;
- staff satisfaction and well-being;
- healthcare-associated infection—urinary tract infection;
- staffing skills mix;
- sickness rates;
- the use of restraints.

There is growing evidence that the use of measurable quality indicators can significantly improve the quality of care. So what does this mean in practical terms? If a metric were used in relation to falls for example, it would be likely to include such aspects as the following.

How a falls assessment metric works

Assessment on admission

- All patients will receive a falls risk assessment on admission to the trust, which is dated and signed by the assessing nurse.
- Care plans to minimize falls will then be completed for all patients assessed as being at risk.
- A further assessment will be undertaken for all patients identified as being at risk.
- All risk assessment documentation will provide details of ward, patient name and date of birth, hospital number, and date.
- A bedrail assessment should be undertaken on all of those patients identified as at risk.

Management of the process

This will include procedures such as monitoring of the clinical results on a monthly basis.

- This would ensure a minimum of 50 per cent of all patients would be monitored.
- It would then be reported and used as feedback to clinical areas and charge nurses/matrons.

- Finally it would be used as feedback 'up' the organization by reports to governance committees, for example.

Outcomes

The hoped for outcomes of this would be:

- a reduction in patient falls;
- resulting in improved quality of care and reduced length of stay if in an acute hospital;
- improved patient/client satisfaction and feedback;
- compliance with NICE and the National Patient Safety Agency (NPSA).

Theory into action

Considering the areas mentioned above, can you consider how a metric might 'look' in relation to medication errors or staff satisfaction, for example? With your mentor, consider such areas using a similar template to the falls metric above.

The Care Quality Commission (formally known as the Commission for Healthcare Audit and Inspection or the Healthcare Commission)

A fundamental aspect of maintaining standards and quality has been the setting up of an organization to *inspect* practice and health services. The history of this role and the organizations set up to fulfil it has included several changes, not least in their names.

Initially, in 2000, this role was undertaken by the Commission for Health Improvement (CHI). The overall aim was to highlight areas in which the NHS was working well and identify areas that needed improvement. Each trust had to ensure that clinical governance systems were in place and recognize and act on targets. Some of these targets were set within NSFs (see below). In 2004, the organization retained its fundamental role in maintaining standards, but changed its name to the Commission for Healthcare Audit and Inspection, or the Healthcare Commission

From 1 April 2009, a new organization, with the same role, called the Care Quality Commission (CQC), was made responsible for regulating health and social care in England. The CQC took over the roles of three organizations:

- the Healthcare Commission;
- the Commission for Social Care Inspection;
- the Mental Health Act Commission.

The latest organization is an attempt to address the need to bring the functions of social care and health services much closer together under one independent regulator. This is now one 'port of call' for people using these services and their carers and families, and one source for information on standards, safety, and the services that are provided. Such bodies have been questioned due to their apparent 'surveillance' and/ or 'controlling' role (Harrison & McDonald, 2008), and their desired impact on the performance of local healthcare organizations has also been questioned (Crinson, 2009). However, as highlighted in *Equity and Excellence: Liberating the NHS* (DH, 2010), there is an intention to further strengthen the role of the CQC as an effective inspectorate of quality provision.

Key points

In the report *Six Lives: The Provision of Public Services to People with Learning Disabilities*, the ombudsman was critical of the failure of trust staff to engage with community staff to ensure that a multi-agency plan was in place for the discharge of Mr Hughes.

Mr Hughes was a 61-year-old man with severe learning disabilities, who had lived in care for most of his adult life. He was admitted to hospital, where he eventually had an operation on his prostate. Post-operatively, Mr Hughes became very unwell and spent 12 days in the intensive care unit. Eventually, he returned to the ward and was subsequently discharged back to the care home at 8 p.m. two days later. The following day, 20 minutes after a meal, Mr Hughes became very unwell and, after an ambulance was called, he was admitted to the emergency department, but died an hour later. Mr Hughes' sister, who complained about some of the care her brother received, felt that staff at the trust 'just did not want him there because he was more difficult', 'wanted rid of him', and 'pushed him out'. She also claimed that some of the healthcare professionals involved in Mr Hughes' care 'thought he wasn't worth saving'. These considerations led, in her opinion, to an inappropriate discharge, which subsequently contributed to her brother's death.

Following investigation, the ombudsman found that neither the doctors nor the nurses acted in accordance with professional standards, as staff on the ward did not take sufficient account of Mr Hughes' needs as a person with learning disabilities and that his discharge was premature and poorly planned.

(The report is available at: **http://www.lgo.org.uk/search/?k=six+lives+Keohane**)

💡 Thinking about

Why do you think it has been seen as essential to bring social care services and health services closer together?

What role do you think nurses have in ensuring that social care staff and healthcare staff work closely together to improve the experience of patients?

A key role of the CQC is to inspect and regulate the services provided for patients and clients, and it thus serves as England's healthcare watchdog. It checks the quality and safety of health care provided by the NHS and independent organizations, and assesses and rates 'performance'. It then provides information about the standard and quality of care and how these might be improved, thereby reducing inequalities and what is often called 'the postcode lottery'.

The functions of the Healthcare Commission were set out in the Health and Social Care (Community Health and Standards) Act 2003, which gave the Secretary of State for Health the power to set standards and clarified the role of the Commission in undertaking an annual review of the provision of health care by each NHS body in England. The government also recognized that legislative changes were necessary to bring the independent sector in line with the NHS to ensure that the independent and NHS sectors were being judged against the same standards. The CQC now operates under this legislation.

The Care Quality Commission's inspection function

Since 2005, the CQC has undertaken the 'Annual Health Check' to assess how well each trust in England is doing. Members of the Commission can also make unannounced visits to check on certain initiatives, such as older people being assisted with their fundamental needs and being treated with respect and dignity.

....

 Theory into action

The Dignity in Care campaign aims to 'stimulate a national debate around dignity in care and create a care system where there is zero tolerance of abuse and disrespect of older people'.

Access **http://www.dhcarenetworks.org.uk/** to discover many of the resources and examples of good practice available.

Discuss with your mentor the initiatives that have been or might be implemented in your placement area.

- What would you consider to be the key issues for nurses in ensuring the dignity of their patients/clients is maintained?
- How might a student nurse contribute to maintaining dignity?

....

Key points

The Dignity Challenge (available at **http://www.scie.org.uk/**)
High-quality care services that respect people's dignity should:

1 have a zero tolerance of all forms of abuse;
2 support people with the same respect that you would want for yourself or a member of your family;

3 treat each person as an individual by offering a personalized service;

4 enable people to maintain the maximum possible level of independence, choice; and control;

5 listen and support people to express their needs and wants;

6 respect people's right to privacy;

7 ensure that people feel able to complain without fear of retribution;

8 engage with family members and carers as care partners;

9 assist people to maintain confidence and a positive self-esteem;

10 act to alleviate people's loneliness and isolation.

According to the DH Care Networks, these are the main challenges to nurses and all other care providers.

Theory into action

In March 2009, the NMC published *Guidance for the Care of Older People*. This document can be accessed at: **http://www.nmc-uk.org/Documents/Guidance/Guidance-for-the-care-of-older-people.pdf**
What does this document say about the nurse's role in maintaining respect and dignity?

The inspection function or review establishes whether all NHS trusts are meeting the appropriate standards and also how they are measuring against certain developmental standards. The inspection or review enables the public to identify the progress of each organization, and if a trust does not meet the standards, it is expected to put together a plan and a set of proposals or 'special measures', which will show how it intends to meet these standards at the earliest possible opportunity.

So why does this matter to you as a student nurse or to other nurses?

You may be surprised to hear that the CQC regulates a wide range of activities, some of which are fundamental to the roles and responsibilities of nurses, such as:

- personal care;
- nursing care;
- accommodation for people who require nursing or personal care;
- assessment or medical treatment for persons detained under the Mental Health Act 1983;
- diagnostic procedures;
- surgical procedures;
- management and supply of blood and blood-derived products.

Patient and public involvement

The CQC also has a significant role in the promotion of patient and public involvement in health care. This includes patient survey programmes and service-user consultations, which may be subsequently included in a trust's overall rating. The CQC attempts to ensure that nurses and other health professionals 'gain a fuller understanding' of the patient experience and what patients need and expect from health care, and to give patients more control over their care. This is indicative of how both patients and carers' expectations of health care and health care professionals have increased significantly over the past decades.

Theory into action

The national NHS patient survey programme includes surveys of inpatients in the NHS undertaken by the CQC. These are available under the 'Publications' tab at:
http://www.cqc.org.uk
Access the survey of your placement hospital.

- What questions are asked that are specific to nurses?
- How did nurses perform in these areas?

The standard questions related to nurses and nursing

- When you had important questions to ask a nurse, did you get answers that you could understand?
- Did you have confidence and trust in the nurses treating you?
- Did nurses talk in front of you as if you weren't there?
- In your opinion, were there enough nurses on duty to care for you in hospital?
- As far as you know, did nurses wash or clean their hands between touching patients?

Clearly, a patient can be involved in their care in many different ways, such as:

- discussing possible treatments with their doctor or nurse;
- exercising choice over which hospital or GP to use;
- giving their views of services by filling in questionnaires about their experiences.

It has been highlighted that patient choice and the implied negotiation and discussion inherent in this can actually undermine patient care, as it allows health practitioners to delve deeper into their patients' personal lives and therefore fail to give adequate attention to the wider social context of health (Taylor & Hawley, 2010). Therefore patient involvement *might* be about much 'bigger questions': for example, how to engage the community as a whole in difficult decisions about service patterns and reconfigurations.

The importance of patient and public involvement has been recognized for a long time; however, the structures to ensure that this happens have changed over the years. The first formal structures to represent the public's interest in the NHS were community health councils (CHCs), which were created in 1974. CHCs were in place for almost 30 years, but were abolished at the end of 2003, with their role being taken over by a number of organizations, including the overview and scrutiny committees (OSCs), the Patient Advice and Liaison Service (PALS), the Independent Complaints Advocacy Service (ICAS), and the patient and public involvement (PPI) forums. In July 2006, the abolition of PPI forums was announced and they were replaced by local involvement networks (LINks). All of these structures essentially have the same purpose: *to ensure a strong voice for local patient and service users.* For example, LINks are there to ask local people what they think about their local healthcare services and also to provide a chance for local people to suggest improvements in services. They may also investigate specific issues of concern to the local community, get information and ensure results by calling local providers to account for their performance, and refer to the local OSC if necessary. LINks aspire to be more representative of the local population than the previous system and provide a strong voice to change aspects of patients' health and social care.

Such networks are attempts to overcome the arguments that the aspiration for greater patient involvement in health care essentially increases inequalities as it simply gives greater credence to the middle classes to further advance their own positions over the more needy sections of society (Dixon & Le Grand, 2006).

....

⮕ Theory into action

What patient liaison groups are you aware of in your various placements areas?
Visit the placement webpage and discover the procedures, timetable of events, and
   minutes of previous meetings if available.
Involvement in such groups is open to all. It could be worthwhile considering future
Involvement in such groups to enhance your understating and ability to maintain high
   standards of care.
Information is available at: **http://www.nhscentreforinvolvement.nhs.uk/index.
   cfm?content=110&Menu=36**

....

Standards for better health and the Care Quality Commission

When the *NHS Improvement Plan* (DH, 2004a) was published, one of its main aims was to 'put patients and service users first through more personalised care'. It was recognized that this also required a change in the way in which improvements in people's health and care were planned and delivered. In *Standards for Better Health* (DH, 2004b), national targets were reduced from the previous processes and a system that attempted to allow greater scope for addressing local priorities was introduced.

The main driver for this was the introduction of standards by which continuous improvement in quality could be measured. It was felt that this would place quality at the forefront of the agenda for the NHS and for private and voluntary providers of NHS care.

The standards were in two different categories:

- core standards;
- developmental standards.

Core standards set out the minimum level of service that patients and service users have a right to expect. They are described as a 'platform' for progress and serve as a marker of where the organization is at that particular moment.

Developmental standards are designed to make clear where trusts need to make progress and provide a framework for improvements in line with increasing patient expectations.

The standards, along with initiatives such as the NSFs and the guidance from NICE, continue to be a major part of the annual review process by the CQC and the Commission for Social Care Inspection (CSCI), and are designed to drive up standards by identifying areas for improvement.

The CSCI looks at the whole picture of social care in England, including social services teams at councils, care homes, and care agencies. It regulates, inspects, and reviews all social care services in the public, private, and voluntary sectors in England, giving a 'star rating' to councils. Its main area of concern is adults services. Since April 2007, social care services for children have been monitored by the Office for Standards in Education, Children's Services and Skills (Ofsted).

These standards thus provide a common set of requirements applying across all healthcare organizations to ensure that health services are both safe and of an acceptable quality. While providing overarching standards defined by the government, they allow scope for staff to determine what works best in the *local* area and therefore have impact on every one who works in health care.

The standards are organized within seven 'domains', which are designed to cover the full spectrum of health care as identified in the Health and Social Care (Community Health and Standards) Act 2003.

The seven domains are as follows.

- Safety
- Clinical and cost-effectiveness
- Governance
- Patient focus
- Accessible and responsive care
- Care environment and amenities
- Public health

First domain: safety

It is essential that all organizations have systems in place to protect patients and identify and learn from patient safety incidents. All staff at the 'front line' need to be fully aware of the latest patient safety advice, not least from NICE and other organizations such as the NPSA with regards the safe use of medical devices.

Similarly, the reduction of healthcare-acquired infections is a central aspect of this domain, with an emphasis on high standards of hygiene and cleanliness. The domain also covers aspects of medicines management, ensuring that all medicines are handled safely and securely.

The requirement for child protection guidance for *all* staff is also covered under this domain

....

⊖ Theory into action

Discuss with your mentor what systems are in place in your placement area to ensure patient safety.

The standard emphasizes a particular need to be aware of risk when patients move from the care of one organization to another. What steps could you, as a newly qualified nurse, take to reduce this risk on transferring a patient?

....

The developmental standard highlights the need to continually review these systems and processes and the need to ensure best practice in all of these areas.

Key points

The emphasis on patient safety is reiterated in the standards of proficiency for pre-registration nursing education, which confirms that for a student to be deemed suitable for entry on to the NMC register, they must be able to identify and actively manage risk (NMC, 2010)

Issues of patient safety are often in the media. As a student nurse, it is important that you keep yourself informed and aware of such newsworthy events. It is quite possible that you might be asked about a high-profile news item at interview. The following is just one example:

'NPSA announces the highest number of in-patient NHS sites rated excellent'—visit **http://www.npsa.nhs.uk/corporate/news/** and search for the news item on 6 July 2009.

Second domain: clinical and cost-effectiveness

This domain is concerned with the evidence base of healthcare decisions and practices and emphasizes the need to recognize NICE guidance, NSFs, and other nationally recognized guidance. It is an attempt to reduce the national differences that have often been referred to as the 'postcode lottery' and also to ensure that treatment and care offered to patients *actually* works. It is concerned with ensuring that all staff are appropriately trained, their skills and knowledge are up to date, and they are supervised accordingly when necessary. This relates both to continuing professional development and recognition of the importance of audit of practice.

....

⊖ Theory into action

You are about to go for an interview. Think of a question that you can ask concerning systems that will be in place to support your continuing professional development.

We have previously discussed audits in which you may be involved and initiatives such as EOC. Revisit this and consider any preparation that you might need to do to be able to answer any related questions at an interview.

How would you discover any recent initiatives that have brought about improvements/ changes in the practice areas?

....

Third domain: governance

We have already discussed the importance of clinical governance and the third domain emphasizes many aspects of this. It is concerned with ensuring that good clinical and managerial leadership is in place, with clear recognition and understanding of accountability in relation to quality, patient safety, and risk management. It also ensures that all staff are appropriately qualified and trained to undertake the job that they are assigned to do. Governance is also concerned with the *culture* of an organization: does the organization encourage openness and honesty, challenge discrimination, and promote equality and respect?

This domain also recognizes the need for organizations to support staff if they feel the need to report on any aspect of care, treatment, or service delivery that they consider to be below standard or to have a detrimental effect on patient care.

'What if I see something that I think is wrong?'

As a student, you will experience a range of different settings in your practice education placements. You will be well placed to question why something is or is not being done. In some cases, you may see a registered nurse or midwife doing something that you feel is inappropriate. Although difficult, you shouldn't ignore the situation. Ask the person or someone else about it.

In some cases, you may be observing what could amount to misconduct. Whether or not this is the case, challenging experienced practitioners' ways of doing things should be encouraged. Doing this will show that you are observing and thinking, and may help a practitioner to improve their own practice. This also clearly echoes the professional requirement of all nurses in relation to their code of professional practice (NMC, 2008a). However, nursing—perhaps like life—is never simple! There have been a few high-profile cases in which whistleblowing by nurses and other staff has resulted in outcomes far from simple and occasionally very controversial. For example, access **http://www.nursingtimes.net** and search for the case of 'Nurse Margaret Haywood'.

➡ Theory into action

Read the example given in the text above and discuss and compare your thoughts with those of your mentor and other colleagues.

In the NMC standards of proficiency for pre-registration nursing education (2010), it is emphasized that nurses must ensure that a safe environment is maintained. This is done by adopting fundamental quality assurance and risk management strategies. The document can be accessed at: **http://www.nmc-uk.org**

Fourth domain: patient focus

Health care is seen as a partnership with patients, their carers, and relatives, respecting patients' diverse needs, preferences, and choices. User and carer feedback is encouraged, giving clear and accessible information about how to make a complaint and a commitment to act on such complaints and any areas of concern generally. Like many other current initiatives, ensuring dignity and respect for patients and ensuring confidentiality and **informed consent** are key aspects of this domain.

The emphasis is also on the necessity for close partnership with other organizations, especially social care organizations the services of which impact on patient well-being.

➡ Theory into action

Below is a quote from a patient that is included in the DH document *Confidence in Caring* (DH, 2007: 15):

> I expected people to know about me—what my problems were and what help I needed. Having a label stuck on your bed is not the same as communicating.

The document suggests many actions that should be taken and the many skills that nurses are required to have to ensure 'partnerships with patients' and improving communication and so on.

Access the document at **http://www.dh.gov.uk/** by searching for 'Confidence in Caring'. Reflecting on your experience on placement, have you witnessed examples of staff offering such good practice? What specific skills do you think they had?

Releasing Time to Care: The Productive Ward (NHS Institute for Innovation and Improvement, 2008) focuses on improving ward processes and environments to help nurses and therapists to spend more time on patient care, thereby improving safety and efficiency. Information can be found at: **http://www.institute.nhs.uk**

Watch 'Episode 1' of the video documentary in the 'Productive Ward' section. Considering your experiences on placement, are there any changes that you felt could be made to 'release time to care?'

Fifth domain: accessible and responsive care

Feedback from patients and the public consistently emphasizes that they want to be able to make choices in accessing services that are convenient and prompt and are not delayed. This is at the heart of all policies, from *The NHS Plan* (DH, 2000) to *Equity and Excellence* (DH, 2010). This domain again emphasizes the crucial role of patients, carers, and service users in the whole range of quality issues. It is expected that their views are taken into consideration in every aspect of care, from the designing and planning, to the delivering and subsequent improving of healthcare services.

⊙ Theory into action

Consider your most recent placement experience.

- Was there any opportunity for users/carers to give feedback to staff about their own care or the care received by their relatives?
- What methods do you know of encouraging such feedback?
- Go to **http://www.which.co.uk** and search for the news article 'Survey reveals health complaints concerns'. How can nurses ensure that patients are able to complain if they feel that they have not received high-quality care?

Sixth domain: care environment and amenities

It is essential that care is provided in environments that promote patient and staff well-being and respect for patients' needs and preferences. This inevitably relates to the need to provide as much privacy as possible in well-maintained and clean wards and departments.

- 'There was a sweet wrapper on the floor for ages. If they don't do anything about those sweet wrappers, what else are they missing?'
- 'Patients see the ward environment as being a direct indication of how attentive staff are.'

These quotes are again from *Confidence in Caring* (DH, 2007). What strategies designed to create a clean and well-maintained environment are suggested in this document:

- for the organization/unit/department?
- for the care team?
- for the individual health professional?

Seventh domain: public health

More and more, the emphasis in health care is changing from acute care to primary care. The seventh domain recognizes that health care needs to be delivered appropriately to the community that it serves. This requires collaboration with several relevant organizations and communities to promote protect and improve the health of all of the population and reduce the inequalities that presently exist. General practitioners have a key role in this through the provision of disease prevention and health promotion programmes, such as reducing obesity through action on nutrition and exercise, and programmes on smoking, substance misuse, and sexually transmitted infections.

⊙ Theory into action

Access your local primary care services website.
- What services does it provide?
- Does it provide health promotion programmes?
- What key role do you think you will play in health promotion as a qualified nurse?

The National Institute for Health and Clinical Excellence

NICE has a crucial role in quality improvement. Prior to its establishment, there were no set clear standards of care within the NHS and there was occasional inconsistency and slow uptake of effective treatments. NICE (then known as the National Institute for Clinical Excellence) was originally established in February 1999 to review clinical and cost-effective evidence to support healthcare practice, and to provide advice and guidance to NHS organizations, healthcare professionals, and also the public (Talbot-Smith & Pollock, 2006). In 2005, NICE absorbed the function of the Health Development Agency, which originally had a key role in public health and the prevention of ill health, and took on the extended title of National Institute for Health and Clinical Excellence (although the acronym remains the same).

NICE consists of a group of experts who make decisions about various treatments based on perceived longer-term benefits versus cost implications. NICE then provides health professionals and the public with authoritative and reliable advice on evidence-based 'best practice'. NICE and the decisions that it has made have often been controversial and the subject of media scrutiny and criticism. This might be to an extent inevitable with the finite resources in health care and the high cost of modern interventions, equipment, and drugs. Clearly, the NHS cannot fund all treatment and all interventions for all people. Several of the criticisms levelled at NICE were discussed in *High Quality Care for All: NHS Next Stage Review* (DH, 2008a), in which it was accepted that NICE appraisal guidance on newly licensed drugs had often taken too long to become available—on occasions up to two years. NICE has now put in place a faster appraisal process for key new drugs, which enables it to issue authoritative guidance within a few months of the launch of a drug in the UK.

However, as we have previously discussed, this is not without criticisms and the cost–benefit evaluation of new technologies and drugs by NICE remains controversial. This means that it becomes possible to only invest in those innovations that produce the most cost-effective results, and as Bradshaw and Bradshaw (2004) point out, this sometimes is seen to be denying potentially effective treatments to certain patients simply because they are not seen to be good value for money. It appears certain, however, that the role and function of NICE will continue to be reformed and developed, with the aspiration of maintaining its independence and extending its remit to social care (DH, 2010).

....

➡ Theory into action

NICE (**http://www.nice.org.uk**) emphasizes the importance of contributions from the public—people like you and me. Do you think that you might consider contributing to the working of NICE?

Why not attend a meeting if there is one in your area or even consider suggesting a topic?

You can also sign up for the regular newsletters and e-alerts from NICE that will help you to keep up to date with regards to resources that may help you to maintain standards of care.

....

National service frameworks

The NSFs, which were introduced in 1999, are evidence-based programmes that set minimum quality standards and also specify services that should be available for a particular condition or care group across the whole of the NHS. They are intended to eradicate local variations in standards and services, raise standards generally, promote collaboration between organizations and contribute to improving public health. Each NSF identifies key interventions, puts in place a strategy to support implementation, and establishes an agreed timescale for the implementation. Each NSF is developed with the assistance from an external reference group of health professionals, service users and carers, health service managers, and others to ensure that the whole picture is considered. In addition, various protocols for care delivery have also been developed—for example, the **integrated care pathways (ICP)**—which are designed to complement the NSFs and clinical governance structures in general to ensure that acceptable standards of both nursing and medical treatment are achieved (Williamson et al., 2008).

....

➡ Theory into action

- Can you name the NSFs that are currently in force?
- Consider where you intend to apply for a job. Which NSF is most relevant to that clinical area and specialty?
- Access the NSF and explore the standards within it. What is the role of the nurse in delivering these standards?
- What is an ICP?

  Access **http://www.medicine.ox.ac.uk/bandolier/painres/download/whatis/ What_is_an_ICP.pdf** to find an explanation of what an ICP is and examples of an ICP for management of meticillin-resistant *Staphylococcus aureus* (MRSA).

....

The NHS constitution: the NHS belongs to us all (2009)

In 2009, the first ever constitution for the NHS in England was launched, which set out the rights that patients have to care while also stating their responsibilities. Although it was criticized in some areas for being a series of optimistic pledges without making clear the consequences for not meeting these pledges (The Patients' Association, 2009), the constitution has much to say in relation to standards and quality. It is also proposed that a report will be published every three years on how the NHS constitution has impacted on the care of patients, the work practices of staff, and the experiences of carers and members of the public (DH, 2010).

The third of the seven principles in the NHS constitution states:

> the NHS aspires to the highest standards of excellence and professionalism—in the provision of high-quality care that is safe, effective and focussed on patient experience; in the planning and delivery of the clinical and other services it provides; in the people it employs and the education, training and development they receive; in the leadership and management of its organisations; and through its commitment to innovation and to the promotion and conduct of research to improve the current and future health and care of the population.

With regards to quality of care and environment:

> You have the right to be treated with a professional standard of care, by appropriately qualified and experienced staff, in a properly approved or registered organisation that meets required levels of safety and quality.

> You have the right to expect NHS organisations to monitor, and make efforts to improve, the quality of healthcare they commission or provide.

The NHS also commits:

> to continuous improvement in the quality of services you receive, identifying and sharing best practice in quality of care and treatment.

And under the heading 'NHS Values: Commitment to Quality of Care':

> We earn the trust placed in us by insisting on quality and striving to get the basics right every time: safety, confidentiality, professional and managerial integrity, accountability, dependable service and good communication. We welcome feedback, learn from our mistakes and build on our successes.

....

💡 Thinking about

The constitution also includes expectations that reflect how staff should play their part in ensuring the success of the NHS and delivering high quality care.

- Why do you think it was felt that an NHS constitution was needed?
- List the legal and professional duties that you think should be included in the constitution.

Check your answers by visiting **http://www.dh.gov.uk** and searching for 'NHS constitution'.

....

Summary

In this chapter, we have explored the role of the nurse in maintaining standards and ensuring quality of care. It is clear that every nurse needs to have an awareness of their unique and individual contribution to this vital area of health care. We explored what is often called the 'quality agenda', and the changing responsibilities and expectations of nurses and the public. This 'quality agenda' is here to stay and it is important that, as nurses, we recognize the essential role played by organizations such as the CQC and NICE, the importance and relevance of policies such as the NHS constitution, NSFs, EOC, and crucially the increasingly lead role that nurses are expected to take in delivering a service that ensures patient safety, quality, and dignity. More and more, health care is seen as a partnership between health professionals and patients, and increasingly nurses will be called to account for the care that they provide and will be judged against such measures as nursing metrics. The chapter offered an overview of many of these challenging, but exciting, initiatives and changes, and an insight into a nurse's current and future role.

In this chapter, we have looked at:

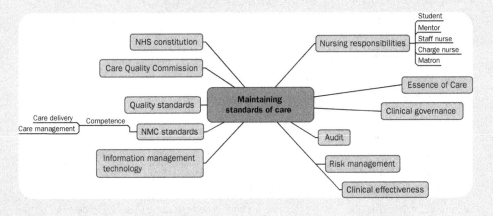

Figure 2.1

Online Resource Centre

 This textbook is accompanied by an Online Resource Centre which provides interactive learning resources and tools to help you prepare for the transition from student to fully qualified member of staff. After you have completed each chapter and whenever you see this icon please go to the ORC at your earliest convenience. If you have not done so already, save the ORC web address in to your Favourites: **http://www.oxfordtextbooks.co.uk/orc/burton**

References

Appleby J & Harrison A (2006) *Spending on Health: How Much is Enough?* King's Fund, London.

Ayres P (1999) Clinical governance: setting the scene. *Hospital Medicine*, **60**(7): 505–8.

Bradshaw PL & Bradshaw G (2004) *Health Policy for Health Care Professionals*. SAGE, London.

Childs L, Coles L & Marjoram B (2009) *Essential Skills Clusters for Nurses: Theory for Practice*. Wiley-Blackwell, London.

Crinson I (2009) *Health Policy: A Critical Perspective*. SAGE, London.

Currie L, Morrell C & Scrivner R (2003) *Clinical Governance: An RCN Resource Guide*. RCN, London.

Department of Health (1992) *The Patient's Charter and You: A Charter for England*. DH, London.

Department of Health (1997) *The New NHS: Modern and Dependable*. DH, London.

Department of Health (1998) *A First Class Service: Quality in the New NHS*. DH, London.

Department of Health (2000) *The NHS Plan*. DH, London.

Department of Health (2003) *The Essence of Care: Patient-focused Benchmarking for Health Care Practitioners*. DH, London.

Department of Health (2004a) *NHS Improvement Plan*. DH, London.

Department of Health (2004b) *Standards For Better Health*. DH, London.

Department of Health (2007) *Confidence in Caring: A Framework for Best Practice*. DH, London.

Department of Health (2008a) *High Quality Care for All: NHS Next Stage Review*. DH, London.

Department of Health (2008b) *Framing the Nursing and Midwifery Contribution: Driving Up the Quality of Care*. DH, London.

Department of Health (2010) *Equity and Excellence: Liberating the NHS*. DH, London.

Dixon A & Le Grand J (2006) Is greater patient choice consistent with equity? The case of the English NHS. *Journal of Health Service Research Policy*, **11**(3): 162–6.

Goodrich J & Cornwell J (2008) *Seeing the Person in the Patient*. King's Fund, London.

Griffiths P, Jones S, Maben J & Murrells T (2008) *State of the Art Metrics for Nursing: A Rapid Appraisal*. National Nursing Research Unit, King's College, London.

Halligan A & Donaldson L (2001) Implementing clinical governance: turning vision into reality. *British Medical Journal*, **322**: 1413–17.

Harrison SR & McDonald ER (2008) *The Politics of Healthcare in Britain*. SAGE, London.

Healthcare Commission (2008) *The Annual Health Check 2008/09. Assessing and Rating the NHS*. Commission for Healthcare Audit and Inspection.

Healy J & Spencer M (2007) *Surviving Your Placement in Health and Social Care: A Student Handbook*. McGraw-Hill, London.

Hicks N (1997) Evidence-based healthcare. *Bandolier*, **4**(39): 8.

HM Government (2010) *The Coalition: Our Programme for Government.* HMSO, London.

Kennedy I (2001) *Learning from Bristol: The Report of the Public Inquiry into Children's Heart Surgery at the Bristol Royal Infirmary 1984–1995.* CM 5207. HMSO, London.

Lansley A (2010) *Secretary of State for Health, Speech to Patients and Patient Organisations.* 8 June 2010. Available at: **http://www.dh.gov.uk/en/MediaCentre/Speeches/ DH_116643**

Leatherman S & Sutherland K (2008) *The Quest for Quality: Refining the NHS Reforms. A Policy Analysis and Chartbook.* The Nuffield Trust, London.

Maben J & Griffiths P (2008) *Nurses in Society: Starting the Debate.* National Nursing Research Unit, King's College, London.

National Health Service Institute for Innovation and Improvement (2008) *Releasing Time to Care:The Productive Ward Series.* NHS Institute, London.

Nursing and Midwifery Council (2010) *Standards of Proficiency for Pre-registration Nursing Education.* NMC, London.

Nursing and Midwifery Council (2007) *Essential Skills Clusters.* NMC, London.

Nursing and Midwifery Council (2008a) *Code: Standards of Conduct, Performance and Ethics for Nurses and Midwives.* NMC, London.

Nursing and Midwifery Council (2008b) *Standards to Support: Learning and Assessment in Practice.* NMC, London.

The Patients' Association (2009) *NHS Constitution.* Available at: **http://www.patients-association.org.uk/News/254**.

Prime Minister's Commission (2010) *Front Line Care: The Future of Nursing and Midwifery in England—Report of the Prime Minister's Commission on the Future of Nursing and Midwifery in England 2010.* HMSO, London.

Rogers A, Kennedy A, Nelson E & Robinson A (2005) Uncovering the limits of patient-centeredness: implementing a self-management trial for chronic illness. *Qualitative Health Research,* **15**(2): 224–39.

Royal College of Nursing (2009) *Breaking Down Barriers, Driving Up Standards.* RCN, London.

Smith C (2001) Trust and confidence: possibilities for social work in 'high modernity'. *British Journal of Social Work,* **31**: 287–305.

Stevenson F, Barry C, Britten N, Barber N & Bradley C (2000) Doctor–patient communication about drugs: the evidence for shared decision making. *Social Science and Medicine,* **50**: 829–40.

Talbot-Smith A & Pollock A (2006) *The New NHS: A Guide.* Routledge, Oxford.

Taylor G & Hawley H (2010) *Key Debates in Health Care.* Open University Press, Maidenhead.

Williamson G, Jenkinson T & Proctor-Childs T (2008) *Nursing in Contemporary Healthcare Practice.* Learning Matters, Exeter.

3

Accountability and ethical decision-making

Graham Ormrod and Nichola Barlow

The aims of this chapter are to:

➔ provide a review of the concept of accountability;

➔ discuss the accepted definitions of accountability;

➔ specifically explore the *professional*, *personal*, and *ethical* contexts of accountability;

➔ discuss the use of a recognized framework to assist in ethical decision-making;

➔ explore how this relates to nursing practice for students and registered nurses.

We have also included scenarios highlighting issues of accountability and investigating the nurse's role in the decision-making process with regards to subsequent choices, actions, and patient care.

Issues of accountability will also be discussed further in Chapter 4, allowing you to revisit your understanding of accountability more specifically from a legal point of view.

Introduction

Before considering what the literature tells us about accountability, what do you think the term means?

....

➔ Theory into action

You have almost completed your course as a student and have applied for a post as a registered nurse. During the interview, one of the interviewers asks: 'In your answers you've talked quite a bit about your accountability. What does this term mean to you?'

Before reading any further, write down a couple of sentences about your own understanding and definition of accountability. We will return to your definitions later.

....

As a final-year nursing student, you will have encountered the concept of accountability before and you may think: 'Hey, I know this!' If you do, great—but are you clear exactly how your accountability changes on registration? Reading this chapter will help you to revisit the issues around this concept in a new light; for those who have not really considered accountability before, fear not—this chapter will also provide a good introduction to what you need to know at this stage of your career. It is important to remember that, to be deemed proficient for entry to the **Nursing and Midwifery Council** (NMC) professional register, all students must demonstrate that they are able to manage the delivery of care services within the sphere of their own accountability (NMC, 2010)

Definitions of accountability

As you may have found in the exercise above, the concept of accountability is very hard to define. In fact, Jacobs (2004) claims that nobody is really sure what it means. Similarly, Sinclair (1995) described accountability as chameleon-like, multiple, fragmented, and subject to continual reconstruction.

The Nursing and Midwifery Council (2008c), in its publication *Advice on Delegation for Registered Nurses,* defines accountability as 'the principle that individuals, organisations and the community are responsible for their actions and may be required to explain them to others'. One point that is clear, however, is that *all nurses are accountable for their practice*. This means that they can be asked to *justify* their practice or be held to account by others for any actions and/or omissions resulting from their individual practice.

According to Dimond (2008), the registered nurse is accountable to:

- the public, through criminal law;
- the patient, through civil law;
- their employer, through a contract of employment;
- their profession, through the NMC via such documents as *The Code: Standards of Conduct, Performance and Ethics for Nurses and Midwives* (NMC, 2008a).

....

➔ Theory into action

Consider, from your experience in practice, what the major differences and similarities are between the accountability of a registered nurse and a student nurse. Write your thoughts in the table below.

Similarities	Differences

The differences in accountability are very likely to be the basis of *at least* one question that you will be asked when you go for a job interview, and it is therefore essential that you have a clear understanding of them.

. . . .

Caulfield (2005) argues that accountability is a key part of the very foundation of nursing. Guidance for student nurses in the UK states that although as a student nurse you are not professionally accountable to the NMC, you are accountable to the patient and public through the law and also to your university (NMC, 2009). This is also corroborated by the NMC Code (NMC, 2008a). The professional dimensions of care are identified throughout the Code and the nurse's responsibilities to those in his or her care are clearly identified, along with the standards of behaviour required from those on the NMC register. Each individual practitioner is reminded that they are accountable for *all* aspects of their practice including that which they delegate to others. This has significant relevance not only for the nurse delegating a task, but also for the person to whom the task is being delegated, which is often the student nurse.

Indeed, the NMC (2010) emphasizes in the standards of **proficiency** for entry to the register that people must be able to trust that the newly qualified nurse will always safely delegate to others and also respond appropriately when a task is delegated to them. Fundamentally, if a registered nurse has a clear understanding of accountability and acts within boundaries of the Code (NMC, 2008a), they will be able to ensure their professional practice remains ethical, legal, and in line with their professional body requirements.

Caulfield (2005) argued that if accountability is simply seen as being responsible for actions, then this can lead to a negative influence on practice, with practitioners purely concerned with *taking the blame* when things go wrong. Generally, however, definitions of accountability do speak in some way of *justifying* practice. For example, one definition speaks of an acceptance of the *obligation to disclose* what you have done and also the *possible consequences* of that disclosure (Duff, 1995). This disclosure involves making all decisions explicit so that others can evaluate them. These others include:

- patients;
- relatives or carers;
- colleagues;

- regulatory bodies such as the NMC;
- employers;
- representatives of the law.

The obligation to disclose or *answerability* and need to offer *justification* of practice is at the heart of the concept of accountability. Every nurse needs to be aware that they may be asked 'Why did you do that? or 'Why did you do that in that particular way?'. This comment from a third-year student might capture the feelings of many:

> What worries me the most about being qualified is holding the keys and being left on my own.

The idea of 'holding the keys' and thereby being ultimately responsible for drug administration, for example, in some ways encapsulates this image of 'answerability' and very powerfully highlights one of the major differences between being a student and being a qualified nurse, irrespective of the field of nursing that you have chosen.

....

➡ Theory into action

Imagine that you are now working as a registered nurse and part of your responsibilities is to administer medications prescribed by a doctor who usually only visits the care home once a day.

When you come to administer the day's medications, you realize that two of the drugs are known to interact. What would you do and why?

....

Points to consider

Remember that the NMC publishes standards and offers guidance with regards to medicines management generally in the document *Standards for Medicines Management* (NMC, 2007) and you should understand the implications of these standards for your practice. For example, they include the directive:

> you must contact the prescriber or another authorised prescriber without delay where contra-indications to the prescribed medicine are discovered.
>
> NMC (2007: 7)

Bearing such guidance in mind, your options would be as follows.

1 Do not give the drugs.
2 Discuss this further with the prescribing doctor, as soon as possible, highlighting the drug interaction and asking for the prescription to be changed.
3 Subsequently administer the medications *only* when you are sure the prescription is correct and appropriate for the patient and the presenting condition.
4 Document events accordingly.

The NMC reports that many queries that it receives arise from nurses' 'uncertainty or lack of awareness about their accountability' (Savage & Moore, 2004: 4). In the example above, the nurse is accountable for their actions in relation to drug administration regardless of advice from other healthcare professionals (NMC, 2008a). They also have a duty to challenge the doctor's, or indeed any other health professional's, decisions in relation to patient care, if they are concerned that another approach would be more appropriate (NMC, 2008a). This could be described as 'professional accountability'.

Professional accountability

Accountability is intrinsically linked to the concept of professionalism, whereby there is a requirement to answer to an external governing body. The NMC has had this role in the UK since its establishment in 2002. Its key role is the protection of the public by establishing standards of education, training, conduct, and performance, and the maintenance of a professional register that includes the names of all those entitled to be called a registered nurse. Professional accountability gives the NMC the power to control entry onto the register and also regulates a nurse's right to remain on the register by imposing professional standards and ensuring the nurse's **fitness to practise**.

The obligations of accountability contained in the NMC Code (NMC, 2008a) can essentially be grouped around a central theme: an obligation *or duty of care* to patients (Jacobs, 2004). Professional accountability maintains the patient's trust in the individual nurse and support for the nursing profession as a whole (Caulfield, 2005). Those nurses who meet the minimum standards for registration also have the power to decide whether to remove an individual from the register for misconduct, lack of competence, or ill health. Public protection is the key aspiration of the council, therefore those on the register must have achieved and maintained the appropriate levels of educational and practical expertise.

The NMC (2009) guide for students of nursing and midwifery explains the role of the NMC as one of protecting the public through the establishment and improvement of nursing and midwifery standards of care. This identifies your accountability in relation to the university and through the law, but not professionally to the NMC until your education is completed and you have been accepted on to the NMC register as a qualified nurse.

....

⊖ Theory into action

The public, employers, and registrants can access information on the NMC's website (**http://www.nmc-uk.org**) and search the register to check whether an individual is registered to practise. This webpage also provides access to NMC publications and guidelines.

Access the website and explore the information available. Think about how the content relates to the idea of professional accountability.

....

Similarly, the International Council of Nurses (ICN), a federation of 128 countries worldwide, which aims to bring nurses together on a global level, provides nursing advice and influences health policy, and publishes a code of ethics for nurses (ICN, 2006), which identifies the nurse's accountability for nursing practice and the maintenance of competence through continuing professional development. The ICN code of ethics identifies the groups to whom the nurse may have some level of accountability, including people requiring care, the profession, and also co-workers; these are similar groups to those identified previously by Dimond (2008).

....

⊙ Theory into action

The International Council of Nurses (ICN) also has a website (**http://www.icn.ch**) that contains important and relevant information, guidance, and fact sheets that you may find of interest in the area of accountability, as well as other areas. Access the website and consider how the content relates to the idea of professional accountability.

....

Personal accountability

The NMC Code (NMC, 2008a: 1) states that:

> As a professional you are personally accountable for your actions and omissions in your practice and must always be able to justify your decisions.

This means that you are answerable for your actions and omissions, regardless of advice or directions from another professional. This highlights again the differences in accountability that you will experience on qualification and registration with the NMC.

Prior to qualification

The NMC guidance on professional conduct for nursing and midwifery students (2009) emphasizes how important it is that a student conducts themselves professionally at all times in order to justify the trust that the public places in nurses. It also confirms that behaviour and conduct, inside and outside of the university, and clinical placement and personal life, may impact on the student's fitness to practise and ability to complete the nursing programme.

After qualification

Ultimately, each nurse must answer for their own actions; it is no defence to claim that they were acting on someone else's orders or advice. Nursing is not simply concerned with carrying out tasks, but also involves a process of decision-making informed by specific and/or specialist knowledge. It is necessary for the nurse not only to understand the reasons for the care and treatment given, but also to understand the anticipated outcome. This means that the 'accountable' nurse will not only understand the practical aspects of undertaking a skill, for example, but will also understand the rationale behind it, recognize the possible outcomes of carrying out the related task, and also have the knowledge to assess its relative benefits.

Delegation and accountability: implications for students and qualified nurses

If a qualified nurse delegates any aspect of care or any task to someone else, especially if that individual is not registered with the NMC, whether a support worker or you as a student nurse, it is the individual, registered nurse's responsibility to make sure that the person is suitably competent, has sufficient knowledge, and is supervised appropriately. The NMC indeed offers specific advice on delegation and emphasizes that delegation must always take place in the best interests of the person for whom the nurse is caring and the decision to delegate must always be based on an assessment of the patient's individual needs (NMC, 2008c).

According to Burnard and Chapman (2005), the above discussion means that while a student, for example, may be *responsible* for care given to a patient, as a learner, it may not be appropriate to expect them to be *accountable* because this implies a certain level of necessary knowledge or skill that may not yet have been acquired. However, it is important to recognize that this does not absolve all responsibility from those undertaking the duties. As a student nurse performing any care, you still have a responsibility to the patient and are personally accountable for your actions. Therefore, as a student nurse, you have a responsibility not to take on duties that you are not fully competent to perform, and also have a responsibility to express your lack of competency to the delegating nurse.

Storey (2002) clarifies that registered nurses' accountability rests on the notion that the task has been *appropriately* delegated. The student nurse would be responsible for the task, and they must be adequately prepared and work within the employer's guidelines and protocols, and have the *authority* delegated by the registered nurse. Consider Scenario 3.1.

There is more advice with regard to this occasionally daunting aspect of professional practice in Chapter 7.

Accountability and patients/clients

Patients/clients and also family members may ask you what you have done and why, and they are obviously entitled to an explanation with regards to nursing care.

Scenario 3.1

You are caring for a client with profound learning disability in their own home and you are asked by your **mentor** to administer medication via a percutaneous endoscopic gastrostomy (PEG) tube, after having checked the medications together. Your mentor tells you to administer them via the tube, saying 'Use a 10 ml flush'.

In such scenarios, the delegating nurse must be sure that you have the appropriate knowledge, competency, preparation, and skill to undertake the task in line with the employer's guidelines/policy and ensuring patient safety.

Having received the authority from the delegating staff nurse, you, as the student nurse, are said to be accountable for your actions.

Where possible, of course, you should also gain consent from the patient.

The NMC (2010) states that the ability to delegate duties to others, as appropriate, while ensuring that those delegated to are supervised and monitored is one of the overarching principles of being able to practise as a nurse. It emphasizes that this involves delegating and supervising care safely and appropriately, while remaining accountable.

Historically, this has been described as being accountable 'for' rather than accountable 'to'. For example, Watson (1992) suggested that nurses were not accountable to patients because they have what he describes as an 'informal' relationship. However, the culture in health care has changed significantly over the years and is now more one of partnership and equality (Department of Health, or DH, 2004), whereby it is now a legitimate expectation of all patients/clients to be able to call nurses, or any other individual, including student nurses, to account for their care. Consider Scenario 3.2.

Scenario 3.2

You are part of the nursing team caring for a 12-year-old child who has been diagnosed with cancer. She appears very optimistic when you and your mentor meet with her and her parents to discuss the options for care management. She and her parents have researched her condition on the Internet and found a website promoting a combination of complementary and alternative therapies as a potential cure. Her parents are less convinced, but do not want to upset their daughter and have not broached this with her. They are told by the consultant that the healthcare team will provide the 'best possible' care and do 'everything' that it can to help her. The girl now wants to know when she can commence her chosen therapies and is convinced that aggressive chemotherapy is not the best approach. As a registered nurse and recognizing your accountability to the patient, what would you do in this situation?

This type of scenario raises many key issues for the student to learn from. As the standards of proficiency (NMC, 2010) state, students must accept the differing cultural traditions and beliefs of their clients when planning care. However, this apparently straightforward aspiration can generate complex dilemmas in practice where the 'rights and wrongs' of the scenario are difficult to discern. It can be even more difficult in the case of children. What is clear in these often very emotional and complicated cases is that a multidisciplinary team approach is essential, with sensitive input and engagement from experts, family, and most importantly the individual child concerned, to manage the complexities of such legal and ethical dilemmas (NMC, 2010). Ultimately, if it is clear that the patient *really* knows the implications of her request, and **capacity** is accepted, then her decision needs to be respected. Issues of capacity and decision-making, including the implications of young people and children, will be further discussed in Chapter 4.

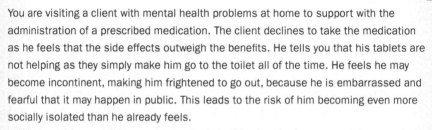

Scenario 3.3

You are visiting a client with mental health problems at home to support with the administration of a prescribed medication. The client declines to take the medication as he feels that the side effects outweigh the benefits. He tells you that his tablets are not helping as they simply make him go to the toilet all of the time. He feels he may become incontinent, making him frightened to go out, because he is embarrassed and fearful that it may happen in public. This leads to the risk of him becoming even more socially isolated than he already feels.

What would you expect your mentor to do in this situation?

You would need to consider both her (and your) accountability and how this impacts on the role as **advocate**.

A possible course of action would be as follows.

1 Listen to his concerns.

2 Discuss your patient's condition and how his medication is helping to treat it.

3 Talk to the prescribing doctor about the patient's concerns to facilitate any possible changes to the medication regimen to reduce any unwanted impact on the patient and his lifestyle. This may include a change of medication or changes to the frequency and administration times.

You have had the opportunity to explore several aspects of the concept of accountability and we have reiterated key principles with regards to the nursing profession—aspects of practice, delegation, and so on. We will now look more specifically at the ethical aspects of accountability.

Accountability and ethical decision-making

Ethical considerations can sometimes seem to have little to do with day-to-day practice, and any discussions of the ethical principles that underpin practice or any moral component of practice can seem more of an *academic* pursuit rather than an underpinning context for everyday practice. However, your modules at university will have confirmed to you that recognition of the ethical values that inform professional practice is as important now as ever. As Mason and Whitehead (2003) confirm, it is no longer acceptable to leave ethical decisions solely to the medical profession as might have historically been the case. When you qualify, you will immediately confirm your role as a patient advocate and very quickly may have to take a lead role within the multidisciplinary team; both then and in the future it will be necessary for you to have the knowledge and insight to offer informed views on certain potentially complicated ethical dilemmas.

The role of the nurse is constantly changing, as are the views and expectations of the public and society (Maben & Griffiths, 2008). This change both in role and expectations brings with it a greater likelihood of dilemmas for the nurse. Fundamental questions can be raised such as 'What is *good* nursing care?' and 'What *ought* a nurse to do for a patient?'. Being described as 'a *good* nurse' might even change as the context of nursing changes. For example, Florence Nightingale identified a number of essential nursing duties, which predominately consisted of actions associated with physical care and the environment, while also identifying the importance of nurse education both in the sciences and in human ethics and morals (Bostridge, 2008); Pugh (1944) described the nurse's most important duty as that of obedience to the physician. The NMC Code (2008a) states that nurses have a duty to work collaboratively within the healthcare team, recognizing the contributions and expertise of others while also recognizing the importance of referring to another practitioner when it is in the best interests of the patient. This may mean challenging the decisions of other professionals including doctors, and these potential challenges indicate the changing context in which nursing is viewed.

Each one of the decisions that you are expected to make requires consideration of certain information. Some of this information may be classed as 'factual'—for example:

- the patient's past medical and nursing history;
- the results of any diagnostic tests or medications prescribed;
- the specific name by which the client would prefer to be called.

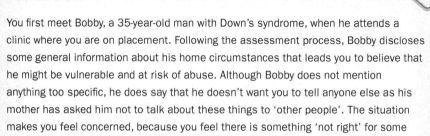

Scenario 3.4

You first meet Bobby, a 35-year-old man with Down's syndrome, when he attends a clinic where you are on placement. Following the assessment process, Bobby discloses some general information about his home circumstances that leads you to believe that he might be vulnerable and at risk of abuse. Although Bobby does not mention anything too specific, he does say that he doesn't want you to tell anyone else as his mother has asked him not to talk about these things to 'other people'. The situation makes you feel concerned, because you feel there is something 'not right' for some reason—although you cannot quite put your finger on it.

  Such feelings can point to a real dilemma. How should you respond to such a situation? Should you disclose any information about Bobby to someone, and, if so, to whom? This type of scenario highlights how purely 'factual' information can only help the decision-making process to an extent. What you, as the nurse involved, *should* do or what you *ought* to do inevitably lead us to different considerations.

Points to consider

Points that you may consider in relation to the disclosure of information that you have about Bobby and his home life will include the following:

1 As a vulnerable adult is Bobby at risk of harm or neglect?
2 How does Bobby feel about this information being shared with others, such as health and social care professionals?
3 What does Bobby expect you to do with this information?
4 What would the consequences be of disclosure or of non-disclosure?
5 Which course of action would be in Bobby's best interests?
6 What does the law say? (This will be further discussed in Chapter 4.)

In 2009, the UK ombudsman highlighted the tragic results that can occur when the rights and needs of vulnerable clients are ignored. The document *Six Lives* criticized organizations and individuals for failing to live up to human rights principles, especially those of dignity and equality of persons with learning disabilities. (To read the full story, see **http://www.lgo.org.uk/** and search for 'Six Lives'.)

Also in the UK, the Royal College of Nursing in various publicity campaigns has emphasized putting dignity at the heart of all nursing care by recognizing the importance of compassion and emotional support as opposed to simply delivering 'technical' nursing.

The NMC (2008b), in a series of focus groups consulting on pre-registration nursing education, also stresses that fitness to practise is not just about giving out the wrong drugs, for example, but can be equally applied to staff who are disrespectful to patients and neglect to treat patients with respect and dignity. Particularly vulnerable groups according to the NMC are the elderly, children, people with mental health problems, and the transient population, such as the homeless and asylum seekers.

Within the endeavour to ensure respect and dignity is recognition of an individual's core ethical and cultural values. A member of the focus group convened by the NMC (2008b) highlighted the case in which staff were unaware of the distress caused as they shaved off the beard of a Sikh patient who, due to language difficulties, was unable to prevent it.

💡 Thinking about

Have you ever experienced care being provided that you felt compromised a client's values in relation to equality and diversity?

Reflect on your experience and training in equality and diversity. Do you feel prepared to deal with such situations in your practice?

Discuss with your mentor the availability of other sources of information and support that might assist you. Are there resources such as booklets that might help to provide a greater understanding of some core cultural issues?

The NMC (2008b) feels that while nurses cannot be expected to know everything about each diverse group, they should have enough basic information available to them to understand the different cultural needs of their patients. Understanding and compassion should be at the heart of all nursing practice, and therefore training and guidance may not necessarily be enough to change attitudes and prejudice. However, feedback from the focus groups set up by the NMC highlighted the need for further training around areas such as:

- diffusing difficult situations, including:
  - how to cope with a situation in which a patient is being racist toward a staff member;
- greater understanding of mental health issues for general nurses in particular, in order to:
  - help staff to recognize mental health symptoms better;
  - reduce the risk of discrimination due to their behaviour;
  - subsequently help staff to cope better;
- greater understanding about specific issues affecting some people with disability.

You might be thinking: 'So why does this matter and what has it got to do with ethics?' It is essential to remember that *every* interaction between you and any service user has ethical implications—implications that carry with them the need to justify practice ethically. In other words, you have to be prepared to be called to account *ethically*.

What is seen to be ethically acceptable is informed by any individual's beliefs and values, which have themselves been influenced by the culture within which they live.

These values might be those that are important to the nurse, or the individual patient, or colleagues or society at large, and may well change over time. However, as indicated by the discussion above, there are certain fundamentals, such as equality, fairness, non-discriminatory practices and attitudes, and the support and protection of the vulnerable, which are held as integral and essential to professional practice. So if you recognize the importance of such considerations, how might you help to ensure that these fundamentals are considered in your daily practice? One strategy might be the use of a theoretical framework to focus your thinking and ensure the consideration of each aspect of the specific scenario or dilemma.

A framework to support ethical decision-making

Caulfield (2005) believes that while an *ethical framework* might not provide all of the answers to the complex ethical problems that a nurse might face, what it *can* do is to at least provide the basis for 'principled discussion'.

The four principles approach as a framework

There are several different frameworks designed to help to support discussion and decision-making in relation to ethical dilemmas. One such framework was put forward by Beauchamp and Childress (2001) to help to examine the ethical dilemma raised by a specific situation and thereby facilitate decision-making and ethical practice.

> ### Key points
>
> Nursing students, like all health professionals, are regularly confronted with ethical dilemmas and the framework is useful in this relatively early stage in your career to clarify your thinking, help to resolve dilemmas, and also provide justification for your decisions.

Let us explore further the potential use of a framework to help to clarify our thinking when confronted with dilemmas. The framework suggested by Beauchamp and Childress (2001) suggests that thinking about moral matters can be broken into four interrelated levels of thinking, as follows.

- Level 1: judgements
- Level 2: rules
- Level 3: principles
- Level 4: theories

Let's look at this in more detail.

Level 1: judgements

When *any* situation arises, not necessarily in the healthcare field, those involved, as well as those who witness it or simply hear or read about it, make an initial *judgement* about that situation. This judgement may be quite difficult to articulate: it might simply be a 'gut reaction', or a feeling that something is either 'not quite right', or conversely that something is right or good.

....

💡 Thinking about

Imagine an occasion recently on which you heard about something that made you feel uneasy or worried—that you feel should not have happened. This may be something that involves a patient or client for whom you have cared or that you have heard about from a fellow student or simply something you have heard on a news report.

How did this make you feel? Why do you think you felt this way? What made you think something wasn't 'quite right'?

....

Consideration of the following clinical example may help to further clarify your thinking.

You are asked to assist in the taking of a venous blood sample from a patient for analysis. The patient is very frail and in the last stages of life. The patient's veins are difficult to find. From handover, you know that the patient is to be treated 'conservatively', and that their care is following an 'end-of-life pathway' (Liverpool End-of-Life Care pathway, 2009, available at **http://www.mcpcil.org.uk/liverpool-care-pathway/index.htm**). You ask the registered nurse who is undertaking the procedure why it has been requested and she responds by saying that although they are routine blood tests, on this occasion they have been asked for specifically by the doctor in charge of the patient's care.

Some questions that you may ask yourself are:

- what benefit are these tests to the patient at this time?
- will the results change the way in which the patient is treated and cared for?

If the answer to these questions is that there is no benefit and no change in patient management and that the patient may experience unnecessary pain, you may make the judgement that to proceed would be inappropriate or even *wrong*. According to the proposed framework, the judgements that are made in such situations are due to the existence of certain *rules* that state what should or should not be done and thereby provide justification for level 1 *judgements*.

Level 2: rules

So what are these 'rules'?

According to Beauchamp and Childress (2001), there are four main 'rules' that generate our judgements. Although these rules are related and in some ways overlap, they can also be discussed individually.

The first rule: always tell the truth

This is sometimes known as the principle of **veracity**, a principle defined as the obligation to tell the truth and not to lie or to deceive others (Fry & Johnstone, 2002).

A situation may make you feel uncomfortable simply because you realize that there has been some deception and you intuitively feel this to be wrong. This is because the 'truth-telling rule' has been broken.

Telling the truth in a clinical situation is clearly very important. Any therapeutic relationship requires *trust* and telling the truth goes some way to reinforcing that trust. Trust in a relationship means that everyone concerned will act and perform as expected. Patients should be able to trust that the nurse caring for them is not only competent and working in their best interests, but also open and honest. Therefore when someone asks a direct question about proposed treatment or care, the nurse is under a moral duty not to lie. Telling the truth is fundamental to the trust within that relationship. Similarly, nurses must also be able to trust that a patient will be truthful and fulfil their responsibilities, so the nurse can be confident that any information given is correct and truthful. If this is not the case, then their ability to help might be compromised.

....

💡 Thinking about

1 Is it ever legitimate to tell a lie?
2 How might you justify this ethically?
3 Is there a difference *ethically* between telling a lie and simply avoiding the question?

....

To help you to answer these questions, let us consider the following example.

Patient: *Nurse—am I going to die?*
Nurse: *What makes you ask me that question?*

What, if any, is the difference between a response such as this and simply lying to the patient? For example, if the nurse, respond were to: *No you are not going to die.*

Let us explore this further by looking at an example from practice (Scenario 3.5).

Scenario 3.5

You are working on a children's ward and a boy, Jamie, aged 13, who has Down's syndrome, asks you what the doctor is saying to his mother and asks if he can go with them to the consulting room. You are aware that the doctor is informing the child's mother of the recent test result, which indicates that he has leukaemia.

You tell Jamie that he can see his mother later and try to distract him by taking him to the day room to watch a film. You realize that you have not been completely honest with the boy, having deliberately withheld information from him about his condition and the purpose of the meeting between his mother and the doctor, even though he has asked you a direct question.

How could you justify not following the 'truth-telling' rule in this case?

Points to consider

1 You might argue that informing the boy may have caused more distress and do 'more harm than good'. You were therefore acting in his best interests.

2 You might recognize that the best situation would be for his mother to inform him or at least be with him when he is informed.

3 You might feel that due to both his age and Down's syndrome, he would not be able to understand what you are telling him. This might be particularly problematic, especially in the context of the discussions concerning equality and diversity in the previous section.

Issues such as competence and mental capacity will be further discussed in Chapter 4. You may wish to return to this question later to reaffirm your understanding.

The second 'rule' : everyone is deserving of privacy

No one should intrude on the personal space of another, either physically or in relation to their business or personal information. In healthcare settings, privacy is often very difficult to promote and maintain. We know that people highly value their privacy and current campaigns in health care emphasize this, including the *Essence of Care* (DH, 2003) and the *Chief Nursing Officer Report on Privacy and Dignity* (DH, 2007). Consider the following examples, which might take place in a hospital ward.

Doctors' rounds or reviews are sometimes undertaken when personal care is being delivered. This can make it difficult to ensure that personal space is not intruded upon either due to the environment or the activity of others in that area.

Similarly, when personal issues are discussed with the patient or between staff at the bedside or on the telephone, others may hear private/personal information and details.

Following the rule of promoting 'privacy', therefore, the nurse must do everything possible to minimize these risks by taking the patient away from the bedside to a private area whenever possible. This might be a bathroom, office, or private day room, for example. On the occasions on which examinations and conversations have to take place at the bedside, those who are able to leave, such as visitors, should be asked to do so with due regard always given to the sensitivity of this request and the potentially negative response of those being asked to leave.

Issues of privacy should not be underestimated in any environment, however. These might be equally as problematic in the person's home as in an acute clinical environment, depending on what the home circumstances are.

Remember that issues of dignity and privacy are not only of concern in hospitals or care homes. Below are some examples of feelings highlighted by clients, which could be equally applicable in any care environment, not least in the client's own home.

- Feeling neglected or ignored while receiving care
- Being made to feel worthless or a nuisance
- Being treated more as an object than a person
- Feeling their privacy was not being respected during intimate care
- Perceiving a disrespectful attitude from staff or being addressed in ways they find disrespectful, for example by their first name
- Generally being rushed and not listened to

The third 'rule': we should always maintain confidentiality

According to Mason and Whitehead (2003), confidentiality is possibly the single most revered principle in healthcare ethics and forms the basis of the professional–patient relationship. Nurses have a duty to protect confidential information and:

> the person who is in the care of a nurse or midwife has a right to believe that information given to them in confidence is only used for the purposes for which it was given and will not be disclosed to others without permission.
> NMC (2008A)

Does this make you reconsider any of your thoughts with regards to Jamie, the boy with Down's syndrome in Scenario 3.5? The NMC is clear that this duty to maintain confidentiality is not necessarily all-encompassing and that there are certain 'exceptional circumstances' in which confidentiality might be broken and information disclosed.

> For example you must disclose information if you believe someone may be at risk of harm in line with the law of the country in which you are practising.
> NMC (2008A)

However, it is emphasized that should a nurse decide to disclose any information without the permission of the individual concerned, then they are fully accountable for this decision and will need to be able to justify their actions as being in the best interests of the public. The legal aspects of confidentiality and the responsibilities of the nurse are further discussed in Chapter 4.

Thinking about

1   Have you ever felt that you ought to break a confidence?
2   Under what circumstances might this be appropriate?
3   Who might support you in this decision-making process?

Scenario 3.6 may help you to answer these questions.

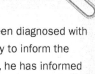

Scenario 3.6

You are aware that one of the men whom you are looking after has been diagnosed with a condition that may impact on his ability to drive. While he has a duty to inform the Driver Vehicle Licensing Authority (DVLA) of the changes in his health, he has informed you that he has no intention of giving up his licence, as he feels that this will seriously affect his independence and impact negatively on his lifestyle.

What might you do?

1   In the first instance, you may try to explain the potential consequences of his choice not to inform the DVLA.
2   However, if you fail to persuade him to inform the authority himself, following discussion with others in the multidisciplinary team, it may be decided to inform the authority, because breaking a confidence may be deemed as being for 'the greater good'. However, this decision should never be taken lightly. Breaking the confidentiality of a person calls into question the whole ethos of the caring relationship and must be undertaken only following significant consideration, appropriate consultation, and with recognition of individual accountability. You also have to tell the patient of your plans to break the confidence.

The fourth 'rule': always keep promises

This is sometimes called **fidelity** and is concerned with an obligation to keep promises and remain faithful to your commitments. More broadly, it might be seen as upholding principles at the heart of the patient–nurse relationship. Implicit within this relationship are certain promises, including promises to work in the best interest of the patient, maintain confidentiality, obtain **informed consent**, be honest, be responsive to their needs, and take on the role of advocate (Bosek & Savage, 2007).

One fundamental rule might be that 'breaking promises is wrong'. However, it is possible to argue that it is morally acceptable to break promises when the breaking of the promise produces more good than if the promise is kept. Similar to the professional commitment to confidentiality, it is sometimes argued that breaking promises is morally acceptable when the welfare of a third party is put at risk by the keeping of that promise.

 Thinking about

1 Is it ever legitimate to break a promise?
2 Under what circumstances might you break a promise to a patient?
3 Has this ever happened to you?

Use the following example to help you to answer these questions
You are undertaking a drug round with your mentor when a patient says: 'I don't need any pain killers at the moment, but I will need them before physiotherapy. You must promise to bring them at 10 a.m.' At 9.50 a.m., a patient at the other end of the ward becomes emotionally distressed when told that she cannot go home that day as she expected. At 10.30 a.m., you see the patient mobilizing with the physiotherapist. As he passes you, he says angrily: 'You broke your promise.' This comment implies the need for you to justify your behaviour. In other words, you are being called to account.

Any justifications would include the fact that you had acted in a way that reflected your priorities at the time and, in weighing up the conflicting needs of both patients, had addressed the dilemma by assessing where the greatest need lay and acted accordingly—a series of actions that are perfectly justifiable ethically. It is likely that, following an explanation, the person concerned is also likely to agree that your priorities had changed as they are likely to view the situation from the same ethical context.

Therefore, according to Beauchamp and Childress (2001), society generally believes that we should all abide by the rules of:

● telling the truth;
● maintaining privacy;
● maintaining confidentiality;
● keeping promises.

It also becomes clear that our original *judgements* about a particular situation are made, almost instinctively on occasions, due to the fact that we hold these rules to be true.

So what underpins these rules? Where did these rules come from?

Level 3: the principles

This particular framework offered by Beauchamp and Childress (2001) indicates that the rules are supported by certain key *principles*, of which there are four.

Autonomy

The first principle is respect for **autonomy**. The concept of autonomy implies personal liberty and relates to ideas of independence, self-reliance, freedom of choice, and the ability to make decisions. It does not mean, however, that we can do exactly what we want because it is based on rational thought or reason rather than simply desires or wants. It is worth recognizing that the idea of personal choice is central to current health care and health care policy and the support of a patient's autonomy coincides with this philosophy (DH, 2008).

Nurses contribute to the autonomy of their patients in a number of ways, not least giving necessary information to promote *informed consent.*

Historically, John Stuart Mill, a British philosopher of the nineteenth century, argued that the only permissible reason to remove a person's social or personal autonomy is to prevent harm to others (Rumbold, 1999). However, you may have experienced a situation in which a person has been advised to have treatment and yet decides to refuse this treatment—a decision that may seem illogical, potentially dangerous, and indeed not in their *best interest*.

....

➡ Theory into action

What does 'in the patient's best interest' mean?

Is it:

1   care/treatment that the health professional considers to be the best for them?

Or:

2   care/treatment that ultimately respects the individual's autonomy?

....

Scenario 3.7 may help you to further consider these issues.

Scenario 3.7

You are caring for a patient who is known to have an alcohol abuse problem; he has been admitted to your unit on a number of occasions following falls at home. He is now mobilizing quite well following his fall and his other chronic health problems are being managed. It is time to clarify the plans for his future care and discharge him from the unit.

The patient's daughter and a number of the members of the team feel that it would not be safe to discharge him to his home, because previously he has continued to drink, and this could result in further falls and the risk of further injury or being left undiscovered for a long period of time. The patient, however, is insistent that he goes home.

Should the man in Scenario 3.7 be 'allowed' home?

Some of the considerations the team may discuss are as follows.

1 Ethically:
   - one should always respect the person and promote their autonomy;
   - one should act in a way to promote well-being and good (known as the concept of – **beneficence** – see below);
   - one should always attempt to ensure that no harm is caused (known as the concept of **non-maleficence** – also see below);
   - one should ensure that the consideration of others is recognized with regards appropriate use of resources, staff support, and so on.
2 Professionally:
   - the NMC directs the registered nurse to act as the patient's advocate, providing person-centred care, maintaining dignity, and showing respect (NMC, 2008a).
3 Legally (as we will see in further detail in Chapter 4):
   - no one has the power to take away this patient's right to freedom (Human Rights Act 1998);
   - nor under the Mental Capacity Act 2005 do you have the right to override the decisions of a competent person.

So what should you do in such situations? Clearly, there are many different aspects to consider, however, the key thing for any nurse is that, when called to account, they can justify their decisions with sound ethical, professional, and legal reasoning.

Non-maleficence

Another principle is known as non-maleficence. According to the *Oxford English Dictionary* (Seanes & Stevenson, 2009), maleficence can be defined as follows.

1 Evildoing; an act of evildoing
2 Malefic character; harmfulness

Non-maleficence is therefore the 'absence or lack of' harm or evil.

This concept is generally considered to be the foundation on which healthcare delivery rests, as nurses and other healthcare workers have a duty not to harm patients or clients. On the surface, this seems obvious and even self-evident.

....

💡 Thinking about

Can you think of any aspects of nursing care that might be described as 'harmful'? Most procedures carry with them some element of risk of harm, don't they?

Who is best placed to define what counts as harmful?

Is the patient or client always the best person to decide this?

Use the following example to help you to answer these questions.

....

You are being assessed by your mentor on your competence at administering medication by intramuscular injection. This procedure carries a number of risks. Some potential risks to consider include:

- correct drug;
- correct dose;
- correct patient;
- correct time;
- correct route and site;
- any issues of informed consent, especially in your role as a learner with relatively limited experience;
- pain that will inevitably be inflicted;
- potential for adverse reaction.

Health and safety issues include:

- the potential for a needle-stick injury;
- correct and safe sharps disposal;
- the reduction of infection risk;
- any issues of insufficient or poor supervision.

It soon becomes clear that the advice to 'at least do no harm' is far more complicated than might be first thought. It seems almost impossible to avoid doing at least *some* type of harm while attempting to promote, maintain, or restore health. Some of this 'harm' might be quite subtle in relation to the needs and preferences of that individual. It might be psychological and relate to threats to the patient's independence. It may concern an individual's ability to make free choices due to incapacity, for example, or the disclosing of confidential information about a person that may result in distress and failure to respect a person's autonomy.

The question then is: how far does this principle of non-maleficence extend? If it is fair to say that every drug administered has the potential for harmful side effects and if we were to take this principle to its logical conclusion, we would never administer any medication to anyone.

Beneficence

According to the *Oxford English Dictionary* (Soanes & Stevenson 2009), beneficence can be defined as follows.

1 Doing good, the manifestation of benevolence or kindly feeling, active kindness
2 A benefaction, a beneficent gift, deed, or work

This therefore promotes an obligation to 'do good' and act in ways that promote the well-being of others (Davis et al., 2006).

However, the principle also brings with it potential problems. It highlights that you should always do what is in the best interest of the patient and that the good of the patient may be put before one's own needs as a nurse (Rumbold, 1999), thus emphasizing the difference between nursing and many other professions or jobs. There seems to be an implied obligation for *self-sacrifice* for the nurse that may not be expected in other walks of life, which is why, for example, you may have felt the obligation, and indeed the willingness, to stay late after your shift officially ended to help a patient or to complete some aspect of care.

Within nursing, beneficence also relates to considerations of the practical outcomes for the individual concerned, and the balancing of benefits and costs (Beauchamp & Childress, 2001). However, as with the other ethical principles, this is not always self-evident and it is often difficult to determine exactly what will benefit another person most.

Rumbold (1999) claims that beneficence is not an independent principle, but is inextricably related to non-maleficence, and it is this relationship that justifies care being delivered that might be, *on first glance*, inappropriate due to the harm that it causes. The administration of medication via a hypodermic needle is clearly harmful in some way, but if the result of non-intervention means certain death from infection, then the morally justifiable act is that which causes the least harm and the most good.

The concept of best-interest decision-making is underpinned by the ethical principles of beneficence and non-maleficence.

Justice

Justice is notoriously difficult to define. It involves ideas of fairness and treating people equally. It relates to giving people what they deserve and/or what they have a right to. However, applying this principle in specific circumstances can be very problematic, as decisions may appear to 'depend on the specific situation'.

Ideas of justice, however, are used to guide our decisions globally, nationally, and locally. Justice might be aspired to through government policy decisions and the equal provision of resources nationally. This attempts to ensure that everyone has equal access to services when they need them. These types of consideration also impact on the relationship between individual nurses and individual patients, assuming that all people have the right to be respected and also assuming that all decisions are made on principle rather than emotion.

· ·

 Thinking about

If two people require the same or similar treatment, who should receive the treatment first?

How might you justify your decision to prioritize?

· ·

Scenario 3.8 highlights some areas that you might consider.

Scenario 3.8

You are undertaking a placement in a health centre and a mother brings her baby to see the health visitor as she is concerned about her development. During the conversation, you get the impression that she is feeling low in mood and has intimated that she has recently experienced suicidal thoughts. When you are asked to make an appointment for her to see the counsellor, you find that the practice nurse also wants the last available appointment with the counsellor for a 72-year-old man. The practice nurse is concerned that, since the death of his wife and with no children close by, the patient is struggling to cope and has expressed a wish to die.

The person who does not get the available appointment may have to wait as long as two months to be seen.

Possible approaches

1 First come, first served: whoever arrived at reception first to make the appointment gets it.
2 According to merit: who deserves this most? The woman who has a long life in front of her and a baby, or an older man who has no one close left and no one who relies on him, but who has worked hard and contributed to society all his life?
3 According to need—that is, medical need: who needs this appointment most to prevent harm coming to them? Judging this is clearly very difficult.
4 According to outcome: whoever will benefit most from the appointment, is given the appointment.

As previously discussed, each of these approaches *may* be legitimately defended; however, the ethical principles and the overriding ethical theories behind the decision-making are the essential issues in relation to the accountability of the nurse.

Level 4: ethical theories

According to Beauchamp and Childress (2001), the whole framework of ethical decision making is underpinned by two main ethical theories generally known as **deontology** and **consequentialism**. A specific type of consequentialism called **utilitarianism** is also often described.

- Deontology
  - Deontology speaks of a person acting according to certain given principles— that which is their *duty*. An act is good or bad simply by the fact that it conforms to a set of rules that lay down our duty or obligation. Therefore the consequences of the act are almost immaterial.

- Consequentialism
  - Consequentialism, on the other hand, judges the rightness or wrongness of an act only on the grounds of whether its consequences produce more benefits than disadvantages. It promotes a calculation of the benefits and disadvantages of the consequence of an action.
- Utilitarianism
  - Utilitarianism, put simply, is a type of consequentialism in that a person ought always to act in a way that produces the *greatest amount of good for the greatest amount of people.*

These ethical theories are very complex. What might these fundamentally theoretical standpoints mean in practice? How might they help your decision-making in the *real world*?

Let us revisit a previous example. You are undertaking a drug round with your mentor when a patient says: 'I don't need any pain killers at the moment, but I will need them before physiotherapy. You must promise to bring them at 10 a.m.' At 9.50 a.m., a patient at the other end of the ward becomes emotionally distressed when told that she cannot go home that day as she expected. At 10.30 a.m., you see the patient mobilizing with the physiotherapist. As he passes you, he says angrily: 'You broke your promise.'

How might the 'rights and wrongs' of this situation be assessed from the point of view of the ethical theories?

1 Deontology
2 Consequentialism

A *deontologist* may argue that the rule of keeping promises overrides other considerations. Therefore they might feel obligated and would have a duty to maintain their promise. Clearly, this becomes less straightforward in reality as they may also hold the belief that you should always help someone in distress. Two 'rules' or 'obligations' clash here and create a *dilemma*.

A supporter of *consequentialism* would justify their practice by working out the alternatives first and the *consequences* of each alternative. Their decision-making would be driven by assessing which action resulted in the best consequences for those concerned.

Such discussions show how integral ethical thinking in the form of principles and theories are to nursing practice. As we shall see in the next chapter, the law and/or professional advice such as the NMC Code (2008a) will not necessarily offer you the specific answers to the complex dilemmas that you will inevitably face as a nurse. Dilemmas that raise questions about whether a nursing intervention is morally acceptable and ethically right require thorough exploration and analysis to help to provide clarity and rationale and justification for practice.

Summary

- There are significant differences in the accountability of students and registered nurses.
- Nurses have a key role as advocates for patients and in their lead role within the multidisciplinary team. This inevitably involves them in certain ethical dilemmas.
- An ethical framework can provide the basis for 'principled discussion' and subsequent action.
- *Rules* that state what should or should not be done provide justification for level 1 *judgements*.
- These rules are supported by four main ethical principles: autonomy; beneficence; non-maleficence; and justice.
- The whole framework of ethical decision-making is underpinned by two main ethical theories: deontology and consequentialism.

In this chapter, we have looked at:

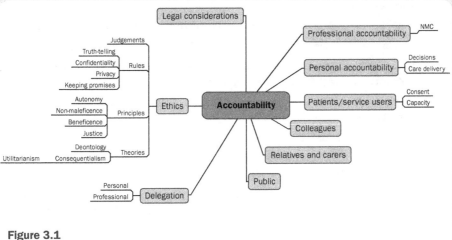

Figure 3.1

Online Resource Centre

 This textbook is accompanied by an Online Resource Centre that provides interactive learning resources and tools to help you to prepare for the transition from student to fully qualified member of staff. After you have completed each chapter and whenever you see this icon, please go to the ORC at your earliest convenience. If you have not done so already, save the ORC web address into your favourites: **http://www.oxfordtextbooks.co.uk/orc/burton**

References

Beauchamp TL & Childress JF (2001) *Principles of Biomedical Ethics*, 5th edn. Oxford University Press, Oxford.

Bosek DeWolf S & Savage TA (2007) *The Ethical Component of Nursing Education: Integrating Ethics into Clinical Experience*. Lippincott Williams & Wilkins, Philadelphia, PA.

Bostridge M (2008) *Florence Nightingale: The Woman and Her Legend*. Viking, London.

Burnard P & Chapman C (2005) *Professional & Ethical Issues in Nursing*, 3rd edn. Bailliere Tindall, London.

Caulfield H (2005) *Accountability*. Blackwell Publishing, Oxford.

Davis A, Tschudin V & De Raeve L (eds) (2006) *Essentials of Teaching and Learning in Nursing Ethics: Perspectives and Methods*. Churchill Livingstone, Edinburgh.

Department of Health (2003) *Essence of Care: Patient-focused Benchmarking for Health Care Practitioners*. HMSO, London.

Department of Health (2004) *Choosing Health: Making Healthy Choices Easier*. HMSO, London.

Department of Health (2007) *Chief Nursing Officer Report on Privacy and Dignity: Mixed Sex Accommodation in Hospitals*. DH, London.

Department of Health (2008) *High Quality Care for All: NHS Next Stage Review*. DH, London.

Dimond B (2008) *Legal Aspects of Nursing*, 5th edn. Pearson Longman, Harlow.

Duff L (1995) Standards of care, quality assurance and accountability. In: R Watson (ed) *Accountability in Nursing Practice*. Chapman and Hall, London.

Fry ST & Johnstone M (2002) *Ethics in Nursing Practice: A Guide to Ethical Decision Making*, 2nd edn. Blackwell Publishing, Oxford.

Human Rights Act 1998. HMSO, London.

International Council of Nurses (2006) *ICN – International Council of Nurses*, Geneva, Switzerland. Available at: **http://www.icn.ch/**

Jacobs K (2004) *Accountability and clinical governance in nursing: a critical overview of the topic*. In: S Tilley & R Watson (eds) *Accountability in Nursing and Midwifery*, 2nd edn. Blackwell Publishing, Oxford, 21–37.

Liverpool End of Life Care pathway (2009). Available at: **http://www.mcpcil.org.uk/liverpool-care-pathway/index.htm**

Maben J & Griffiths P (2008) *Nurses in Society: Starting the Debate*. National Nursing Research Unit, King's College, London.

Mason T & Whitehead E (2003) *Thinking Nursing*. Open University Press, Maidenhead.

Mental Capacity Act 2005. HMSO, London.

Nursing and Midwifery Council (2010) *Standards of Proficiency for Pre-registration Nursing Education*. NMC, London.

Nursing and Midwifery Council (2007) *Standards for Medicines Management*. NMC, London.

Nursing and Midwifery Council (2008a) *The Code: Standards of Conduct, Performance and Ethics for Nurses and Midwives*. NMC, London.

Nursing and Midwifery Council (2008b) *Focus Group Consultation Report on Have Your Say on Equality and Diversity.* NMC, London. Available at: **http://www.nmc-uk.org/Documents/ Consultations/RPNE/RPNE%20Phase%201/RPNE%20Phase1%20consultation%20 focus%20group%20report.pdf**

Nursing and Midwifery Council (2008c) *Advice on Delegation for Registered Nurses and Midwives.* NMC, London. Available at: **http://www.nmc-uk.org/Nurses-and-midwives/ Advice-by-topic/A/Advice/Delegation/**

Nursing and Midwifery Council (2009) *Guidance on Professional Conduct for Nursing and Midwifery Students.* NMC, London.

Pugh WTG (1944) *Practical Nursing including Hygiene and Dietetics*, 4th edn. Blackwood and Sons, London. In: McClarey M. Quality measures in health care: have they always been with us? (2009) *Journal of Research in Nursing*, **14**: 291–3.

Rumbold G (1999) *Ethics in Nursing* Practice, 3rd edn. Bailliere Tindall, Edinburgh.

Savage J & Moore L (2004) *Interpreting Accountability.* Royal College of Nursing Institute, Oxford.

Soanes C & Stevenson A (eds) (2009) *Concise Oxford English Dictionary*, 11th edn. Oxford University Press, Oxford.

Sinclair A (1995) The chameleon of accountability: forms and discourses. *Accounting, Organisations and Society*, **20**: 219–37. In: S Tilley & R Watson (eds) (2004) *Accountability in Nursing and Midwifery*, 2nd edn. Blackwell Publishing, Oxford.

Storey L (2002) The 'crackerjack' model of nursing and its relationship to accountability. *Nurse Education in Practice*, **2**: 133–41.

Watson R (1992) Justifying your practice. *Nursing*, **5**(3): 11–13.

Accountability, decision-making, and the law

Graham Ormrod and Nichola Barlow

The aim of this chapter is to:

- ➔ specifically explore the legal context of accountability and its relevance for student nurses in their transition to becoming staffs nurses;
- ➔ review specific legal concepts and definitions;
- ➔ explore the differences between criminal and civil law;
- ➔ further investigate the concept of negligence and its relevance to nurses;
- ➔ discuss the concepts of consent and capacity in a legal context;
- ➔ confirm the practical and everyday relevance and importance of the law to the nurse's role.

Introduction

In the previous chapter, we explored the concept of accountability, particularly from an ethical point of view, and highlighted the importance of this in everyday nursing practice.

The ethical context of society can change, and the things that society deems good, right, or proper can change as years pass. The law might change accordingly, as the law represents the rules that reflect the values of a society at that particular time in its history. The function of the law, therefore, clearly relates in some way to the current moral context of society. The law can, for example, state what is acceptable as *good* behaviour and also place *duties* on individuals to act in the best interests of others. It also requires individuals to behave in a *fair* way and insists on equal treatment of every member of the community. These points have obvious *moral* components and similarities.

. . . .

 ## Theory into action

How do you think *ethical* accountability is related to *legal* accountability?

How do you think the ethical values of society relate to the laws that govern that society?

. . . .

To help you to answer these questions, consider Scenario 4.1.

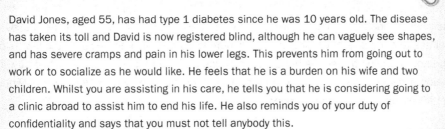

Scenario 4.1

David Jones, aged 55, has had type 1 diabetes since he was 10 years old. The disease has taken its toll and David is now registered blind, although he can vaguely see shapes, and has severe cramps and pain in his lower legs. This prevents him from going out to work or to socialize as he would like. He feels that he is a burden on his wife and two children. Whilst you are assisting in his care, he tells you that he is considering going to a clinic abroad to assist him to end his life. He also reminds you of your duty of confidentiality and says that you must not tell anybody this.

As a student nurse, what would you do? How might this differ from when you are a registered nurse?

Such scenarios indicate how legal, ethical, and professional issues are invariably intertwined. They indicate some of the difficult moral questions about modern life and the potentially changing moral landscape both nationally in the UK and also internationally. Only time will tell if this ongoing *ethical* debate will eventually be reflected in *legal* changes.

Professionally, however, it is worth remembering that the **Nursing and Midwifery Council** (NMC, 2010), while confirming the need for the student to ensure confidentiality, also emphasizes that it is essential that a student consults and refers to a registered nurse when clinical decisions need specialist knowledge. Similarly the NMC (2009a: 12) counsels that, as a student, you should 'seek advice from your mentor or tutor before disclosing information if you believe someone may be at risk of harm'.

Similarly, in 2009, following the publication of the Crown Prosecution Service (CPS) guidelines, *Interim Policy for Prosecutors in Respect of Cases of Assisted Suicide*, the NMC felt it necessary to reiterate its statutory duty and remind nurses that *the law on assisted suicide has not changed.*

Key points

The web links below give examples of emotional and impassioned 'real-life' stories that indicate how incidences in society can eventually result in changes in the law.

http://news.bbc.co.uk/1/hi/health/7898816.stm

http://www.dignityindying.org.uk/

http://www.guardian.co.uk/society/2009/jul/30/scotland-considers-assisted-suicide-law

What is the law?

Let us first review a few fundamentals. You might think that the healthcare context is more *litigious* or *legalized* than in the past, as there may appear to be an increasing number of healthcare cases being heard in court. An understanding of the law as it relates to nursing is becoming more and more important, as knowledge of the law helps in understanding the scope of nursing practice and the responsibilities that come with being a registered nurse, as well as providing insight in how to prevent any potential legal problems before they happen.

Key points

It is essential, however, not to get too anxious about the possibility of becoming embroiled in legal action! From your discussions with colleagues during your training, you may have come to the conclusion that every nurse knows of 'someone' who has been sued for negligence and 'struck off' or removed from the NMC register. Rest assured that this is far from the truth: as we shall see, it is still very rare for nurses to become involved in legal processes and the vast majority of nurses go through their career without such an unfortunate experience.

According to Caulfield (2005), the law is a set of rules and penalties agreed by society. Another definition claims that the law is the framework that a society develops to limit lawlessness, thus allowing it to function in a way that is predictable and acceptable to its members (Jones & Jenkins, 2004).

Scottish law

Scotland has a different court system from that of England and Wales. Scots law is the law of Scotland. It is a unique system with ancient roots and has a basis in Roman law, combining features of both civil law and common law. Thus Scotland has what is called a pluralistic legal system. Since 1707, Scotland has shared legislature with the rest of the UK, but both Scotland and England retained their fundamentally different legal systems, although there is some English influence on Scots law. In recent years, Scots law has also been affected by European law.

The Court of Session is the supreme court and the Sheriff Courts are the regional courts. The main division in Scots law is between *public law*, involving the state, and *private law,* in which only private persons are involved. Public law covers, among other areas, criminal law. Private law or the 'law of persons', including children and adults, is often simply part of the law of the land: for example, murder and theft are not defined in statute as offences, but are dealt with under common law. The majority of discussion within this chapter will relate to English law, but, reference will be made appropriately on occasions to the differences in the two countries.

The two main types of law

The two main types of law that affect nurses and to be discussed in this chapter are *criminal* law and *civil* law. What are the main differences between criminal law and civil law? According to Dimond (2008: 12):

> 'a breach of the criminal law can be followed by prosecution in the criminal courts, whereas liability in civil law is actionable in the civil courts and may or may not be a crime. There is no necessary moral difference between the two.'

Let us explore the differences a little further.

Criminal law

Criminal law is concerned with the relationship between the *state* and the *individual* (Caulfield, 2005). This type of law essentially settles disputes between individuals and society as a whole. It deals with offences that transgress rules of society and is a means of enforcing society's rules on an individual. To break the laws of the land allows the state to punish the offender by means of arrest by the police and prosecution by the state in the name of the Queen as head of state. Guilt under criminal law invariably results in some form of punishment. Punishment can be in the form of:

- fines;
- probation (which can include conditions such as attendance at a training centre or hospital order under various sections of the Mental Health Act 2007 or Mental Health (Care and Treatment) (Scotland) Act 2003);
- community service;

- suspended sentence (with or without supervision);
- prison.

One of the main differences between criminal law and civil law is what is known as the *burden of proof*. In criminal law, the prosecution has the burden of proving to the satisfaction of the jury that the accused is guilty 'beyond all reasonable doubt'.

Civil law

Unlike criminal law, civil law regulates relationships between *individual citizens* rather than between the *state* and an individual. An action is brought by a person, who has suffered harm, known as the claimant or plaintiff, against another person or organization, known as the defendant. This is often the area of the law that concerns nurses most as they feel they may be accused of *negligence* and of causing harm to a patient or client.

The *burden of proof* in cases of civil law rests on 'on the balance of probabilities' rather than 'beyond reasonable doubt'. What this means in practical terms is that the accusation has to be deemed more likely to be true than not. If an accusation of negligence is proved 'on the balance of probabilities', then, again unlike in criminal law, this wrong is redressed by awarding *damages*, and financial compensation is given in place of punishment such as imprisonment, for example (Dimond, 2008).

Vicarious liability

It is important to recognize and understand the concept of *vicarious liability* at this point. Vicarious liability is defined as the indirect liability of an organization for negligence by its staff while acting in the course of employment. An employer has certain responsibilities to their staff: a National Health Service (NHS) trust, for example, has responsibilities towards the nurses whom it employs. These responsibilities may include creating an environment in which the general working conditions are appropriate and equipment is available and working properly. Similarly, the employer has a responsibility to ensure that staffing levels are adequate and staff are competent and know what they are doing. This all relates to the concept of vicarious liability. As the employer is responsible for the environment and ultimately the competence of its employees, it is invariably the employer/trust that is sued if any employees are accused of negligence. Therefore, the employer would take on any liability *vicariously* as long as the nurse were working within an appropriate scope of practice and within any appropriate guidelines. It is also true to say that your employer will undoubtedly have more money than you!

Theory into action

Do you know how to access relevant guidelines, policies, or procedures in your placement area?

It is important, and could be very interesting, to find some of the key policies within your current placement.

Do you know of any that specifically relate to students while undertaking placement learning?

For example: what is the policy in relation to student involvement in the administration of controlled drugs?

Find this policy, read it, and discuss any implications for your learning experience with your **mentor**.

It is worth remembering that the NMC standards of **proficiency** (NMC, 2004/2010) stress that students must be able to apply relevant principles to ensure the safe administration of therapeutic substances.

Elements in an action of negligence

Let us look a little more closely at the concept of negligence, which can cause such anxiety for nurses. Put simply, the elements involved in any action of negligence can be summed up in three key points (Dimond, 2008), as follows.

- A *duty of care* is owed by the defendant to the plaintiff.
- There is a breach in the *standard* of the duty of care owed.
- This breach has caused *reasonably foreseeable harm*.

Duty of care

Theory into action

What is your understanding of the term 'duty of care'?

How does this relate to the relationship between a nurse and a patient/client?

Make a list of to whom you feel the nurse may owe a duty of care.

Discuss this with your mentor and/or personal tutor.

Did their list match yours?

It is not always easy to decide when a nurse owes a duty of care to another person. For example, if you are looking after a child, you clearly owe that child a duty of care. However, where does the duty of care lie in relation to the parents, both mum and/or dad? This might not be quite so clear, especially if there is disagreement with regards to which treatment is in the child's best interest. This may be further complicated by the rare, but tragic, 'right to life' decisions, which can generate opposing views from the mother and father, for example, in the case of the mother and father who opposed each other in court over whether life support for their severely ill son should be turned off (see **http://news.bbc.co.uk/1/hi/health/8339078.stm**).

This is just one example of where things may not be as clear as may be initially thought. Remember that the plaintiff or claimant must show that a duty of care was owed for any accusations of negligence to be further pursued.

The standard test of duty of care in law was laid down in the case of *Donoghue v Stevenson* (1932) AC 562 and enshrines the philosophy of the 'good neighbour principle'. Famously, the specifics of this case were that, having bought and drunk half a bottle of beer, someone (the eventual claimant) claimed to have discovered the decomposed remains of a snail in the bottle and then chose to sue the manufacturer, rather than the cafe owner interestingly enough, arguing that it owed a duty of care to the consumer who bought their products to ensure that such a thing should not happen.

Lord Atkin subsequently pronounced:

> You must take reasonable care to avoid acts or omissions which you can reasonably foresee would be likely to injure your neighbour. Who then in law is my neighbour? The answer seems to be persons who are so closely and directly affected by my act that I ought reasonably to have them in contemplation as being so affected when I am directing my mind to the acts or omissions which are called in question.
>
> CITED IN DIMOND (2008: 40)

Put simply, this means that a duty of care exists if you can see that your actions are reasonably likely to cause harm to another person. Therefore, simply by virtue of your relationship with a patient, you owe a duty of care to them.

Key points

In Scots law, *delict* – a Latin word sometimes translated as 'a wilful wrong' – is, among other things, the responsibility to make reparation caused by breach of a duty of care, whether deliberate or accidental. Scots law is different in many respects and concentrates more on general principle and less on specific wrongs. However, the landmark decision in this area for Scotland as for the rest of the UK, is the Scottish case of *Donoghue v Stevenson* (1932) AC 562.

So do you have a duty of care to other service users and carers, relatives, and so on? This may become less clear in the complex healthcare situations in which you become involved. What about situations that arise outside work, for example?

Duty of care outside of work

Presently in the UK, there is no *legal* duty to volunteer help in such circumstances, as there is no *pre-existing* duty of care. It is interesting, however, that this is not necessarily the case in all other countries. Morally, it might be argued, you have a duty of care to assist. If we agree that *all* individuals ought to adhere to the principles of **beneficence**, **non-maleficence**, justice, and **autonomy** as discussed in Chapter 3, then, within a civilized society, it might be argued that such a duty of care is owed simply by virtue of being a fellow human being.

Therefore ,in such circumstances, the nurse owes no greater duty of care than anyone else who might be at the scene. From a professional point of view, the NMC has previously insisted that the nurse should stop and assist as best they can with regards to their competence, although this is slightly less explicit in the current Code (2008). However, in the two advice sheets on 'Duty of care' (**http://www.nmc-uk.org/aArticle. aspx?ArticleID=4011**) and 'Providing care in an emergency situation outside the work environment' (**http://www.nmc-uk.org/aArticle.aspx?ArticleID=4007**), the NMC clarifies that 'although the nurse has no legal duty to stop and give care, she does have a professional duty'. Although, depending on the circumstances, it might be reasonable to expect the 'nurse to do no more than comfort and support the injured person and to reduce the potential for further harm', it is clear that if a nurse 'chooses to walk away from an emergency situation they could be called to account for this'.

So if you do stop and become involved, then you thereby take on a duty of care and would be expected to employ an appropriate professional standard of care. You would be judged against what could reasonably be expected from someone with your knowledge, skills, and abilities when placed in those particular circumstances and would have to demonstrate that you had acted in the person's best interests.

As Dimond (2008) points out, if you move the victim in a car accident and this causes spinal injury, then you could be sued for any further injuries that you has caused. It would have to be shown that you should have anticipated the dangers of moving a person when a spinal injury was possible and also that the victim was not in greater danger by being left where they were.

....

➡ Theory into action

The examples above highlight the complex issues of the nurse's role and responsibility while off duty. It might be interesting to discuss such issues further with colleagues and friends.

For example, should a nurse stop at the scene of an accident? Should this be a *legal* requirement or is it more of an ethical or professional responsibility?

How might this differ from the responsibilities of a member of the general public?

Would you expect the response to be different from nursing students, qualified nurses, and your friends who aren't nurses?

....

One thing that is clear is that 'being a nurse' brings with it certain responsibilities that many other careers do not. Nurses have an obligation to be of good health and good character, and part of the ways of assuring this is the necessity to undergo a Criminal Records Bureau (CRB) check.

The Criminal Records Bureau

The CRB allows organizations such as hospitals, schools, and universities, in which staff, volunteers, or students work with children or vulnerable adults, to check police records and, where appropriate, information held by the Independent Safeguarding Authority (ISA). The two levels of CRB check are:

- standard disclosure;
- enhanced disclosure.

Both are available in cases in which an employer is entitled to ask exempted questions under the Exceptions Order to the Rehabilitation of Offenders Act (ROA) 1974.

Standard disclosure checks show current and spent convictions, cautions, reprimands, and warnings held in the police national computer system. Enhanced disclosure, as in the case of student nurses, is the highest level of check available to anyone working in regulated activity with children or vulnerable adults. This disclosure contains the same information as the standard disclosure, but with the addition of:

- any relevant and proportionate information held by the local police forces;
- a check of the new children and/or vulnerable adults barred lists where requested.

Similar systems are in place in Scotland. Disclosure Scotland has a role in enhancing public safety by providing employers or organizations with criminal history information about individuals applying for posts. More information can be found at: **http://www. disclosurescotland.co.uk/what-is-disclosure/**

The NMC (2009a) leaves no doubt that the behaviour and conduct in a student's personal life may have an impact on:

- **their fitness to practise;**
- their ability to complete their programme;
- the willingness of the university to sign the declaration of good health and good character that enables the student to become a registered nurse.

The examples of inappropriate behaviour offered by the NMC include such wide-ranging issues as aggressive, violent, or threatening behaviour, cheating on course work or plagiarism, and misuse of the Internet and social networking sites. The latter example indicates the ever-changing areas deemed as inappropriate behaviour that can have such a profound and negative effect on a student's career aspirations and also that these obligations continue after registration.

Standards of care

So if we now have greater clarity with regards to the duty of care, let's explore a little further the second element in any accusation of negligence: the concept of *standard of care*. The test to decide whether the standard of care has been broken is based on 'the reasonable man'. (You will note that discussions with regards to the law are often very gender-specific—that is, the law often appears only interested in 'men' and also often relates to specific professions, such as medicine. Unfortunately, or fortunately, however, the law relates equally to us all!) So the 'reasonable man' in the case of nurses means that the nurse acted to the standard expected of a *hypothetical* reasonable nurse in that same situation, or behaved to the standard expected of a reasonable student at that point in their training. It is interesting to note that the law does not speak of acting as the *best* nurse might have done or even a *good* nurse, but simply a reasonable nurse.

This test of the standard of care is often known as the *Bolam test,* after *Bolam v Friern Barnet Hospital Management Committee*: [1957] 1 WLR 583. Any nurse would be deemed to have acted appropriately if they had:

> Acted in accordance with the standard of ordinary skilled man exercising and professing to have that special skill.
> CITED IN DIMOND (2008: 44)

In other words, the *Bolam* test means that where a nurse acts in a way that would be supported by other nurses as being appropriate or *reasonable* practice at that time, it is likely that the court will find that the nurse did not act below the standard of care expected. The court would only deem that the nurse had 'failed' the *Bolam* test if this was seen as '[a] failure to act in accordance with a practice accepted as proper by a responsible body of medical men skilled in that particular art' (Dimond, 2008: 47).

This does not mean that if a nurse chose in very particular circumstances to deviate from standard and 'normal' practice, this would automatically be deemed negligent or wrong, as there may well be appropriate reasons for this in very specific circumstances. This decision to act outside normal practice may have been made following great consideration and delivered subsequently in a most careful or caring way, even though it unfortunately resulted in harm to the patient. However, the great wealth of policies and procedures that support nursing practice are there for a very good, hopefully evidence-based, reason and nurses choosing to take actions outside any standard guidance do so on the understanding that they might well be asked to defend their practice as 'reasonable' in the future.

This standard will have implications for you throughout your career especially if you are eventually in a role that requires extended practice. Nurses working at a 'higher level of practice, such as nurse specialists or nurse consultants, for example, will be judged against the standard expected of others working at that level of practice. This may therefore result in a nurse being judged against the standards of care traditionally delivered by a doctor.

In a climate of changing public and professional expectations and the continuing blurring of professional boundaries and responsibilities, standards will inevitably change accordingly. This reinforces the importance of ensuring competence and proficiency before undertaking any aspects of care, no matter how experienced you are.

As the NMC guide for students of nursing and midwifery emphasizes, you should always recognize and work within your limits of competence and 'work only under the appropriate supervision and support of a qualified professional and ask for help from your mentor or tutor when you need it' (NMC, 2009a: 14).

⊜ Theory into action

Have you ever been put in a position in which you felt that you were working outside your level of competence or felt inadequately supervised?

Such situations can sometimes have tragic consequences, as seen in the case of a student who misunderstood the instruction of her supervising nurse, resulting in a fatal drug error: **http://news.bbc.co.uk/1/hi/england/merseyside/7664404.stm**

How would you advise a more junior student to handle such a situation?

The NMC offers lots of advice for what to do in lots of different situations. Reading and understanding such advice will be useful for you to gain further insight. See **http://www.nmc-uk.org/Nurses-and-midwives/Advice-by-topic/A/**

It is also important to ask your mentors and staff from the university for advice if you find yourself in a situation in which you feel that you lack proficiency or do not know what you are doing. The golden rule is do not put patients at unnecessary risk.

It is extremely important that you inform your mentor or university lecturer immediately if you believe that you, a colleague, or anyone else may be putting someone at risk of harm (NMC, 2009a). Just as for qualified nurses, you have a responsibility to report poor practice and/or abuse. This is often called 'whistleblowing' and can cause significant upset and anxiety for the student nurse. The Royal College of Nursing (RCN) in the UK recognized the seriousness of poor standards going unreported in its initiative *Raising Concerns, Raising Standards* (RCN, 2004), which includes a helpline for members, including students, who have concerns over clinical and staff safety in the workplace or on placement.

The nurse's responsibility in highlighting poor practices again indicates the importance of recognizing and understanding local policies and procedures for safeguarding and protecting the vulnerable in your care and whistleblowing if necessary to ensure that agencies such as social services or the police are involved as appropriate. As the RCN states, serious concerns should initially be disclosed 'internally'. This means discussing with your mentor or tutor first. This may not always be possible, especially if the poor practice involves your mentor or a senior member of staff, and in such cases clearly your university tutor will be the obvious option for support. In the unlikely event that this remains an inappropriate option, talking through with a trusted independent person will help you to clarify whether further action needs to be taken. Available policies for whistleblowing will support and perhaps clarify your thinking and you should always be mindful of the potential for breaking confidentiality in such difficult and often traumatic circumstances. Indeed, according to Gallagher (2010), balancing the obligation to report concerns that prevent further harm to patients with the obligation to maintain confidentiality is one of the most challenging ethical issues in relation to whistleblowing.

Key points

The key point is always that you have a duty to protect those in your care from harm.

So let us get back to the law. It is important to recognize that, fundamentally, the law does not see inexperience as any justification for poor standards of care. A student nurse providing care is judged, legally, by the same standards as an experienced nurse. On first glance, this may seem a little unfair. However, we would all agree that a learner driver is not allowed to drive on the pavement simply due to their inexperience! Certain levels of competence and standards of proficiency are still legitimately expected.

Professionally, as far as the NMC is concerned, it is the registered nurse who is working with you, who is professionally accountable for the consequences of your actions and omissions (NMC, 2009c), and this is why, as a student, you must always work under appropriate supervision. The NMC does reiterate, however, that you can always be called to account by your university or by the law for the consequences of your actions or omissions as a student.

It seems fair to say that patients are entitled to be cared for in a competent way at all times irrespective of whether they are being cared for by a student on their first day or a staff nurse of 20 years' experience. This again emphasizes the importance of:

- only undertaking care when you are competent;
- ensuring appropriate supervision at all times;
- calling for assistance if you are unclear about any aspect of care.

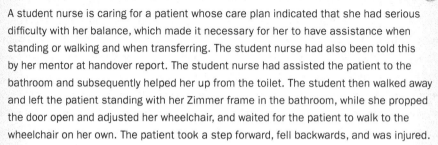

Scenario 4.2

A student nurse is caring for a patient whose care plan indicated that she had serious difficulty with her balance, which made it necessary for her to have assistance when standing or walking and when transferring. The student nurse had also been told this by her mentor at handover report. The student nurse had assisted the patient to the bathroom and subsequently helped her up from the toilet. The student then walked away and left the patient standing with her Zimmer frame in the bathroom, while she propped the door open and adjusted her wheelchair, and waited for the patient to walk to the wheelchair on her own. The patient took a step forward, fell backwards, and was injured.

1 What do you consider to be the main legal issues here?
2 Is the student nurse negligent?
3 What is the legal position of the mentor?

Points to consider
Some points that may help you to answer the above are as follows.

- From a legal point of view, any negligence claim would undoubtedly be made against the trust or care home rather than the individual nurse.
- Failing to give proper appropriate attention to a patient's need for assistance while ambulating is negligence.
- The healthcare facility would be held to the same legal standard of care for a student nurse's error or omission as for the same error or omission by a registered nurse.
- Had the student received training to assist patients with ambulation and transfer?
- Testimony from appropriate colleagues might establish that it is reasonable to expect a nursing student to have the competence and experience to safely support a patient in these circumstances.
- It might be deemed reasonable to expect a student to have had mandatory moving and handling training, for example.
- The nursing student's mentor may be called to testify with regards to her delegation, supervision, communication, and record-keeping. Should the student have known whether the patient needed someone close with her at a safe distance at all times to ambulate?

Caulfield (2005) does acknowledge that the courts will accept that junior staff who have articulated any concerns about their levels of proficiency, competence, and inexperience—for example, if you ask a more senior member of staff to check your work—are more likely to be recognized as having met their expected standards of care. This also highlights the continuing need for all nurses to assertively challenge instructions that they believe to be inappropriate or incorrect.

Reasonably foreseeable

One of the basic principles of the law of negligence is that precautions can be taken only against reasonably known risks (Dimond, 2008). A case of negligence would only be successful if the claimant could prove that what happened could have been foreseen or predictable. The court will ask whether a reasonable person in the defendant's position would have foreseen that the claimant might be injured. If they could not have foreseen injury or damage to the claimant, then the claim will inevitably be unsuccessful.

· ·

➡ Theory into action

In Scenario 4.2, in which the patient fell while being cared for by a student nurses, was the fall 'reasonably foreseeable'?

In such cases, considerations would include the following.

● What was included in the patient's care plan? As emphasized by the NMC (2009b), good record-keeping is an integral part of nursing practice, and is essential to the provision of safe and effective care.

● Had a mobility assessment been undertaken?

● Had advice been taken from physiotherapy colleagues if appropriate?

● Was the patient appropriately confident and aware of the proposed plan?

● What was the student's previous experience and level of proficiency?

● Was the level of supervision sufficient?

● Was delegation appropriate in such circumstances?

Exploration of the above and other aspects of the scenario would help to confirm whether this unfortunate accident was, indeed, 'reasonably foreseeable' or not.

· ·

Cause

Not only has the outcome to be reasonably foreseeable, but a *causal* link between the actions of the nurse and the harm suffered by the plaintiff has also to be proven. Put rather bluntly in the eyes of the law, unlike the NMC, it may not matter how badly a nurse behaves as long as there is no injury. The law is not only interested in the behaviour of the nurse, but crucially also the consequence of that behaviour. This is often known as the 'but for' test. In other words, *but for* the action of the nurse, acting in a way that breaks the standard expected, then no harm would have been caused (Dimond, 2008).

Is the injury measurable?

The final consideration in negligence cases is whether the injury is measurable in some way. This is to enable calculation of the financial compensation if required. In many cases of healthcare negligence, as with many patients who complain about their care, the claimant is often simply asking for an apology or an assurance that such practice will not be repeated. However, should financial damages be deemed appropriate, they are essentially an attempt to place the victim, as far as is possible, in as close a position as that in which they would have been had the incident not happened (Caulfield, 2005).

Accountability: consent and capacity

As was discussed in the previous chapter, the underpinning ethical principle of consent is the promotion of autonomy. The concept of consent is at the heart of the nurse–patient relationship and, on a day-to-day basis, this relationship is often developed on the assumption of *implied consent*. However, as a qualified nurse, you will need to be continually mindful of the many difficult issues associated with gaining appropriate consent. For example, any mentally competent adult has the right in law to consent to any touching of their person. If they are touched without consent or other lawful justification, then they have the right of action in the civil courts of suing for trespass to the person, under section 18 of the Offences Against the Person Act 1861, which relates to grievous bodily harm. In fact, those who provide treatment without consent are more usually prosecuted under the offence of battery, which is a relatively less serious crime. There is no requirement for proof of damage, and any non-consensual touching can result in a case being brought (Tingle & Cribb, 2007). The gaining of consent will usually prevent a successful action for trespass (Dimond, 2008).

The role of the registered nurse in ensuring appropriate lawful consent

So what is the registered nurse's role in ensuring that they act in a legally appropriate manner in line with the NMC Code (2008)? How might this differ from your role when you are a student?

As we have seen, the International Council of Nurses (ICN) and the NMC identify the importance of obtaining consent from patients before conducting any type of intervention or care activity (ICN, 2006; NMC, 2008). Moreover the NMC (2009a) informs student nurses that they should not only always make sure that people know that they are a student, but also emphasize the importance of respecting the wishes of patients and clients and of their right to refuse to allow student nurses to participate in their care. This confirms that the rights of patients and clients override any rights that students may have to knowledge and experience.

In relation to the registered nurse, the NMC (2008) states that, as a registered nurse, you must obtain consent before engaging in any aspect of treatment and care and that it is important that registered nurses always respect the patient's right to decline any treatment offered. As a registered nurse, you must be able to demonstrate that you have acted in the patient's best interest in any situation, particularly in an emergency.

The principle of patient autonomy means that every competent adult has the right to refuse treatment. A person who acts autonomously is self-directed, free from the interference of others, and is able to process information, understand, deliberate, and reason, enabling them to make independent choices (Beauchamp & Childress, 2001). This highlights the crucial consideration of **capacity** in all aspects of consent.

Patients who lack capacity *can* be treated without consent, although slightly different rules apply depending on the reason for the patient's incapacity. The introduction of the Mental Capacity Act 2005 means that statute law rather than common law now governs the treatment of some of these patients.

The Mental Capacity Act 2005

The Mental Capacity Act 2005 provides healthcare professionals with a clear legal framework for ensuring that consent obtained from patients is valid. It also highlights the required course of action when the patient may be temporarily or permanently unable to provide consent. (Figure 4.1 provides an overview of the Act's main areas.)

The Mental Capacity Act 2005 provides a set of good practice principles that encompass all aspects of consent (see Figure 4.2).

Obtaining consent

Consent can be obtained in a number of ways, all of which are equally valid. It may be given in an expressed way, either through word of mouth or written, or it may be implied—that is, the actions of a patient will suggest that they are consenting to the treatment to be given. However, written consent is considered the best evidence in proving that consent was given (Dimond, 2008).

It is important to remember that consent must always be gained for *all* nursing interventions, assessment, and care, and not simply limited to those procedures that constitute medical treatment.

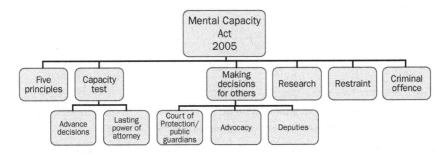

Figure 4.1 The Mental Capacity Act 2005: overview and structure (adapted from Richards & Mugal, 2006)

Always assume that an adult has
capacity unless otherwise established
(Burden of proof lies with those
making the assessment)

All possible efforts must be made
to promote capacity

What appears to be an unwise decision must not
lead to an assumption that a person lacks capacity
(respecting the views and beliefs of others)

When making decisions or acting on behalf of a person who lacks capacity

Any act done or decision taken under this Act must be
a 'best interest' decision

Acts and decisions must be those that ensure that the
restrictions of a person's rights and freedom of action are
minimized

Figure 4.2 The principles within the Mental Capacity Act 2005 (adapted from Richards &
Mugal, 2006: 5)

➡ Theory into action

Think of examples when you might have obtained:

1   implied consent
2   verbal consent
3   written consent

Examples of the various types of consent are given below.

1   **Implied consent:** You approach a patient to take a blood pressure recording and,
    as you approach, he rolls his sleeve up and holds out his left arm ready for you to
    take the measurement. His action therefore *implies* consent.
2   **Verbal consent:** When you wish to take a urine sample from a patient, you might
    obtain verbal consent from the patient by simply explaining why you need the
    sample and asking if they understand.

3 **Written consent:** This type of consent is usually obtained prior to an invasive procedure such as surgery. The consent will be obtained on the form chosen by the organization providing the treatment and requires that the person taking consent explains the procedure and the possible benefits, risks, and alternatives, thereby allowing the patient to make an informed decision prior to signing the consent form.

Key points

To make an informed decision, it is important that the person fully understands the implications of this consent. This is often called **capacity**. When obtaining consent, *capacity* to give this consent always needs to be assessed.

Where there is any doubt about the person's capacity, then a test for capacity must be performed. This test is performed by the person requiring consent unless this is disputed for some reason (see Figure 4.3). In such circumstances, it may be taken to the Court of Appeal.

Where a person is found to have capacity, their wishes must be respected unless others are put at risk. Wherever possible, there is a duty to support the person in the decision-making process to facilitate autonomous decision-making. This support might include:

- ensuring that information is provided in a format that the person making the decision understands;
- providing all of the appropriate information in order that they can weigh the variety of probabilities;
- ensuring the provision of time and support for deliberation;
- answering any further questions appropriately;
- that a means of communicating the decision must also be facilitated—for example, if a person no longer has the ability to express their decision verbally, other means may be used to support communication, such as picture boards, using closed questions, allowing for nods of the head or hand-squeezing in response, etc;
- the use of interpreters, which is recommended as appropriate, as is the use of specialist hearing equipment if required;
- the provision of written information, which can also help the patient to retain the information long enough to make the required decision.

As the patient's **advocate**, the nurse may need to play a central role in support of this process.

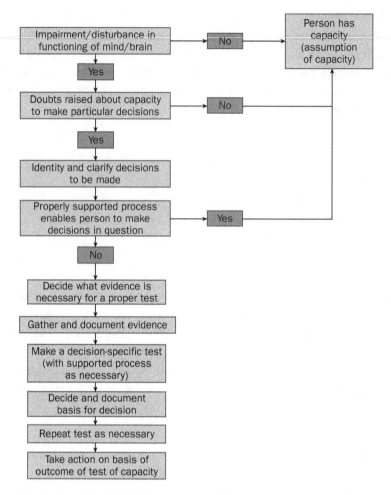

Figure 4.3 Flow chart of the assessment of capacity (taken from Church & Watts, 2007)

Best-interest decisions

Where the person is found *not* to have capacity, then a 'best-interest decision' is made. The Mental Capacity Act 2005 provides clear guidance of how this decision should be made, including that:

- all relevant circumstances must be considered;
- whether the person might have capacity in the future and if so when;
- the person's previously expressed and present wishes;
- the person's significant and relevant beliefs and values;
- factors that the person would consider if able to do so;
- consultation of significant others if possible and appropriate (which might include family, religious leaders, social workers, who can provide information on the person's known beliefs and views);
- encouragement and support to enable the person to participate if possible.

once all circumstances have been considered the least restrictive option must be preferred.

Scenario 4.3

You wish to provide care that you know will help improve a patient's condition and have a positive impact on his life. He, however, reports that he will not accept the treatment as he believes the treatment has been tested on animals and his conscience would not allow him to consent to this.

As a student nurse, what would you do in this situation? Would your actions change as a registered nurse?

Points to consider

Here are some points that may help clarify your decision-making in Scenario 4.3.

1   The NMC Code (2008) states that, as a registered nurse, you must respect the patient's beliefs and values. The Mental Capacity Act 2005 emphasizes that a decision that might be considered by some as an unwise decision does not mean that the individual concerned does not have the capacity to understand the consequences of that decision.

2   If, however, there is doubt about the patient's ability to understand the information provided and the consequences of the decision, then the test for capacity may be applied and if they are deemed to have capacity, then you must respect the decision. If the patient is found not to have capacity, then a 'best-interest decision' may be made.

The use of restraint

Key points

Any decisions made on behalf of another person must always be the least restrictive option available and the consequences should be kept to a minimum. Physical restraint should be used only in very specific circumstances.

Patients/clients refusing treatment is a very difficult situation to deal with and can be very distressing for all concerned, especially for less-experienced staff or students. This is particularly the case if restraint has to be used. While these situations are inevitably upsetting, it is not acceptable that employers allow nursing students to be put in a position of making decisions about restraint because of a lack of qualified nurses (RCN, 2008: 2). The definition of restraint offered by the RCN is 'stopping a person doing something they appear to want to do'. Restraint may be justified in certain circumstances according to the RCN—for example, when the individual is:

- displaying behaviour that is putting themselves at risk of harm;
- displaying behaviour that is putting others at risk of harm;
- requiring treatment by a legal order, for example, under the Mental Health Act 2007.

It is important to recognize that these decisions may need to be made in many different settings, whether that be in a mental health or forensic environment, critical care, continuing care, or care delivered within the community in someone's own home. It is interesting that the use of certain devices of restraint that might be quite common in other countries is presently seen as unacceptable in the UK, although the debate about their appropriateness continues (Morgan, 2010).

Also, as the RCN (2008) guidance points out, there is evidence that indicates even clients who were confused when restrained later remembered and valued nurses' explanations of what was happening to them and particularly with regards to the reassurance that the nurses were trying to keep them safe. Therefore, if a client cannot give **informed consent**, you should always explain the rationale behind what you are doing, helping to achieve understanding and agreement as far as possible.

> **Key points**
>
> If you suspect that restraint is being used inappropriately, you should report this immediately to your mentor and/or your personal tutor.

Advanced directives

Advanced directives are directives made by individuals when they still have full decision-making capacity and they give guidance to those providing care as to the present or future wishes of that individual should certain specific circumstances occur.

> **Key points**
>
> It is important to recognize that nothing can override an appropriately written and legally sound advanced directive.

However, a directive can only be viewed as legally binding in very specific circumstances. For example, if the directive expressly refers to long-term care following a stroke (when the patient may no longer be able to communicate their decisions and wishes), then it will not apply in relation to long-term care or treatment where the person has dementia. It will, however, indicate the person's fundamental values and beliefs and therefore will contribute to discussions prior to the making of any best-interest decision.

Where the advanced directive relates to life-sustaining treatment, this must be documented very clearly and unequivocally. The directive must be signed and also witnessed by another person. It is also important to recognize that advanced directives can be withdrawn and altered at any time while an individual has capacity.

Scenario 4.4

You are caring for a woman who has been admitted following a road traffic accident, and her family provide you with an advanced directive that she had asked them to give to the hospital staff if she were ever admitted to hospital in a condition in which she was not able to make her own decision. The advanced directive states that when the degenerative disease that was diagnosed four years ago becomes so advanced that she cannot care for herself, or if she is unable to eat or drink, then she does not want her life to be prolonged or any attempt to resuscitate to take place.

While in your care, the patient suffers a cardiac arrest. What would you do?

In such situations, unless a decision regarding resuscitation has been agreed upon by the healthcare team and the patient, if able to participate, resuscitation would need to be commenced. In this instance, the advance directive is in relation to the specific disease and there is no indication that her condition is such that her quality of life has deteriorated to the extent detailed in the advanced directive.

Key points

It may be a good point here to recognize the potential upset and anxiety that such scenarios can cause for students. As the NMC (2009a) states: 'Don't be afraid to ask for help.' There is a lot of help available if you feel you need it and the golden rule should be to ask your university tutor or clinical mentor straight away, so that they can provide the support and advice you may need. This early support should reduce the possibility of the matter becoming more serious later on. Your university and your clinical placement provider will also provide student support services, such as confidential counselling, occupational health services, advisers, and student groups or unions. The NMC also has a confidential helpline to talk to expert advisers, and the RCN also offers advice and advocacy should you be having a difficult time at university or on placement.

The role of independent mental capacity attorneys

So what happens if someone no longer has capacity? An independent mental capacity attorney (IMCA) (Richards & Mughal, 2006) makes decisions on behalf of an individual who no longer has the capacity to make that decision independently. The IMCA must provide support for the individual concerned and gather any information that is relevant to any decisions. In order to do this, the attorney has the right to see all relevant health and social care records to ascertain the individual's wishes and gain clarity concerning possible alternatives.

There is a statutory duty upon NHS organizations to appoint such an advocate in specific circumstances. These circumstances might include when the person involved has been found not to have capacity to make decisions related to:

- any serious medical treatment, including the taking of a biopsy;
- any intention to detain the individual in hospital for greater than 28 days, or eight weeks in the case of a care home;
- any change of accommodation to another hospital where the stay will be greater than 28 days, or eight weeks in the case of a care home, and the person has no relatives, friends, or unpaid carer, who is appropriate to consult in determining their best interest (Dimond, 2007).

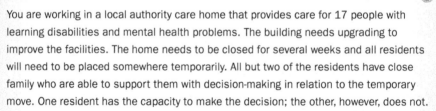

Scenario 4.5

You are working in a local authority care home that provides care for 17 people with learning disabilities and mental health problems. The building needs upgrading to improve the facilities. The home needs to be closed for several weeks and all residents will need to be placed somewhere temporarily. All but two of the residents have close family who are able to support them with decision-making in relation to the temporary move. One resident has the capacity to make the decision; the other, however, does not.

1 What is an appropriate course of action in these two cases?
2 What will your responsibilities be as a registered nurse?
3 Are they any different from those of a student nurse?

Points to consider

- Registered nurse
    As a registered nurse, in the case of the patient who has capacity, the NMC Code (2008) requires you to 'ensure you gain consent'. You can achieve this by ensuring that the patient has all the required information to facilitate informed consent and that you promote their autonomy by *advocating* for them when appropriate.

- Student nurse
  Remember, as a student nurse, you are also both legally and ethically accountable and the NMC (2009a) states that you must treat patients as individuals and respect their dignity. Where the patient does not have the capacity to make the decision, a 'best-interest decision' would be made incorporating the patient's current and previous views if they are known, involving the health and social care team and, if they have no family, perhaps close and long-standing friends of the individual. If these are not available, then the organization that plans to move the patient will be required to appoint an IMCA.

Lasting power of attorney

A lasting power of attorney (LPA) is another means for people to plan ahead and can be appointed by an individual who at the time has capacity and the ability to forward plan in relation to financial management for their future health and social care. The lasting power of attorney only becomes effective when capacity is lost, and the appointed attorney must then be consulted when any health and social care decisions are made. This is to ensure decisions are in the person's best interest.

It is important to recognize the distinctions between the two different lasting powers of attorney.

- **A lasting power of attorney – property and affairs** essentially allows a person to appoint somebody to look after their money and related affairs. This effectively replaces the old enduring power of attorney.

  So while a will ensures that a person's estate can be distributed according to their wishes when they die, a lasting power of attorney – property and affairs protects their assets by authorizing somebody chosen by them to deal with their property and affairs on their behalf, should they become unable to manage them themselves, while they are alive.
- **A lasting power of attorney – personal welfare** allows a person to appoint one or more attorneys to make decisions on their behalf about their personal welfare and health care. This includes whether to give or refuse consent to medical treatment or deciding where they might live, decisions that can only be taken on their behalf when they lack the capacity to make them themselves.

The duties of the attorney include:

- a duty of care;
- a duty not to delegate authority;
- a duty not to take advantage of the position;
- a duty to act in good faith;
- a duty to maintain confidentiality;
- a duty to keep their money separate from that of the person for whom they are the attorney.

Issues of withholding or withdrawing treatment, donation, and best interests

Just as with some of the complex situations mentioned above, some decisions are made *solely* by the courts. These include the withholding or withdrawing of life-sustaining treatment, organ and bone marrow donation, non-therapeutic sterilization, and where there is dispute relating to a best-interest decision.

Decisions relating to the withholding or withdrawing of life-sustaining treatments, for example, occur frequently in healthcare practice, and such decisions require both the consideration of a number of principles and assessment of the possible outcomes of any course of action. Clearly, this can be very complex and is rarely straightforward. Where an individual has capacity, the Mental Capacity Act 2005 requires the individual's autonomy, beliefs, values, and wishes be respected. However, if the individual concerned does not have capacity at this time, then certain processes would be initiated.

In cases of withholding and withdrawing of life-saving treatment:

- an advanced directive in writing and witnessed would take precedence;
- if there is no advanced directive, a lasting power of attorney would be consulted;
- failing these contingencies and depending on the individual circumstances a best-interest decision will be sought *or* application made to the Court of Protection.

Consent, capacity, and children

What about consent and capacity where children are concerned? Consider the following scenario.

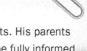

Scenario 4.6

Barney, a 6-year-old boy, is admitted to the ward for insertion of grommets. His parents insist that he is not told any details of the surgery, so he is not able to be fully informed or prepared for theatre.

Such a scenario clearly raises many issues and to resort to the law in such cases appears an overreaction. However, the principles enshrined within the law can help and guide our plans and interventions in such cases.

The Mental Capacity Act 2005 applies to adults—in this case, those over the age of 16 (Dimond, 2007). However, young people under the age of 18 are not able to refuse *life-saving treatments*. They are, however, able to consent or refuse other treatment, as identified within the Family Law Reform Act 1969 or Family Law (Scotland) Act 2006.

Younger children who fully understand what is involved in the proposed procedure can also give consent. '*Gillick* competence' is often the name given to the competence of a minor.

Gillick competence

In 1982, Mrs Victoria Gillick took her local health authority (West Norfolk and Wisbech Area Health Authority) and the Department of Health and Social Security to court in an attempt to stop doctors from giving contraceptive advice or treatment to under-16-year-olds without parental consent. The case went to the High Court, where Mr Justice Woolf dismissed Mrs Gillick's claims. The Court of Appeal reversed this decision, but in 1985, it went to the House of Lords and the Law Lords (Lord Scarman, Lord Fraser, and Lord Bridge) ruled in favour of the original judgment delivered by Mr Justice Woolf:

> whether or not a child is capable of giving the necessary consent will depend on the child's maturity and understanding and the nature of the consent required. The child must be capable of making a reasonable assessment of the advantages and disadvantages of the treatment proposed, so the consent, if given, can be properly and fairly described as true consent.

The eventual outcome was that the consent provided by the young girl was deemed lawful as she was found:

- to understand the doctor's advice;
- not to be able to be persuaded to inform her parents;
- likely to engage in sexual activity, irrespective of the prescription;
- likely to do so without contraception, which might adversely affect her physical and mental health.

Therefore the decision to prescribe contraception was found to be in the child's best interests (Dimond, 2008). It is important to note that while '*Gillick* competence' allows a minor to consent to treatments provided that they are found to have capacity to do so, they are not able to *decline* treatment that is *life-saving*.

Where the child does not have capacity to make the decision, the consent of the parent or legal guardian is sought, and if this is not possible, a 'best-interest decision' is made. Where there is a need for ongoing decision-making or a dispute, a deputy is appointed through the Court of Protection. Similar provision is offered in Scotland under the Age of Legal Capacity (Scotland) Act 1991.

Persons with learning disabilities

Clearly individuals who have learning difficulties will all have different levels of understanding and each case therefore requires individual assessment. If their capacity is in doubt, the 'test for capacity' would be applied.

Persons with mental health problems

Patients detained under a section of the Mental Health Act 2007 are held regardless of their capacity to make decisions. The order under which they are held will be simply to detain them for assessment or to provide treatment in relation to the *specific* mental health problem that they are experiencing. This does *not* mean that they do not have capacity generally. As such, valid consent must be obtained for any intervention other than the conditions set out in the detention order, if the nurse is to act legally, ethically, and within the Code (NMC, 2008).

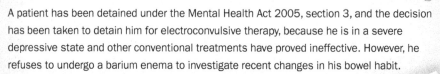

Scenario 4.7

A patient has been detained under the Mental Health Act 2005, section 3, and the decision has been taken to detain him for electroconvulsive therapy, because he is in a severe depressive state and other conventional treatments have proved ineffective. However, he refuses to undergo a barium enema to investigate recent changes in his bowel habit.
  What is the best course of action for you as a nurse?

Points to consider

Remember that although the man is detained under the Mental Health Act 2007, this is not in relation to the condition affecting his bowel and, as such, these investigations and treatments require specific informed consent. You would first need to *ensure capacity*.

If there is doubt with regards to capacity to consent, then the test for capacity should be applied. If it is confirmed that the patient has capacity, information must be provided in a form that he can understand, and time and support given to allow him to consider the information and provide the opportunity for him to communicate his decision. As a nurse, you have the responsibility within the law to facilitate this. As a registered nurse, you are professionally accountable. You must uphold people's rights to be fully involved in decisions about their care (NMC, 2008).

As a student nurse, the NMC guidelines also state that you should treat people as individuals and respect their dignity (NMC, 2009a).

- If the man is found to be lacking capacity, you must first establish if he is likely to recover capacity, and if this is likely following treatment for the depression and intervention is not urgent, *you should wait until capacity is regained.*
- If capacity is not likely to be regained nor it is not possible to wait, then a *best-interest decision should be made.*

Adults with Incapacity (Scotland) Act 2000

The Adults with Incapacity (Scotland) Act 2000 provides a similar framework for safeguarding the welfare and managing the finances of adults who lack capacity due to mental disorder or inability to communicate. It allows other people to make decisions on their behalf subject to certain safeguards. The main groups to benefit from this Act include people with dementia, people with a learning disability, people with an acquired brain injury or severe and chronic mental illness, and people with a severe sensory impairment.

Power of attorney is also a similar means by which individuals, while they have capacity, can grant someone whom they trust the powers to act as their continuing (financial) and/or welfare attorney.

The Act allows treatment to be given to safeguard or promote the physical or mental health of an adult who is unable to consent. The principles apply to medical treatment decisions as to other areas of decision-making.

Principle 1: benefit

Any action or decision taken must benefit the person and only be taken when that benefit cannot reasonably be achieved without it.

Principle 2: least restrictive option

Any action or decision taken should be the minimum necessary to achieve the purpose. It should be the option that restricts the person's freedom as little as possible.

Principle 3: take account of the wishes of the person

In deciding if an action or decision is to be made, and what that should be, account must be taken of the present and past wishes and feelings of the person, as far as this may be ascertained.

Principle 4: consultation with relevant others

Take account of the views of others with an interest in the person's welfare.

Principle 5: encourage the person to use existing skills and develop new skills

Further information can be gained here: **http://www.scotland.gov.uk/Topics/Justice/law/awi**

Research and the issues of capacity and consent

You may think: 'Why include this section in this book?' While you are unlikely to begin undertaking research in the early stages of your nursing career, research and

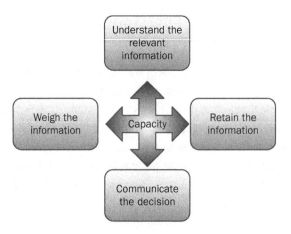

Figure 4.4 Components of capacity (MCA, 2005).

evidence-based practice play a central role in professional practice. Similarly, you may be caring for a patient who has been asked to be involved in research, and they may ask for your guidance and advice. The following information will help you to protect the rights of the patient and give you an insight into pertinent considerations should you be interested in pursuing research yourself in the future.

All research that involves human participants, including cases in which tissues or organs are intended to be retained for research or education, requires ethical approval from local and/or national ethics panels. This includes identifying how freely given and informed consent will be obtained from the participants. To be deemed to have capacity to consent to be involved in research, like consenting for any other procedure, a partici- pant must be able to demonstrate the four aspects shown in Figure 4.4.

For further information, see **http://www.myresearchproject.org.uk**

This site requires you to log in, however it is possible to access the 'help' section, which contains interesting and relevant information.

Particular complications occur when research subjects no longer have, or may never have had, capacity to consent to participate in research. These are often groups of the most vulnerable people, such as children or those who have learning disabilities and mental health problems. Despite the difficulties, however, it would be morally wrong to avoid research that involves these groups, as research is crucial to continuously improve and develop health and social care practice (Dimond, 2007). Moreover, as we have seen, the NMC Code (2008) identifies the importance of delivering care that is based on the best available evidence and ensuring that any healthcare advice is evi- dence based.

The Mental Capacity Act sets out seven precise conditions for research involving participants who do not possess the required capacity to consent. The purpose of these conditions is to protect the welfare of the individuals involved (Dimond, 2008).

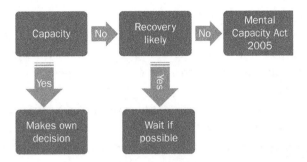

Figure 4.5 When to consult the Mental Capacity Act 2005

These conditions are that:

1 the research is related to their condition;
2 their condition is an impairment or disturbance of the brain;
3 there is reasonable belief that the research would not be as effective if carried out on those with capacity;
4 the research must have potential to benefit the individual and not impose a burden that is disproportionate.

Or that:

5 it is intended to provide knowledge of the cause or treatment;
6 if point 5 applies, but not point 4, the risks to the individual are reasonably believed to be negligible;
7 there reasonable arrangements in place for ensuring that the requirements of consulting carers and additional safeguards are met.

The decision-making path for patients/clients whom you consider may not have capacity, and therefore when the Mental Capacity Act may be invoked, is shown in Figure 4.5. It is very likely that you will be involved in caring for people who need to consent for certain interventions or treatments.

Summary

This chapter has explored various aspects of the law in relation to professional practice and how this may impact on your current and future experience. You should now understand the major differences between criminal law and civil law. We explored in detail the area of negligence that can cause such anxiety for students, explaining the *elements* in any accusation of negligence. These include proof, *on the balance of probabilities*, that a duty of care was owed, that the standard of that duty of care was not breached, and if it was, that this breach did indeed cause reasonably foreseeable harm.

The complex issues of consent were further discussed—particularly in relation to those deemed to be without capacity, and how ensuring informed consent is paramount in providing good health and social care while acting within the law. Essentially, the underpinning principle that informs this and other current healthcare practice and the law is having respect for persons.

You must always assume that those for whom you are caring have capacity unless it is proved otherwise using the test for capacity. The Mental Capacity Act 2005 is a structured legal framework to protect those who are vulnerable and may not have capacity to make all of their own decisions, while also providing each person with the opportunity to plan for the future when, for whatever reason, capacity may be temporarily or permanently lost.

Here is a recap of some of the main points that you will need to consider.

- No treatment may be given to an individual unless the patient has consented to treatment.
- If nurses proceed with treatment without the patient's consent, they are vulnerable to an accusation of battery. However, this assumes certain circumstances.
- For consent to be valid, the individual must have capacity and understand what is involved in the proposed treatment.
- They must also be fully informed of the advantages and disadvantages of the proposed treatment, including the risks involved, whether any alternatives are available, and the possible consequences of the treatment.
- Consent must be given freely without coercion or under real or implied threat.
- If the person were unable to offer valid consent, the principle of 'best interest' would be utilized. This is a complex concept, but includes such considerations as the welfare, interests, values, and known wishes of that person.
- The decision-making must take into account the patient's values and preferences when competent, their well-being and quality of life, and relationships with others family, carers, and friends.

In this chapter, we have looked at:

Online Resource Centre

 This textbook is accompanied by an Online Resource Centre that provides interactive learning resources and tools to help you to prepare for the transition from student to fully qualified member of staff. After you have completed each chapter and whenever you see this icon, please go to the ORC at your earliest convenience. If you have not done so already, save the ORC web address into your favourites: **http://www.oxfordtextbooks.co.uk/orc/burton**

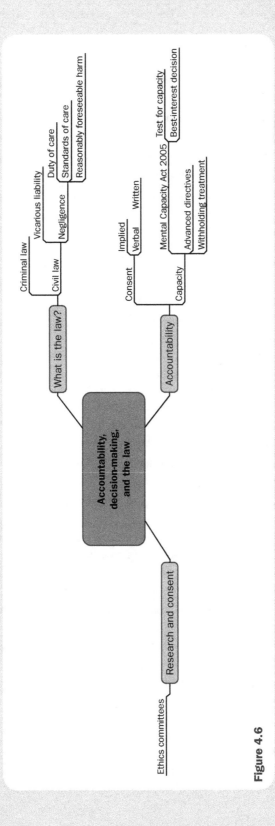

Figure 4.6

References

Beauchamp TL & Childress JF (2001) *Principles of Biomedical Ethics*, 5th edn. Oxford University Press, Oxford.

Caulfield H (2005) *Accountability*. Blackwell Publishing, Oxford.

Church M & Watts S (2007) Assessment of mental capacity: a flow chart guide. *Psychiatrist* **31**: 304–7. Available at: http://pb.rcpsych.org/cgi/content/full/31/8/304

Dimond B (2007) *Legal Aspects of Mental Capacity*. Blackwell Publishing, Oxford.

Dimond B (2008) *Legal Aspects of Nursing*, 5th edn. Pearson Longman, Harlow.

Director of Public Prosecutions (2009) *Interim Policy for Prosecutors in Respect of Cases of Assisted Suicide*. Available at: http://www.cps.gov.uk/consultations/as_consultation.pdf

Donoghue v Stevenson (1932) AC 562. In: Dimond B (2008) *Legal Aspects of Nursing*, 5th edn. Pearson Longman, Harlow.

Family Law Reform Act 1969. HMSO, London.

Family Law (Scotland) Act 2006. Available at: http://www.opsi.gov.uk/legislation/scotland/acts2006/asp_20060002_en_1

Gallagher A (2010) Whistleblowing: what influences nurses' decisions on whether to report poor practice? *Nursing Times*. Available at: http://www.nursingtimes.net/nursing-practice-clinical-research/acute-care/whistleblowing-what-influences-nurses-decisions-on-whether-to-report-poor-practice/5010979

International Council of Nurses (2006) *Nurses and Human Rights*: ICN Position. International Council of Nurses, Geneva, Switzerland.

Jones S & Jenkins R (2004) *The Law and the Midwife*, 2nd edn. Blackwell Publishing, Oxford.

Mental Health Act 2007. HMSO, London.

Mental Health (Care and Treatment) (Scotland) Act 2003. Scottish Executive, Edinburgh.

Morgan S (2010) Nursin' USA: Why do UK nurses consider restraints unacceptable? *Nursing Times*. Available at: http://www.nursingtimes.net/forums-blogs-ideas-debate/nursing-blogs/nursin-usa-why-do-uk-nurses-consider-restraints-unacceptable/5016114

Nursing and Midwifery Council (2010) *Standards of Proficiency for Pre-registration Nursing Education*. NMC, London.

Nursing and Midwifery Council (2008) *The Code: Standards of Conduct, Performance and Ethics for Nurses and Midwives*. NMC, London.

Nursing and Midwifery Council (2009a) *Guidance on Professional Conduct for Nursing and Midwifery Students*. NMC, London.

Nursing and Midwifery Council (2009b) *Record Keeping Guidance for Nurses and Midwives*. NMC, London.

Nursing and Midwifery Council (2009c) *Accountability: Nurses and Midwives—Advice by Topic, A*. Available at: http://www.nmc-uk.org/Nurses-and-midwives/Advice-by-topic/A/Advice/Accountability/

Richards S & Mughal AF (2006) *Working with the Mental Capacity Act 2005*. Matrix Training Associates, Hampshire.

Royal College of Nursing (2004) *Raising Concerns, Raising Standards*. RCN, London. Available at: **http://www.rcn.org.uk/_data/assets/pdf_file/0007/157723/003208.pdf**

Royal College of Nursing (2008) *Let's Talk About Restraint*. RCN, London. Available at: **http://www.rcn.org.uk/_data/assets/pdf_file/0007/157723/003208.pdf** (accessed 26 June 10)

Tingle J & Cribb A (2007) *Nursing Law and Ethics*, 3rd edn. Blackwell Publishing, Oxford.

5

Teamwork: working with other people

Graham Thurgood

The aims of this chapter are to:

➡ help you to prepare for the roles and responsibilities of a qualified nurse in relation to working with others within teams;

➡ review definitions of teams and consider the ingredients and skills of an effective team;

➡ identify potential problems of teamworking and how these can be addressed;

➡ assist you in reflecting on your role within teams and help you as a new staff nurse to settle into existing teams;

➡ explore and develop the teamworking skills that a qualified nurse needs.

Introduction to teamwork in nursing

Your role as a qualified nurse will inevitably involve the ability to work effectively in teams with nursing colleagues and other healthcare professionals (NMC, 2010). This chapter seeks to explore the principles of good teamworking and allow you to develop your teamwork skills. Figure 5.1 highlights the many 'teamwork' elements of the nursing role.

As a nursing student approaching qualification, it can seem daunting to work in a new team and know that you will occasionally be expected to lead the team when you are a staff nurse; however, it is important to recognize that you already have considerable experience of working in teams, and that you will be able to utilize this experience in your new role.

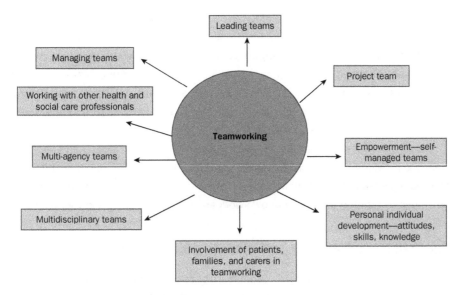

Figure 5.1 The different elements of teamworking in nursing roles

This chapter will help you to consider your current experience by exploring the following areas (Martin & Henderson, 2001: 96–7):

- definitions of teams;
- the types of team in which nurses work;
- theories, concepts, and models of teamwork;
- the types of role that team members play;
- skills required for effective teamworking;
- problems of teamworking and how to solve these;
- planning your personal development.

To start with, let's consider why teamworking is so important to health care, why you are expected to study it, what benefits it provides to staff and patients, and what kind of teams you may work in.

Why will you need to work as part of a team?

Martin and Henderson (2001: 93) state:

> Managing groups and teams – supervising and organising their work so that their talents and resources are deployed efficiently and effectively – is essential to the delivery of health and social care services.

Teamwork in health care is important for several reasons. Firstly, healthcare systems require huge amounts of resources to ensure that patients receive appropriate services and good quality care. These resources include staff knowledge and skill, equipment, time, information, finance, and buildings (Benson & Cunningham, 2006). McBride and Hyde (2006) and Smith et al. (2009) suggest that good teamwork improves performance such as enhanced patient safety and satisfaction, reduced length of stay in acute environments, lowered patient mortality rates, high staff morale, and improved recruitment and retention. Positive teamworking can therefore clearly help to create healthy working environments (Fleissig et al., 2006).

Underperforming team members can reduce the team's performance and affect team morale and individual motivation (Chapman, 2009). So how can we avoid this and ensure that all teams work well? Personally, you can, at least, ensure that you are motivated and have a positive attitude towards your own work and the work of others in your team.

Organizational aspects of working in teams

When we consider the health needs of the variety of patients/clients and the services needed to provide care, we realize that the needs of most patients cannot be met by one profession and that therefore collaborative **interprofessional teamworking** is essential (Freeth, 2001; NHS Confederation, 2003; National Patient Safety Agency, 2008). Figure 5.2 illustrates the number of health professionals a patient can encounter on their health journey in *acute care*. At each stage, nurses work alongside other professionals, which is key for effective teamwork and also illustrates how the patient and their carers are important players in an effective team approach.

Government policy

Government policy has promoted multidisciplinary teamworking, with some evidence suggesting that interprofessional educational opportunities are important for embedding positive attitudes early in the professional's career. This, however, can be problematic (Thurgood, 1992a, 1992b; Henderson, 2009; Mahon et al., 2009; Miller et al., 2009).

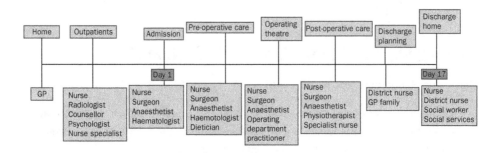

Figure 5.2 Example of a patient's care pathway and relevant team members

Pollard (2009) explored improvements in interprofessional collaboration opportunities for pre-qualifying health and social care students, and identified that:

> few formal interprofessional education initiatives occur in practice settings and little is known about prequalifying students' non-formal learning about interprofessional issues while on placement.
>
> POLLARD (2009: 2846)

The numerous benefits of effective teamwork in relation to delivering quality services are claimed to be (Cook et al., 2001):

- better communication between professionals;
- improved coordination of service delivery;
- prompt referrals between team members;
- less likelihood of clients falling between services;
- a more holistic approach to client need;
- enhanced contribution of different practitioners.

Benefits of multidisciplinary teams (MDTs) include:

- improved record-keeping and communication (Haigh, 2001);
- reduction in delays in treatment via faster and more coordinated treatment (Fleissig et al., 2006);
- good continuity of patient care (Fleissig et al., 2006);
- fewer consultations with doctors (Williams & Laungani, 1999);
- improved communication for hospital and community staff (Fleissig et al., 2006).

Other policy initiatives encouraging interprofessional teamwork include those related to patient safety and vulnerable patients. Examples of these in relation to young people include the Every Child Matters policy (Department for Children, Schools and Families, 2003a), the Victoria Climbié Inquiry (House of Commons Health Committee, 2003b), and the Children Act 2004. The Royal College of Psychiatrists (2007) also considers good teamworking to be essential in reducing the vulnerability of mental health patients.

Why do student nurses need to study teamwork?

The importance of student nurses having an underpinning knowledge of teamwork and the opportunity to practise teamworking skills is clearly stated within the **Nursing and Midwifery Council's** four domains and standards of **proficiency** for nursing (NMC, 2010). As a student nurse, you may be familiar with these, but they are worth revisiting as they provide valuable opportunities for reflection and emphasize the importance of teamworking to your studies.

The NMC and teamworking

The following activities will allow you to explore the reasons why the NMC considers teamworking important and help you to confirm its relevance for you as a future qualified nurse.

....

⊜ **Theory into action**

Here are some examples of standards that student nurses should achieve prior to registration; these are adapted from the NMC standards for pre-registration nursing education (NMC, 2010) and the **Essential Skills Clusters** framework (NMC, 2007). Consider each one based on your experience of nursing so far.

● Registered nurses should be able both to demonstrate knowledge of and to identify examples of effective interprofessional working practices.
● They should be able to identify and subsequently value the roles of others within the health and social care team.
● The nurse should recognize the need to work within the context of a multiprofessional team to enhance the care of patients/clients.
● Each nurse should actively seek and learn from feedback from other members of the team to enhance care and their own professional development, and refer to specialist members of the multidisciplinary team for additional or specialist advice when necessary.
● Taking leadership of the team when appropriate, all nurses should be prepared to review, evaluate, and challenge the practices of themselves and others when necessary.

....

You may have considered these in relation to the following health and social care team members:

● nurses;
● doctors;
● healthcare assistants;
● social workers;
● educational staff;
● teachers;
● local government officers;
● dieticians;
● clinical psychologists;
● managers;
● paramedic/ambulance staff;
● police officers;
● telephonists;

- porters;
- laboratory staff, pathologists, biochemists;
- risk management/audit staff;
- pharmacists;
- administrative support staff;
- ward clerk;
- supplies;
- maintenance staff, electric, water, heating, estates;
- occupational therapists;
- healthcare professional students;
- physiotherapists.

Mansell and Harris (1998), when discussing learning disability nurses and MDT working, identified the following team members: social workers; physiotherapists; speech and language therapists; Mencap support workers; psychiatrists; and team managers.

Establishing and maintaining collaborative working relationships with members of the health and social care team is a large area of teamworking. 'Collaboration' is a skill that nurses can develop by having a willingness to work with others and to share information and knowledge in the best interests of patients. 'Working relations' is a general term suggesting that nurses need to be able to work with others to provide high standards of care. Having an open mind about others with whom you work is an important attitude to develop. This, coupled with confidence in your roles and responsibilities, and effective communication skills, can ensure good working relations and full contribution to the MDT.

Healthcare professionals working together facilitates combined decision-making with regards to assessment, planning, reviewing, and evaluating care. You may have seen this occurring in case conferences or medical ward rounds, as well as during nursing handover reports. Having an underpinning knowledge of patient care gives you confidence to participate in patient-centred decision-making with other professionals.

It is vital to recognize the role of service users/patients and carers in the team and decision-making process to promote patient advocacy and to protect the vulnerable.

....

➡ Theory into action

The NMC's position on interprofessional working is highlighted in the Essential Skills Clusters framework (NMC, 2007). Statements from this framework are given below. Complete the two sentences following the statements, checking your understanding of the terminology and making a list of team members with whom you have worked in practice.

- Nurses must be able to manage care for individuals and groups, coordinate interprofessional care when needed, liaise with specialist teams, and understand the role of other healthcare professionals.

● Nurses must be able to work interprofessionally and autonomously as a means of achieving optimum outcomes for people.

'**Coordinate interprofessional care**' means . . .

'**Works interprofessionally and autonomously as a means of achieving optimum outcomes for people**' means . . .

. . . .

You may have considered some of the following points.

Effective interprofessional working practices means . . .

'Effective' can mean productive, meeting aims and objectives, targets, or standards with available resources. 'Interprofessional working practices' means working with other professionals, demonstrating understanding of your own and others' professional contributions to practice.

Respect and utilize the contributions of members of the health and social care team means . . .

This means respecting other professional's roles and responsibilities, skills, and knowledge by having knowledge and understanding of them and working collaboratively, and using other MDT members effectively to ensure that quality care and services are provided. One of the core knowledge and skills areas all National Health Service (NHS) staff should have is to 'work effectively in teams, appreciating the roles of other staff and agencies involved in the care of patients' (Department of Health, or DH, 2009b). Whyte and Brooker (2001: 26) found that, in effective mental healthcare teams, 'members value the support, knowledge, and professional development that membership offers'.

Teamwork can also include service users, families, and other teams, as effective interprofessional and inter-agency teamworking contributes to service user recovery while also challenging discrimination and inequity (NMC, 2010). Allowing student nurses practical experience of teamworking emphasizes links between theory, practice or attitudes, skills, and knowledge.

Mentors should 'enable students to access opportunities to learn and work within interprofessional teams' (NMC, 2008: 24), which will promote an understanding that 'evidence-based practice, involving patients, clients, carers and other members of the health and social care team, enhances care delivery and learning opportunities' (NMC, 2008: 27).

All nurses need to have a working knowledge and an array of appropriate skills that will allow them to 'work as a member of a multi-professional team, contributing effectively to team working' (NMC, 2008: 50). So there are employment, organizational, policy, and professional reasons why you should study teamworking and consider teamwork theories. There is an underlying presumption that teamworking is beneficial for nurses but there are more cautious and negative views on this that you may wish to follow up with your own reading, such as Finn et al. (2010).

What is a team?

Definitions of what a team is vary from simple to complex. Teamwork can be described as 'A group of 2 or more people whose primary purpose is to facilitate through member interaction, the accomplishment of a common goal' (Bedeian, 1989: 457). However, for the purposes of this chapter, the following definition is used:

> A Team is something more than a group. It is a group with a sense of a common goal or task, the pursuit of which requires collaboration and the co-ordination of activities of its members, who have regular and frequent interactions with one another.
>
> LEWIS & HENDERSON (2000: 6)

....

💡 Thinking about

Consider this definition based on your own experiences of being in a team either on your nursing course, in any jobs you've had, or in social or sport activities.

What do you think are its strengths and weaknesses?

....

The definition asserts that a team is different from a group in having an *aim* that team members work towards. This work requires planning and the activities of team members require an element of control to ensure effectiveness and interaction between team members.

To illustrate the value of considering more than one definition, Katzenbach (1993) stated that a team is a small number of people:

> with complementary skills who are committed to a common purpose, performance goals and approach for which they hold themselves mutually accountable.
>
> CITED IN ROYAL COLLEGE OF NURSING (RCN)/NHS INSTITUTE FOR INNOVATION AND IMPROVEMENT (2007: 3)

It's useful to compare and contrast this definition with that of Lewis and Henderson (2000) above to identify the similarities and differences between them. While they agree on having a common purpose or goal, there are differences, such as an emphasis on ideas of collaboration, coordination, and communication between team members by Lewis and Henderson (2000), whereas Katzenbach (1993) emphasizes the number of team members, skill mix, and accountability.

Types of team in which nurses work

This section will explore the enormous variety of teams in which nurses work and consider their roles within them. It might be useful to take this opportunity to reflect on your nursing experiences and identify the job titles of team members with whom you have worked and indicate their roles and responsibilities.

⊖ Theory into action

List the job titles of members of healthcare teams with which you are familiar or in which you have worked and identify their roles and responsibilities.

	Team member's job title	Roles and responsibilities
1		
2		
3		
4		
5		
6		
7		
8		
9		
10		

You may have worked in various different types of team—for example, teams defined in relation to their make-up/membership:

- unidisciplinary;
- multidisciplinary/interprofessional;
- multi-agency.

Multidisciplinary teams

While and Barriball's (1999) study of qualified and unqualified nurses' views of MDTs found that quality healthcare services need effective teamworking to ensure positive patient outcomes. However, 28 per cent were unfamiliar with the term 'multidisciplinary team' and the same number could not clearly describe the term. Knowledge and understanding appeared to improve with professional experience and changing hierarchical position within the organization (While & Barriball, 1999). Increasing your knowledge of teams may therefore accelerate your ability to contribute to teams effectively.

Teams can also be defined by their function or area of clinical responsibility, such as:

- mental health team or paediatric team;
- community health team or hospital team;
- a specialist team, such as a child and adolescent mental health services (CAMHS) team.

Within health care, many teams are based on the two different categories (their function or area of clinical responsibility), although they can also be combined whereby a mental health team may be unidisciplinary, consisting of nurses only, whereas another mental health team may be multi-agency. Interestingly, Williams and Laungani (1999) noted that unidisciplinary teams tended to be more task-focused and support- ive to peers. An example of a multi-agency team is the CAMHS, which may include psychiatrists, social workers, clinical psychologists, community psychiatric nurses, occupational therapists, play therapists, family therapists, and educational school representatives.

Other teams may be defined by their patient grouping, such as a breast cancer team or a rehabilitation team, whereby a team is centred around a specific service. The former team cares for a specific group of patients with a diagnosis or disease and the latter a wider group of patients with varied diagnostic disorders, but who all need rehabilitation care.

Team members' roles and responsibilities will also vary and be based on their pro- fessional expertise and their expected contribution to the team. This skill mix is one of the most important benefits of working in MDTs.

Molyneux (2001: 29) found three indicators for positive teamworking:

- personal qualities and commitment of staff;
- communication within the team;
- opportunities to develop creative working methods within the team.

The 'personal qualities and commitment of staff' related to their motivation, creative ability, adaptability, flexibility, openness, and willingness to share, cooperate, and support (Molyneux, 2001).

More than one team

The complexity of nursing and healthcare teams is highlighted by the fact that individuals are often members of several teams and by there being 'teams within teams' whereby boundaries of one team may overlap with others (RCN/NHS Institute for Innovation and Improvement, 2007). This is further complicated by teams often consisting of members from different organizations, agencies, or professions.

Figure 5.3 illustrates the fact that you could be a member of several different teams at different levels of an organizational hierarchy, and also a member of different teams, but at the same organizational level. Figure 5.4 highlights the similar phenomenon of the overlapping of roles within a small team.

Consider the example of an elderly person recovering from a hip fracture and receiving rehabilitation care from nurses, doctors, physiotherapists, and occupational therapists. Considerations of priority or the relative contribution of individual members of the MDT will depend upon opinion, experiences, and knowledge of team members' roles and responsibilities. For example, in Figure 5.5, you may believe that the nurse plays a central coordinating role, and that the occupational therapist and physiotherapist are also important players, but that the doctor's role is minimal at this point in the patient's journey.

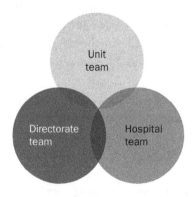

Figure 5.3 Teams at different levels of the organizational hierarchy

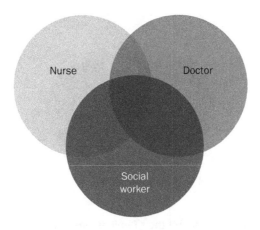

Figure 5.4 A simple example of a multidisciplinary team

Figure 5.6 illustrates that nurses may work within even wider multi-agency teams.

Nurses therefore can work in a variety of interconnected teams and understanding other team members' roles and responsibilities is an important part of being an effective team member (Newson, 2006). Working in different types of effective team gives nurses varied work experiences and job satisfaction. Views on teamwork and its place in health and social care vary and there is some debate about the healthcare team make-up and the use of MDT working.

You will, of course, have considered that central to all of these examples of teams are the patient and family. This is the case for all four fields of nursing and you should

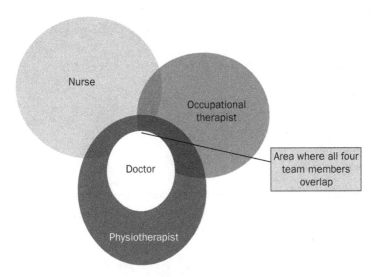

Figure 5.5 An example relating to an elderly person recovering from a hip fracture and receiving rehabilitation care from a nurse, doctor, physiotherapist, and occupational therapist

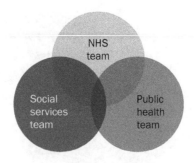

Figure 5.6 A simple example of a multi-agency team

be able to identify how patients and their families are involved in teamworking for your own field of nursing. Having explored what teams are and the types of team in which you may work, we can now review what makes an effective team and the factors that influence team performance.

Qualities of an effective team

 Thinking about

What do you think are the qualities of an effective team?

Consider your initial thoughts on this based on your past experiences and what you have read in this chapter so far.

You may have listed key points such as:

- type of team;
- its size;
- skill mix;
- membership;
- the team's tasks.

Effective teamwork can appear straightforward and in some ways it is; however, as with other human activities, it can sometimes prove complex and problematic.

Handy's determinants of group effectiveness

Handy (1999) provides determinants of group effectiveness under two main headings: the 'Givens' and the 'Intervening factors', as illustrated in Box 5.1. Using this list as a

Box 5.1 Handy's determinants of group effectiveness

1 **The givens**

- **The group**
  - o Size
  - o Membership
  - o Individual objectives and roles
  - o Stage of development
- **The task**
  - o The nature of the task
  - o The criteria for effectiveness
  - o Salience (importance) of task
  - o Clarity of task

- **The environment**
  - o Norms and expectations
  - o Leader position
  - o Intergroup relations
  - o The physical location

2 **The intervening factors**

- **Leadership style**
- **Process and procedures**
  - o Task functions
  - o Maintenance functions
- **Interaction pattern**
- **Motivation**

framework, we will explore each factor in order to help you to understand how you can successfully develop your teamwork skills.

The 'givens'

The group

Group size and membership

The first of Handy's three givens includes group size, membership, individual objectives and roles, and the stage of development of the group. All are seen as important elements and some of these you can influence and others you cannot (for example, group size or membership).

These are important considerations not least because, as Molyneux (2001) suggests, communication is easier in smaller teams than more complex ones; Barr and Dowding (2008) also suggest that the larger the team, the less cohesive it will be. However, King (2009) states that patients can be cared for by up to ten or more different professionals. Evidence also suggests that the more effective teams have *clear objectives* or a vision to which to commit (Williams & Laungani, 1999; Borrill & West, 2002; West, 2004).

'Team roles' is a general term used to describe the roles that individual team members may play in teams or during a team's life. Some roles are played by more than one member, whereas other teams may not have individuals who can play these roles. Teams that include members who possess a mixture of personalities, attitudes, opinions, beliefs, aptitudes, competencies, skills, knowledge, and experience can therefore potentially ensure that the team works more effectively than the individuals alone. The team roles that we play are often either given to us or we evolve into them as we and the team members develop.

So far, we have mainly identified professional roles or roles linked to skill mix and hierarchy. However, there are other ways of viewing team roles and these are discussed next. We will return to Handy's work and what he calls the 'intervening factors' later.

Belbin's principle's for establishing and integrating a team

According to Belbin (Belbin, 1981, 2000a, 2000b, 2003), team members may have at least two roles: their professional role (nursing) and their team role. In addition to reading Box 5.2, you can assess your Belbin team role strengths and weaknesses by visiting the official BELBIN website (Belbin, 2000b).

The team's effectiveness may depend on how members adapt themselves and their contribution to both their professional and team roles. Depending on the team's focus, the team roles will need to be balanced. The personal characteristics of members will fit well for some roles, but stifle their ability in others. Once the team has an appropriate balance of team roles with the correct people in them, it will allow members to contribute effectively. As a sporting example, a football team would struggle to win matches with 11 goalkeepers and a successful team will include varied specialist players with specific skills.

Box 5.2 Belbin's team roles (Belbin, 2000a; 2003)

- The **resource investigator** explores opportunities and develops contacts.
- The **company worker/implementer** turns ideas into practical actions.
- The **coordinator** makes a good chairperson, who clarifies goals, promotes decision-making, and delegates well.
- The **monitor evaluator** can see all options and make accurate judgements.
- The **team worker** is cooperative and diplomatic and helps to avert friction.
- The **professional/specialist/expert** uses expertise and knowledge to help with standard setting and sets an example to others.
- The **shaper** is dynamic, thrives on pressure, and has the drive/courage to overcome obstacles.
- The **completer-finisher** is painstaking/conscientious in searching out errors and omissions, and delivers on time.
- The **plant** is creative, imaginative, and unorthodox, and helps to solve difficult problems.

Team roles	Emily	Melissa	Pat	Andrew	Sarah	Riley	Totals
Plant							0
Resource investigator							1
Coordinator							2
Shaper							1
Monitor evaluator							2
Teamworker							2
Implementer							2
Completer finisher							1
Specialist/expert							1

Figure 5.7 Example grid for team analysis using Belbin's team roles. For each team member, you can plot the two strongest Belbin scores to illustrate the make-up of the team illustrated by the total scores. (Very light grey grids are where individuals have not scored highly.) The dark grey cells indicates each individual's strongest role. The light grey cells indicates each individual's second strongest role. This analysis will reveal the strengths and weaknesses of your team.

Within health care, no formal selection of team members based on roles occurs, with team members being 'thrown together randomly' (Miller et al., 2009). However, Belbin's team roles can aid the analysis of teams and allow teams to problem-solve and find ways of improving their performance, as shown in Figure 5.7. Having this under-pinning knowledge can help you to understand the group dynamics that may occur in your team and give you self-awareness of your own role and contribution within teams. Assessing your Belbin characteristics can allow you to strengthen any weaker roles to give you a more 'rounded' ability in all of the roles and is one form of skill mix that can be important to consider. Thus, this analysis can not only help to identify a team's strengths and weaknesses, but also highlight which team members can offer specific roles or skills.

➡ Theory into action

In due course, return to the Belbin grid once you are in your new team and consider how members fit against it. Would you interact with them differently?

Discussions concerning skill mix within health care are usually linked to profes-sional and occupational roles, pay grading, and levels of experience, and can vary depending upon speciality and patient need. Mansell and Harris (1998) suggested that learning disability nurses contributed five key roles when working in community support teams:

- client-based interventions;
- coordination and planning of care;
- training;
- care management;
- health promotion.

It is therefore not only the individual team member's professional expertise, knowledge, and skills, but also their own personality and personal attributes that can enrich teams; and the effectiveness of any team relies on a clear understanding of each member's roles and responsibilities.

Stages of team development

To become an effective team member, it is also important to understand team evolution and the different stages of team development. Tuckman's (1965) group dynamics theory (cited in Guirdham, 1996) provides a four-stage view of the life of teams. The initial stage of setting up the team and meeting new members is called 'forming'; the second is the 'storming' stage, when members find their feet, test out the water and develop membership hierarchies. This can create particular stresses and conflicts. The 'norming' stage follows allowing the team to get down to the task in hand despite any lingering conflicts and with signs of positive collaborative attitudes emerging. The final 'performing' stage confirms that team members are task-focused and working more efficiently. A fifth stage was added later, 'adjourning', recognizing that some teams come to a natural end.

Knowing that teams may perform differently during their life cycles helps us to understand the dynamics that can occur and has relevance any time you join a new team.

The life cycle of teams: students and new staff

It is usually the case that the teams in which student nurses work are already established in both their membership and functions, although their effectiveness may be variable. Therefore it is probably rare for nurses to experience the full group life cycle. Exceptions might include starting a new team to work on a specific project or when new units, wards, or departments open. However, the lifecycle approach is useful for you to consider, as you essentially join an existing team on each new clinical placement. Similarly, you leaving a team at the end of each clinical placement illustrates how teams continually change in both membership and function. When you qualify, you will join an existing team with all of its embedded behaviours, characters, and skill mix, and you will find your own place within the team.

The provision of induction programmes for new staff allows time to get to know policies and procedures and also to meet new colleagues. **Preceptorship** for newly qualified nurses provides a similar opportunity to help to adjust to a new role. Morrow (2009) identified the need for support and involvement in teamwork when discussing the transition of newly qualified nurses into their role. Some authors argue that if the team member's stage of development allows them to work in a safe, comfortable, trusting environment, they can be creative, innovative, and effective (Molyneux, 2001; Holleman et al., 2009).

So let's return to Handy's 'givens'. The second 'given' is the 'task', which we will now consider further.

The task

The nature of the task

Consideration of the 'nature of the task, its clarity and importance' includes characteristics such as:

- workload;
- specific characteristics of the patient population;
- complexity of patient/client needs and acuity of their health condition;
- frequency of team interactions.

Having a clear view of the task and its impact upon resources is vitally important for all qualified nurses. Across the four nursing fields, there are wide variations in patient needs, which impact on the tasks nurses perform. Caring for an adult with severe learning disabilities in the community, for example, would clearly be a very different task from caring for an adult admitted to a day surgery unit for a hernia repair. The frequency of team interactions within nursing can vary, but it is important that, during a shift, team members have chance to communicate so, that they can report on progress and identify priorities of care. Also, the criteria for assessing the effectiveness of the team need to be clearly stated so that success or failure can be objectively measured. It is important that teams make time for regular formal, or ad hoc informal, meetings to review objectives and ensure that corrective action is taken if deficiencies are found, as the qualified nurse must be able to prioritize care and make clinical decisions related to both patient need and staffing and other resources.

The clarity of the task

For a team to function effectively, there must be a clear vision of what the task is. For nurses, this is generally to provide high-quality patient care with the resources available and may be articulated in ward or departmental objectives or nursing philosophies (Wilson, 2005). A further element to the task is 'task orientation', which relates to having a focus on getting the job done and managing priorities (Williams & Laungani, 1999). This is helped by maintaining your nursing knowledge, skills, and competencies, improving your decision-making skills, and managing your own time well.

The environment

Norms and expectations

The third of Handy's givens is the 'environment' and in relation to this the norms and expectations of the organizational structure and culture should be considered. Nurses need to know their organization's policies, systems, and procedures, as these will need to be followed as part of their employment contract.

Key points

When you start a new job, you will be provided with induction in-service training sessions and advice on organizational policies, systems, and procedures. Make time to read these as they will give you important insights into the environment in which your team works. If you don't read them straight away, you may never do so, because the new job will demand all of your attention!

Intergroup relations

Intergroup relations explore how teams work with each other, which is vital in health care, with its diversity and complexity of teams. Having good communication channels can aid intergroup working and ensure that patient care is continuous and coherent. Improving your knowledge and understanding of the main theories of communication and the skills that you need to be an effective communicator is therefore crucial. Within children's nursing, effective multidisciplinary teamworking has been found to be enhanced by communication and information-sharing, with the team members' location seen as a way of promoting this (Doyle, 2008). Ensuring adequate team meetings, good working practices, and appropriate communication channels can promote effective teamwork (Doyle, 2008). The physical location can play an important part in teamworking and one of the main issues here is the need for an environment that is suitable to facilitate communication.

Having considered Handy's 'givens', we can now explore his 'intervening' factors.

The intervening factors

The first factor Handy highlights is leadership style, which is discussed further in Chapter 7.

Process and procedures

The second intervening factor is 'process and procedures'.

. . . .

⊙ Theory into action

In relation to the four effective teamwork factors below (Canadian Health Services Research Foundation, 2006: i), consider a team in which you have worked recently and make comments on how you think this team rated on a scale of 1–10 (where 10 is 'very competent').

Factors for effective teamwork	Your comments	Score
Good communication		
Coordination		
Protocols and procedures		
Effective mechanisms to resolve conflict		

. . . .

An effective team will always be striving to achieve good communication; however, as we have seen, within teams this can often be problematic. Molyneux (2001) stated that communication was improved by regular team meetings and a common work base or environment. The more frequently team members actually meet face to face and have the chance to discuss issues and work together, the better communication will be (Whyte et al., 2009). However, having meetings too often can be counterproductive and ineffective, although short, frequent meetings might be more useful than long, infrequent meetings. This again highlights the complexity of effective teamworking. Regular monthly or annual meetings may be too far apart to be effective; therefore, to be effective, 'regular' here needs to mean *consistent* so that all team members know when they will occur and frequent enough to ensure effectiveness dependent on the team's purpose and needs. Having a common working base or environment is not always possible. You may have worked in teams that did not have this. The fundamental point here is that effective communication can be facilitated more easily if team members have easy access to each other. However, with improvements in technology such as email, the Internet, teleconferencing, web cameras, and mobile phones, this is becoming less problematic, as even teams who work across quite large geographical areas can communicate effectively via these. However, it is noted that these modes of communication may never replace face-to-face contact in their effectiveness.

Communication can be in various forms including verbal and written. Guidelines and policies in this area can be useful for clarifying responsibilities, highlighting the need for coordination, and generally easing the transition of new staff into teams.

> ### Key points
>
> When you first start your new job, ask when team meetings are held and be sure to attend them where possible. (Ask your manager if it is appropriate for you to reorganize shifts or even training days around these.)

Conflict

Having mechanisms to resolve conflict if it occurs is essential to ensure that teams are effective, cohesive, and not hampered by problems between members. Having an open culture in which team members can express feelings freely is also important in relation to managing conflict (Critchley & Casey, 1984). Jones (2006) suggests that, in mental health areas, having clear role boundaries reduces conflict and enhances patients' needs being met. Conflict inevitably plays an important factor in reducing effectiveness in teams and how to address this is discussed further later in this chapter.

Task functions and maintenance functions

Task functions and maintenance functions are other skills or behaviours required for effective team membership, and each is divided into a number of descriptive categories. 'Task functions' relate to behaviours needed in order to achieve objectives and get the job done, whereas 'maintenance functions' are the behaviours needed to maintain an effective team. The following activity will allow you to make observations from practice to aid your understanding of the practical elements of this aspect of teamwork.

....

➜ Theory into action

This activity can be conducted in a practice setting of your choice with your mentor's permission.

You must be mindful that you need the consent of the patients in the area. Observe a team in action, either a team you are in or one you can observe, and make notes on the 12 behaviours listed below.

- Complete the observation checklist and record specific detail.
- Be objective.
- Be constructive.
- Maintain confidentiality and anonymity in any notes taken.

Roles of group members can be identified under two headings: 'task', meaning the job to be done; and 'maintenance', meaning keeping the group going (Handy, 1993). You may find it useful prior to starting your observations to look up any unfamiliar terms. Do not worry if any of the behaviours are not evident, but record this observation and consider why it is the case.

Task behaviours

1 Initiator

2 Information-seeker

3 Diagnoser

4 Opinion-seeker

5 Evaluator

6 Decision-maker

Maintenance behaviours

1 Encourager

2 Compromiser

3 Peace-keeper

4 Clarifier

5 Summarizer

6 Standard-setter

Summarize your findings on the 'task' and 'maintenance' roles on a separate sheet of paper, and reflect on what this tells you about the skills of effective teamwork that you may want to nurture.

....

You will have noted that the roles in the box are important for effective teamwork and that not all team members display them.

Interaction pattern

'Interaction pattern' is the third of Handy's intervening factors and reminds us that the intergroup relations and the physical location of team members and their accessibility to each other are important for effective communication.

Motivation

Motivation is the fourth and final of Handy's intervening factors. The team needs to be maintained and supported by positive motivation and mutual commitment to achieve the task. Davey et al. (2009) identified that morale, job satisfaction, and work design were all factors in predicting short-term absences of staff nurses working in hospital settings. They identified five other factors related to groups that need considering:

- group commitment;
- group absenteeism;

- work group culture;
- group cohesion;
- group norms.

These five factors clearly suggest that teamwork has a powerful impact on nurse absenteeism. It is not uncommon for team roles to have to manage very quick changes due to colleagues' sickness or absence. Arriving on duty to find that you are in charge due to sickness or absence is a regular occurrence for some nurses. Positive personal qualities and commitment of well-motivated staff, coupled with an ability to see colleagues as equal partners, helps to ensure that teamwork is effective. Having reliable, consistent, and committed members improves the team's effectiveness whilst also promoting a positive environment for all members within the team.

Teamworking problems

Teamworking is not easy and there are numerous problems that can challenge its effectiveness. A general principle is that the more complex the team, the more chance of problems, so, according to this theory, a uniprofessional team may be less likely to develop problems than a MDT or multi-agency team. However, the reasons for an ineffective team are multifactorial.

Membership

Many healthcare teams lack stable membership (Miller et al., 2009). As a student, you will have joined teams for a few weeks and then left, and your temporary membership may have influenced the team in some way. Disorganized teams can emphasize group confusion, with members becoming unmotivated, uncooperative, defensive, or argumentative (Banks, 2002).

Patient safety

Armitage (2009) makes links between teamwork, risk management, clinical governance, and human error theory, suggesting that mistakes occur for a number of interconnected reasons including:

- poor communication;
- teamwork difficulties;
- lack of training;
- team dynamics problems such as 'groupthink'.

When considering interdisciplinary teams and safety, it is suggested that teams make fewer mistakes than individuals (Miller et al., 2009; Parker, 2009). Perhaps one of the most serious nursing concerns is the safe administration of medicines (Brady et al., 2009; Riley, 2009). The complexity of this MDT procedure is problematic and risky unless there are good practices (Armitage et al., 2007).

Within the National Patient Safety Agency's (2004) *Seven Steps to Patient Safety* guide, the principle of 'multidisciplinary responsibility' is addressed, stressing the need for MDTs to be 'open' in relation to identifying risk and preventing errors.

Roles

Another problem linked to teamworking is the overlap of teams or roles of team members. Kennard (2002: 383) identified that 'overlap in competencies between occupational groups' can be problematic to effective MDT working, resulting in duplication of care, role overlap, and lack of role clarity. 'Role blurring' can be a problem if:

- the nature of the team's work is complex;
- membership is large;
- roles are not clearly identified and organized.

This includes, for example, different MDT members repeating patient assessments and recording information in uniprofessional records. To illustrate duplication within MDTs, consider Scenario 5.1.

Scenario 5.1

On arrival at the stroke ward, Mrs Silcox became angry when the staff nurse asked about her husband's medications, stating:

> This is the fourth time I have had to explain which tablets Bill takes and it's getting me down. I have already told the nurse in casualty and the two doctors who saw him there. Why can't you talk to each other? I'm sure the doctor wrote them down.

While confirmation of information and rechecking the patient's story may be important and appropriate—especially when dealing with vulnerable individuals in complex cases—generally if this repetition were to be reduced, it would improve patient satisfaction, increase teamworking effectiveness, and reduce the workloads of the different healthcare professionals.

Ruhstaller et al. (2006) suggests that MDT working can improve clinical outcomes and service coordination such as 'avoidance of the duplication of examinations and investigations'. Williams and Laungani (1999: 22) also discuss the importance of staff having organizational support to be innovative, as exemplified in primary health care, including 'multidisciplinary records for patients so that patients do not have to repeat details about themselves to a variety of health professionals'.

There are current initiatives addressing teamworking problems. The NHS in England has introduced the NHS Care Records Service (NHS CRS), designed to improve the safety and quality of care (DH, 2009a, 2009b), and highlighting:

> Today, all the places where you receive care keep records about you. They can usually only share information from your records by letter, email, fax or phone. At times, this can be slow and sometimes things get lost on the way.
>
> DH (2009c)

These initiatives and others, such as the Electronic Prescription Service, are attempting to improve care by addressing some of the issues of teamworking. Consider Scenario 5.2 and record your thoughts in relation to teamwork.

Scenario 5.2

Mr Womersley had, for several years, attended the outpatients clinic following the discovery of polyps in his bowel. However, having not had an appointment for a number of months, he had presumed this was normal and that he was now not required to attend. Out of the blue, he received a leaflet from the hospital related to bowel cancer alongside a letter with another appointment. This upset him greatly, and he started to worry that he had now got bowel cancer and that this was an urgent appointment.

This is an example of how different parts of the healthcare system can work independently of each other and therefore create duplication and inefficiencies. Lack of collaboration or communication can therefore have serious consequences for patients, but good communication channels can limit misunderstandings and mistakes (Banks, 2002).

Managerial issues

Fleissig et al. (2006) identified ten potential problems with MDT work, as follows.

1 Use of substantial amounts of healthcare professional time
2 Ineffective if key members are frequently absent
3 Insufficient administrative support
4 Too costly
5 Increased bureaucracy
6 Used for all patients instead of those whose care is difficult or complex
7 Increasingly more new referrals
8 The need to respond quickly
9 Advances in diagnosis/treatment mean that teams need to be organized and supported

10 Historical enmities, hierarchical boundaries, and personality styles that are not conducive to harmonious exchange and respect of different viewpoints can make teams dysfunctional, and participation can be stressful

These ten points are important and although they mostly relate to managerial resource issues beyond our scope, some points need addressing here.

You may have considered that effective teamwork requires a lot of time that can detract team members from their other responsibilities. Stark et al. (2002a) found that when groups of mental health professionals worked under stringent financial resources and larger workloads, MDT working was rare. Slevin (2008) found that community learning disability teams (CLDTs) identified poor staffing and high workloads as barriers to effective teamworking. Furaker (2009) recognized that psychiatric nurses spent 38 per cent of their working time with patients and it seemed that the organization of care, including teamwork, tended to fragment work routines, hindering individualized care. To rectify this, nurses must be patient-centred and ensure that care is delivered effectively while working in varied teams.

Team members need to be reliable in relation to attendance, but you may have met a team member who was consistently absent or who came to work, but appeared to make little commitment to the team when they were there. These absent or ineffective team members can be common within some teams and are problematic unless managed appropriately. Therefore, to make yourself an effective team member, you need to attend reliably, and be enthusiastic, hard-working, and willing to contribute to the team.

Healthcare teams work within environments in which changes in technology impact upon their work, and Stark et al. (2002b) discuss the tensions and paradoxes that can create problems for effective teamworking within mental health nursing. Organizational and professional issues of 'historical enmities' show how individuals or organizations can obstruct effective teamworking. Tradition is a strong factor in nursing and can cause resistance to innovation, as identified by Fiddler et al. (2010). You may know people who have 'personality styles that are not conducive to harmonious exchange and respect of different viewpoints' (Fleissig et al., 2006: 941).These individuals can be powerful and greatly affect teams positively or negatively.

To avoid interprofessional jealousy and develop trusting relationships, team members need confidence in their professional role (Molyneux, 2001). Kennard (2002) identified trust and professional role clarity as two important components of effective teamworking. Alongside these there are other points that suggest that effective teamwork requires 'a genuine commitment to working together' (While & Barriball, 1999: 77).

To what extent you have witnessed team members caring for each other in trusting, open, and honest relationships will depend on your unique experiences; however, there is some evidence that, within nursing and health care, this is not always the case, as examples of bullying and group conflicts illustrate (Alspach, 2007; Strandmark & Hallberg, 2007; DH, 2008; Johnson, 2009; Spence Laschinger et al., 2009; Hutchinson et al., 2010).

In relation to MDT and multi-agency teamworking, team members may have different:

● professional perspectives;
● lines of accountability;
● legal and statutory frameworks;
● funding budgets; (Gorman, 1998).

Acknowledging these differences and being proactive in dealing with them, by adopting such strategies as joint appointments of staff or joint funding arrangements for service delivery, can prevent them becoming problematic.

Finally, you may have experienced yourself or seen team members dealing with, reacting to, or suffering from stress as a result of MDT working. Andrews and Wan (2009) considered stress in mental health practice and found coping skills important, with nurses coping better within groups via peer support than when working alone. However, Leiter and Maslach (2009) identified that value conflicts and inadequate rewards occurring within teams in fact increased stress. You may wish to reflect on how nurses can reduce stress or how you cope with stress. As you can see, there is no guarantee of teamwork success. Cleary et al. (2005: 74) found that mental health nurses satisfaction ratings related to teamwork were as follows.

● Nursing teamwork – 73%
● Nursing status within the interdisciplinary team – 57%
● Interdisciplinary collaboration – 55%

These authors further found that one-third of respondents were particularly dissatisfied with the continuity and consistency of nursing work, nursing status within the interdisciplinary team, nurse–patient ratios, and patient continuity of care. They concluded that frameworks that ensure effective consumer, nursing, and multidisciplinary communication may improve teamwork and interdisciplinary collaboration (Cleary et al., 2005). Overall, these considerations indicate that team members can work to overcome challenges that continually confront effective teamworking.

⊖ Theory into action

In the table below, there is a list of barriers to good practice in relation to MDT meetings and membership (adapted from Fleissig et al., 2006: 940). Make some notes on the barriers to good MDT practice and how they may be solved.

Meetings	Your comments
Frequency of MDT meetings	
Day/time of meetings	
Poor information	
Inadequate record-keeping	

Membership	Your comments
Time management	
Travelling commitments	
Varied workload pressures	
Staff establishment	

. . . .

The importance of recognizing these factors means that your underpinning knowledge is increased and there is more chance that you will be able to prevent, solve, or reduce their negative impact. You may have struggled to identify some solutions to these factors, but do not worry: these complex factors illustrate that MDT working is difficult and that getting it right is a challenge for all involved. You may have also identified that some solutions are beyond yours or others' influence: for example, resource capacity and workload demands. But despite all of these potential problems, initiatives are at play to improve teamwork, and you need to be aware of them so that you can use your underpinning knowledge to develop effective team membership skills.

Collaborative working

Collaboration can be seen as a central theme of effective teamworking, and Freeth and Reeves (2004: 43) state:

> Interprofessional and interagency collaboration are essential features of professional practice for effective health and social care.

However, there is a need to make explicit efforts to ensure that collaborative practices are encouraged and facilitated (Tierney & Vallis, 1999), as Barker and Walker (2000), for example, found that the relationship between the MDT and patients and their families did not fully back up the concept of increased collaboration. As highlighted by the NMC Essential Skills Clusters, nurses must engage in person-centred care, empowering people to make choices about how their needs are met when they are unable to meet them for themselves. Similarly, they should act collaboratively with other members of the interprofessional team, people, and their carers to empower them to take a shared and active role in the delivery and evaluation of their interventions (NMC, 2007).

Your contribution to helping, to ensure this happens might involve:

- empowering patients within the care planning process;
- teaching and facilitating patients to enable them to cope with their problems;
- using coping theories and mechanisms;
- working with patients in planning, delivering, and evaluating their care to highlight their value as equal team members;
- assuming responsibility for ensuring effective communication between patients and staff.

➡ Theory into action

Freeth and Reeves (2004: 43–4) identified six competencies needed for effective teamworking. Reflect upon these and make notes of any examples you have seen of them. Assess yourself out of 10 (where 10 is very competent).

Competencies	Reflective comments	Self-assessment score
Describing your roles and responsibilities to other professions		
Recognizing and respecting other professionals' roles, responsibilities and competence		
Coping with uncertainty and ambiguity		
Facilitating interprofessional case conferences and meetings		
Handling conflict with other professions		
Working with other professions to assess, plan, and provide care		

Key points

The competences in the 'Theory into action' box above are useful for you to consider within a personal development plan in preparation for qualifying. Freeth and Reeves (2004: 46) also provide another list of six related terms that may help you to focus your reflections:

● Attitudes
● Perceptions
● Knowledge
● Skills
● Behaviour
● Practice

Roles and responsibilities of a qualified nurse

Preparing to work with other people

When you get your first job as a newly qualified nurse, you will usually join an established team. This is helpful as it can cushion the 'transition shock' of changing from a student to a staff nurse (Duchscher, 2009). But, as a student nurse, your teamworking experiences will have allowed you to develop your own attitudes, skills, and knowledge about teamwork.

....

➜ Theory into action

Consider what attitudes, skills, and knowledge you have to become an effective team member.

Attitude/skill/knowledge	Contribution to making you an effective team member

_____

_____

_____

_____

....

If you have written some notes in the boxes above: well done! Reflecting on your current competencies and proficiencies in such areas will prepare you well for job interviews. This is further explored in Chapter 8.

....

⊖ Theory into action

Morrow (2009: 279) identified eight points that newly qualified nurses felt were important in smoothing the transition to qualified nurse. Review these and record your comments.

- Adequate number of staff to provide care
- Good relationship among multidisciplinary team members
- Support for professional practice
- Lack of fear of criticism when seeking guidance
- Role stress
- Role ambiguity
- Differing expectations and values
- Moral integrity

....

McKenna et al. (2003) identified that newly qualified nurses need to feel part of the team and a means of ensuring that is to provide time for them to get together for peer support (Alspach, 2007). This supportive approach can ensure that there is no fear of criticism when seeking guidance and thereby reduces any role stress or ambiguity. It can also prevent differing expectations and values, so that team members are working together and integrity is maintained. You may have also considered important points such as how to communicate with medical staff—particularly senior doctors such as consultants, with whom some student nurses have little direct contact until they qualify.

Morrow (2009) identified that anxiety about teamworking affects newly qualified nurses in their transition from students, and Caldwell et al. (2006) found that although some newly qualified nurses felt well prepared for their role in their new teams, they were worried about equality of status within the team and subsequent cooperation and conflict resolution. Therefore newly qualified nurses working in teams is a positive way of adapting to their new role. However, this can also create stress and the more you can learn about the attitudes, skills, and knowledge needed to be a confident team member, the better prepared you will be.

Tips for success

During your student experience, ensure that you get as much experience as possible of working in teams by planning learning opportunities in consultation with your mentor, such as participation in case conferences, team meetings, and consultant ward rounds. Interprofessional teamworking can help to facilitate peer review and supervision, and improve patient safety by reducing lone working and protecting vulnerable service users (Field & Pearson, 2010; Mattox, 2010).

. . . .

➲ Theory into action

Consider the following 18 team-related skills. Comment on your understanding of them and rate yourself using a scale of 1–10 (where 10 means very competent).

	Skills	Comments	Self-assessment score
1	Assessment		
2	Prioritizing		
3	Communication		
4	Listening		
5	Interactive		
6	Interpersonal		
7	Collaborative		
8	Negotiation		
9	Small group		
10	Teamworking		

11	Evidence-gathering
12	Questioning
13	Analytical
14	Critical thinking
15	Problem-solving
16	Evaluation
17	Creativity
18	Reflection

List the skills in which you may have scored a 5 or less in the table below and make some provisional action points on how you might improve your score.

Skills	Action points
Assessment	
Prioritizing	
Communication	
Listening	
Interactive	
Interpersonal	
Collaborative	
Negotiation	

Summary

This chapter has considered:

- what teamwork is and the constituents of an effectively functioning team;
- why teamwork is important in health care;
- the type of teams in which nurses can work during their careers;
- what skills team members need and how students can develop these;
- potential problems of teamworking;
- how to assess your teamworking skills and develop a personal development plan to assist you to build up the skills that may require some development.

You should have considered the required attitudes, skills, and knowledge needed for you to become a valued qualified nurse team member. However, you will need to continue your education once you have qualified to keep up to date with future developments. These changes are difficult to predict, but an example of how healthcare teamwork may develop is as follows.

> As service users become more involved in care provision, the notion of a multidisciplinary team may well be superseded by one of partnership teams in which professionals, agencies and service user's work together to achieve shared outcomes. The breaking down of professional barriers in this way can be emancipating for service users but it also requires a paradigm shift in the world views held by many professionals used to working in uniprofessional ways.
>
> SLEVIN (2008: 64)

In this chapter, we have looked at:

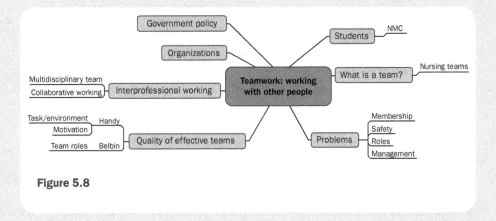

Figure 5.8

Online Resource Centre

 This textbook is accompanied by an Online Resource Centre that provides interactive learning resources and tools to help you to prepare for the transition from student to fully qualified member of staff. After you have completed each chapter and whenever you see this icon, please go to the ORC at your earliest convenience. If you have not done so already, save the ORC web address into your favourites: **http://www.oxfordtextbooks.co.uk/orc/burton**

References

Alspach G (2007) Critical care nurses as coworkers: are our interactions nice or nasty? *Critical Care Nurse*, **27**: 10–14.

Andrews DR & Wan TTH (2009) The importance of mental health to the experience of job strain: an evidence-guided approach to improve retention. *Journal of Nursing Management*, **17**: 340–51.

Armitage G (2009) Human error theory: relevance to nurse management. *Journal of Nursing Management*, **1**(7): 193–202.

Armitage G, Newell RJ & Wright J (2007) Drug errors and their reporting in a British acute hospital trust. *Clinical Governance*, **12**(2): 102–14.

Banks C (2002) Make the most of your team. *Nursing Standard*, **17**(10): 96.

Barker PJ & Walker L (2000) Nurses' perceptions of multidisciplinary teamwork in acute psychiatric settings. *Journal of Psychiatric and Mental Health Nursing*, **7**(6): 539–46.

Barr J & Dowding L (2008) *Leadership in Health Care*. Sage, London.

Bedeian AG (1989) *Management*. Dryden Press, New York.

Belbin RM (1981) *Management Teams: Why They Succeed or Fail*. Butterworth-Heinemann, Oxford.

Belbin RM (2000a) *Beyond the Team*. Butterworth Heinemann, Oxford.

Belbin RM (2000b) *Welcome to the Official BELBIN® Website: Home to the Team-building Work of Dr R. Meredith Belbin*. Available at: **http://www.belbin.com/**

Belbin RM (2003) *Team Roles at Work*. Butterworth Heinemann, Oxford.

Benson A & Cunningham G (2006) *The Clinical Teams Project Evaluation Report*. RCN, London.

Borrill C & West M (2002) *Team Working and Effectiveness in Health Care: Findings from the Health Care Team Effectiveness Project*. Aston Centre for Health Service Organisation Research, Birmingham.

Brady AM, Malone AM & Fleming S (2009) A literature review of the individual and systems factors that contribute to medication errors in nursing practice. *Journal of Nursing Management*, **17**: 679–97.

Caldwell K, Atwal A, Copp G, Brett-Richards M & Coleman K (2006) Team working: preparing for practice—how well are practitioners prepared for teamwork? *British Journal of Nursing*, **15**(22): 1250–4.

Canadian Health Services Research Foundation (2006) *Teamwork in Healthcare: Promoting Effective Teamwork in Healthcare in Canada—Policy Synthesis and Recommendations.* Canadian Health Services Research Foundation, Ontario.

Chapman A (2009) *Adams' Equity Theory*. Available at: **http://www.businessballs.com/adamsequitytheory.htm**

Children Act 2004. HMSO, London.

Cleary M, Walter G & Hunt G (2005) The experience and views of mental health nurses regarding nursing care delivery in an integrated, inpatient setting. *International Journal of Mental Health Nursing*, **14**: 72–7.

Cook G, Gerrish K & Clarke C (2001) Decision-making in teams: issues arising from two UK evaluations. *Journal of Interprofessional Care*, **15**(2): 141–51.

Critchley B & Casey D (1984) Second thoughts on team building. *Management Learning*, **15**(2): 163–75.

Davey MM, Cummings G, Newburn-Cook CV & Lo EA (2009) Predictors of nurse absenteeism in hospitals: a systematic review. *Journal of Nursing Management*, **17**: 312–30.

Department for Children, Schools and Families (2003a) *Every Child Matters.* HMSO, London.

Department of Health (2008) *Bullying of Staff within the NHS*. DH, London.

Department of Health (2009a) *Learning to Manage Health Information: A Theme for Clinical Education—Making a Difference.* DH, Leeds.

Department of Health (2009b) *Connecting for Health.* Available at: **http://www.connectingforhealth.nhs.uk/**

Department of Health (2009c) *NHS Care Records Service*. Available at: **http://www.nhscarerecords.nhs.uk/**

Doyle J (2008) Barriers and facilitators of multidisciplinary team working: a review. *Paediatric Nursing*, **20**(2): 26–9.

Duchscher JEB (2009) Transition shock: the initial stage of role adaptation for newly graduated registered nurses. *Journal of Advanced Nursing*, **65**(5): 1103–13.

Fiddler M, Borglin G, Galloway A, Jackson C, McGowan L & Lovell K (2010) Once-a-week psychiatric ward round or daily inpatient team meeting? A multidisciplinary mental health team's experience of new ways of working. *International Journal of Mental Health Nursing*, **19**(2): 119–27.

Field J & Pearson A (2010) Caring to death: the murder of patients by nurses. *International Journal of Nursing Practice*, **16**(3): 301–9.

Finn R, Learmonth M & Reedy P (2010) Some unintended effects of teamwork in healthcare. *Social Science and Medicine*, **70**: 1148–54.

Fleissig A, Jenkins V, Catt S & Fallowfield L (2006) Multidisciplinary teams in cancer care: are they effective in the UK? *Lancet Oncology*, **7**: 935–43.

Freeth D (2001) Sustaining interprofessional collaboration. *Journal of Interprofessional Care*, **15**(1): 37–46.

Freeth D & Reeves S (2004) Learning to work together: using the presage, process, product (3P) model to highlight decisions and possibilities. *Journal of Interprofessional Care*, **18**(1): 43–56.

Furaker C (2009) Nurses' everyday activities in hospital care. *Journal of Nursing Management*, **17**: 269–77.

Gorman, P (1998) *Managing Multi-disciplinary Teams in the NHS*. Kogan Page, London.

Haigh C (2001) Contribution of multidisciplinary team to pain management. *British Journal of Nursing*, **10**(6): 370–4.

Handy C (1993) *Understanding Organisations*. Penguin, London.

Handy C (1999) *Understanding Organisations*, 4th edn. Penguin, London.

Henderson A (2009) Commentary on Pollard K (2009) Student engagement in interprofessional working in practice placement settings (*Journal of Clinical Nursing*, **18**: 2846–2856). *Journal of Clinical Nursing*, **18**: 2916–17.

Holleman G, Poot E, Mintjes-de Groot J & van Achterberg T (2009) The relevance of team characteristics and team directed strategies in the implementation of nursing innovations: a literature review. *International Journal of Nursing Studies*, **46**(9): 1256–64.

House of Commons Health Committee (2003b) *The Victoria Climbié Inquiry Report*. HMSO, London.

Hutchinson M, Wilkes L, Jackson D & Vickers M (2010) Integrating individual, work group and organizational factors: testing a multidimensional model of bullying in the nursing workplace. *Journal of Nursing Management*, **18**(2): 173–81.

Johnson SL (2009) International perspectives on workplace bullying among nurses: a review. *International Nursing Review*, **56**: 34–40.

Jones A (2006) Multidisciplinary team working: collaboration and conflict. *International Journal of Mental Health Nursing*, **15**: 19–28.

Katzenbach JR (1993). In RCN and NHS Institute for Innovation and Improvement (2007) *Developing and Sustaining Effective Teams*. RCN, London.

Kennard J (2002) Illuminating the relationship between shared learning and the workplace. *Medical Teacher*, **24**(4): 379–84.

King N (2009) *Macmillan Research*. Available at: **http://www2.hud.ac.uk/news/research_profiles/hhs/nigel_king.php**

Leiter M & Maslach C (2009) Nurse turnover: the mediating role of burnout. *Journal of Nursing Management*, **17**(3): 331–9.

Lewis P & Henderson E (2000) *Managing in Health and Social Care, Module 2: Managing People; Book 2: Managing Performance*. Open University Press, Milton Keynes.

Mahon A, Walshe K & Chambers N (2009) *A Reader in Health Policy and Management*. Open University Press, Maidenhead.

Mansell L & Harris P (1998) Role of the registered nurse learning disability within community support teams for people with learning disabilities. *Journal of Intellectual Disabilities*, **2**(4): 190–4.

Martin V & Henderson E (2001) *Managing in Health and Social Care*. Routledge, London.

Mattox E (2010) Identifying vulnerable patients at heightened risk for medical error. *Critical Care Nurse*, **30**(2): 61–9.

McBride A & Hyde P (2006) Human resource management in healthcare. In: K Walshe & J Smith (eds) *Healthcare Management*. Open University Press, Maidenhead, 239.

McKenna BG, Smith NA, Poole SJ & Coverdale JH (2003) Horizontal violence: experiences of Registered Nurses in their first year of practice. *Journal of Advanced Nursing*, **42**(1): 90–6.

Miller K, Riley W & Davi S (2009) Identifying key nursing and team behaviours to achieve high reliability. *Journal of Nursing Management*, **17**(2): 247–55.

Molyneux J (2001) Interprofessional teamworking: what makes teams work well. *Journal of Interprofessional Care*, **15**(1): 29–35.

Morrow S (2009) New graduate transitions: leaving the nest, joining the flight. *Journal of Nursing Management*, **17**: 278–87.

National Patient Safety Agency (2004) *Seven Steps to Patient Safety: Full Reference Guide*. Second print. National Patient Safety Agency, London.

National Patient Safety Agency (2008) *Teamwork for Safety: Why We Need it and How We Do it*. Available at: **http://www.npsa.nhs.uk/nrls/improvingpatientsafety/humanfactors/teamworking/**

Newson P (2006) Participate effectively as a team member. *Nursing & Residential Care*, **8**(12): 541–4.

NHS Confederation (2003) *Creating the Virtuous Circle: Patient Safety, Accountability and an Open and Fair Culture*. NHS Confederation, London.

Nursing and Midwifery Council (2007) *Introduction of Essential Skills Clusters for Pre-registration Nursing Programmes*. NMC Circular 07/2007. NMC, London.

Nursing and Midwifery Council (2008) *Standards to Support Learning and Assessment in practice. NMC Standards for Mentors, Practice Teachers and Teachers*. NMC, London.

Nursing and Midwifery Council (2010) *Standards of Proficiency for Pre-registration Nursing Education*. (Standards 2010). NMC, London.

Parker D (2009) Managing risk in healthcare: understanding your safety culture using the Manchester Patient Safety Framework (MaPSaF). *Journal of Nursing Management*, **17**: 218–22.

Pollard K (2009) Student engagement in interprofessional working in practice placement settings. *Journal of Clinical Nursing*, **18**: 2846–56.

Riley W (2009) High reliability and implications for nursing leaders. *Journal of Nursing Management*, **17**: 238–46.

Royal College of Nursing and NHS Institute for Innovation and Improvement (2007) *Developing and Sustaining Effective Teams*. RCN, London.

Royal College of Psychiatrists (2007) *Vulnerable Patients, Safe Doctors. Good Practice in our Clinical Relationships*. Royal College of Psychiatrists, London.

Ruhstaller T, Roe H, Thurlimann B & Nicoll JJ (2006) The multidisciplinary meeting: an indispensable aid to communication between different specialities. *European Journal of Cancer*, **42**: 2459–62.

Slevin E (2008) Community learning disability teams: developments, composition and good practice—a review of the literature. *Journal of Intellectual Disabilities*, **12**(1): 59–79.

Smith P, Pearson PH & Ross F (2009) Emotions at work: what is the link to patient and staff safety? Implications for nurse managers in the NHS. *Journal of Nursing Management,* **17**: 230–7.

Spence Laschinger HK, Leiter M, Day A & Gilin D (2009) Workplace empowerment, incivility, and burnout: impact on staff nurse recruitment and retention outcomes. *Journal of Nursing Management,* **17**(3): 302–11.

Stark S, Skidmore D, Warne T & Stronach I (2002b) A survey of 'teamwork' in mental health: is it achievable in practice? *British Journal of Nursing,* **11**(3): 178–86.

Stark S, Stronach I & Warne T (2002a) Teamwork in mental health: rhetoric and reality. *Journal of Psychiatric & Mental Health Nursing,* **9**: 411–18.

Strandmark KM & Hallberg LRM (2007) The origin of workplace bullying: experiences from the perspective of bully victims in the public service sector. *Journal of Nursing Management,* **15**(3): 332–41.

Thurgood G (1992a) Let's work together, let's learn together. *Journal of Advances in Health and Nursing Care,* **1**(4): 51–77.

Thurgood G (1992b) Let's work together, let's learn together. *Journal of Advances in Health and Nursing Care,* **1**(5): 13–40.

Tierney AJ & Vallis J (1999) Multidisciplinary teamworking in the care of elderly patients with hip fracture. *Journal of Interprofessional Care,* **13**(1): 41–52.

Tuckman BW (1965) Developmental sequences in small groups. *Psychological Bulletin,* **63**: 384–99. In: M Guirdham (1996) *Interpersonal Skills at Work.* Prentice Hall, London, 476–7.

West MA (2004) *Effective Teamwork: Practical Lessons from Organisational Research,* 2nd edn. British Psychological Society and Blackwell Publishing, Leicester/Oxford.

While A & Barriball KL (1999) Qualified and unqualified nurses' views of the multidisciplinary team: findings of a large interview study. *Journal of Interprofessional Care,* **13**(1): 77–89.

Whyte L & Brooker C (2001) Working with a multidisciplinary team in secure psychiatric environments. *Journal of Psychosocial Nursing and Mental Health Services,* **39**(9): 26.

Whyte S, Cartmill C, Gardezi F, Reznick R, Orser BA, Doran D & Lingard L (2009) Uptake of a team briefing in the operating theatre: a Burkean dramatistic analysis. *Social Science and Medicine,* **69**: 1757–66.

Williams G & Laungani P (1999) Analysis of teamwork in an NHS community trust: an empirical study. *Journal of Interprofessional Care,* **13**(1): 19–28.

Wilson V (2005) Developing a vision for teamwork. *Practice Development in Health Care,* **4**(1): 40–8.

Further reading

Skill mix

Flynn M & Mckeown M (2009) Nurse staffing levels revisited: a consideration of key issues in nurse staffing levels and skill mix research. *Journal of Nursing Management,* **17**(6): 759–66.

Greenhalgh and Co (1991) *Using Information in Managing the Nursing Resource (The First Rainbow Pack)*, Mersey Regional Health Authority, Greenhalgh, Macclesfield, Skill Mix Management, Cheshire, 9–10, 12, 16.

Mullins LJ (1996) *Management and Organisational Behaviour*. Pitman Publishing, London.

Groups, teams, and membership

Barr J & Dowding L (2008) *Leadership in Health Care*. Sage, London.

Onyett S (1999) Community mental health team working as a socially valued enterprise: Tensions in mental health policy? Working together in adult community mental health services: an inter-professional dialogue. *Journal of Mental Health*, **8**(3): 245–51.

Primary healthcare teamwork

Bennett-Emslie G & Mcintosh J (1995) Promoting collaboration in the primary health care team: the role of the practice meeting. *Journal of Interprofessional Care*, **9**: 251–6.

Quinlan E (2009) The 'actualities' of knowledge work: an institutional ethnography of multi-disciplinary primary health care teams. *Sociology of Health and Illness*, **31**(5): 625–41.

Robison J & Wiles R (1994) *Teamwork in Primary Care: Do Patients Benefit?* Institute for Health Policy Studies, Southampton.

Teamworking

Borgatti S (2004) *Manual for Working in Teams*. Available at: **http://www.analytictech.com/mb021/teamhint.htm**

Life cycles of teams

Robbins H & Finley M (1998) *Why Teams Don't Work: What Went Wrong and How to Make it Right*. Orion Business, London.

6

Teaching, mentoring, and assessing

Rob Burton

The aims of this chapter are to:

- ➔ identify the teaching, mentoring, and assessment responsibilities of the newly qualified nurse;

- ➔ explore the NMC (2008b) standards to support learning in practice;

- ➔ explore theories of learning and teaching, and help the reader to learn how to apply them in practice;

- ➔ explore mentoring and assessment, and help the reader to learn how to apply them in practice.

Introduction

Qualified nurses need to possess a wide variety of skills. These include: the clinical skills needed to care for their patients/service users; recognition of policy and procedures; their professional mandate for accountability and standard-keeping; leadership and management; teamworking on a number of levels; and the ability to teach, train, and educate others, particularly other nurses. As they further their career, there are also expectations that the nurse will need to closely **mentor** student nurses and also assess them in relation to their progressive competencies and their final **proficiency** to practise. Indeed, a large professional responsibility of a qualified nurse is related to the development of themselves and others around them. As a final-year student or recent student, you will hopefully appreciate the huge input that qualified nurses have had in your nursing education and the value that a good mentor has made to your placement experiences.

As a newly qualified nurse, you will not become a mentor overnight, but you will need to be involved in some teaching, and this chapter is designed to help you to prepare for teaching, mentoring, and assessing others. We will look at setting learning outcomes, identifying learning needs, and taking action to meet them. Learning opportunities present themselves in practice every day and it is up to the nurse to seize those opportunities readily when they arise. Therefore, theories of learning, managing learning environments, and teaching strategies will be discussed so that the nurse can understand their role in developing others more clearly. The **Nursing and Midwifery Council** (NMC) produced a document in 2006 (updated in 2008) on the standards of teaching, mentoring, and assessing in practice. The main aspects and requirements of this document will be explored, as well as its application to practice.

The NMC standards

To begin, the *Standards to Support Learning and Assessment in Practice* (NMC, 2008b) sets out exactly what the nurse's responsibilities are. First, they highlight, in a developmental framework, four levels of practice that align with the career development of nurses. These levels are as follows. (NMC 2008b: 16)

1 **Nurses and midwives**: these standards are aimed at the newly qualified nurse who has attained proficiency and registered with the NMC. It reflects that the Code of Conduct (NMC, 2008a) highlights the need to facilitate the learning of students in developing their competence.
2 **Mentor**: these standards are applicable to those nurses who have completed relevant training and education, and supports their role in supervising and mentoring student nurses. A *local* register is also maintained to record the names of these mentors and assessors.
3 **Practice teacher**: these standards are applicable to those involved in teaching and assessing, and those wishing to have roles such as specialist public health nurses or other specialist practice qualifications (SPQs) on NMC-approved courses. These nurses are also similarly registered at local level.
4 **Teacher**: these standards apply to those nurses wishing to become nurse teachers and contribute to the development of nurses and midwives or specialist community public health nurses. This qualification is recorded with the NMC.

In addition, the standards are underpinned by five principles (NMC, 2008b: 16), as follows.

1 The nurse should be on the same part of the register as that which the students with whom they are involved wish to enter.
2 The nurse should have demonstrated some continuing professional development.
3 The nurse should hold professional qualifications equal to or higher than those of the students whom they are supporting.

> ### Box 6.1 NMC domains for supporting learning in practice (NMC 2008b: 10)
>
> - Establishing effective working relationships
> - Facilitation of learning
> - Assessment and accountability
> - Evaluation of learning
> - Creating an environment for learning context of practice
> - Context of practice
> - **Evidence-based practice**
> - Leadership

4 The nurse should have been prepared for their role, including support for interprofessional learning.

5 Those completing an NMC teacher preparation programme can record their qualification with the NMC.

At each of the four levels of practice, there are outcomes set, based on content related to eight domains. These get progressively more complex and numerous at each level. The eight domains are given in Box 6.1.

The nurse's role in maintaining standards of care (that is, contributing to the clinical practice area to make sure that standards of practice are maintained and developed, thereby creating a stimulating learning environment), the use of evidence in practice, and leadership are dealt with extensively in other chapters in this book. This chapter will focus on the educational aspects of which a newly qualified nurse will need to be aware and develop as they progress with their career.

Establishing effective working relationships

The subject of teamwork is discussed in detail elsewhere in this book, so here we will look at how team relationships are used to facilitate and support learning of junior staff (and in some cases senior staff), students, and other team members.

Cable (2002) pointed out that fundamental differences in the approach of professionals in care services could impact on the development of interprofessional relationships. However, as there is a developing culture of 'lifelong learning' for all professionals working in the healthcare services, there can often be a wide range of those considered to be students or learners, from those on pre-registration courses to those on post-registration courses (Quinn & Hughes, 2007). Therefore the needs of all of these professionals will need to be addressed in such environments. A nurse may find themselves acting as a supervisor, teacher, mentor, or assessor to a more junior student while being supervised, taught, mentored, and assessed by others in their own environment. It also means that, in the context of this chapter, 'student' will normally mean a pre-registration nursing student, but can also refer to those whom newly qualified nurses will often teach, including a new member of staff, a junior member of staff, or a student of any healthcare profession. Scott (2008) suggests that teamworking and interprofessional approaches to health care are now the focus for providers, and that nurse education needs to have an emphasis on partnerships with other professionals and service users to maintain and expand professional relationships. Therefore, the care environment needs to be one in which all groups of staff can be educated together.

Muijs and Reynolds (2005) suggest that the 'climate' of the environment is a very important aspect in developing working relationships between those considered as teachers and their students. This does not mean 'climate' in the sense of temperature and physical environment (although this is important, as will be discussed later), but actually relates to the climate of the relationships formed within it, such as how 'warm' or 'cool' the relationship between the parties is. This can be observed in the formality or informality placed on the learning/teaching relationship, the nature of support that is fostered, and the nature of trust in the person's knowledge skills, authority, and approach. Young and Maxwell (2007) suggest that there is a shift in professional education away from a style whereby expert knowledge is passed to students in a distant manner and the student is a passive recipient of this, towards more student-centred approaches whereby they are more actively engaged. This approach helps to develop their confidence and skills in lifelong learning, problem-solving, and critical thinking. In order to engage students in identifying their own learning needs (while maintaining standards), an important basis will be the nature of the relationship developed between the two parties involved: the educator and the learner.

....

➡ Theory into action

Consider your experience as a student thus far. Identify your most positive experiences of learning in practice and how your mentor/supervisor established a positive working relationship. What steps did they take to develop and maintain this?

....

A good beginning: getting to know your student

Race (2001) proposes that successful learning comprises wanting, needing doing, feedback, and digesting. Therefore, to facilitate this process, the mentor/supervisor should take steps to find out the learning needs of the student and what they want and need in relation to their experience and requirements. This includes knowing the curriculum of the course they are on, their level of experience, their learning styles, and specific requirements related to their placement. A carefully planned programme of activities is then needed, in which they can be involved, with regular opportunities for learning formally and informally, and an opportunity for regular feedback on their performance.

Rapport

One of the key approaches to effective relationships is ensuring that **rapport** occurs. 'Rapport' derives from the French verb *porter*, which means *to carry*, and rapport means *to carry back*. Therefore, in the sense of building relationships, rapport occurs when information is carried back to the original person, or, more accurately, *matched*. This includes the matching of non-verbal, vocal/tonality, and verbal content. On a basic level, the words that are understood by the student should be used to create a basis of the relationship that should then be developed from there. This principle also fits with the notion of **advanced organizers**, as suggested by Ausubel (1968): that the best starting point is to begin from where and what the student already knows. This requires the mentor/supervisor to listen carefully and observe, and have conversations with the student, in order to ascertain this.

O'Connor and Seymour (1990) argue that communication is a loop, and that it is essential, as an educator or practitioner, to establish atmospheres in which trust, confidence, participation, and the opportunity to respond freely are crucial components. In order to do this, a student should find their mentor/supervisor approachable, therefore early contact and intervention is essential, at which ground rules are negotiated and a plan of action set out so that outcomes can be met.

Practical tip
Ground rules can be set as follows.

- Provide a clear induction to the practice environment including its physical layout, the team members, and the policies and procedures that guide it.
- An induction pack should be printed including helpful information about the practice environment and its purpose.
- Introduce the student to all members of the care team.
- The initial conversation should include questions to ascertain the student's previous experiences, knowledge, and requirements for their placement with you.
- Highlight opportunities to observe and be involved in working with nursing staff and other multiprofessional team members.

Finally, it is important to ensure equity for students with diverse needs and recognize their differing learning needs.

Facilitation of learning

The word 'facilitation' derives from the French *facile*, which means 'easy'. Therefore a straightforward translation in this context is: making it easy for the student to learn. In order to do this, there is a need for the facilitator to understand the nature and theories of learning, which can be a complex issue. Although there are several different schools of thought and theories related to learning, and there are many overlapping principles, there are similar concepts with differing names and different concepts with similar names. Three main schools will be considered here:

- the behavioural school of learning theory;
- the cognitive school of learning theory;
- the humanistic school of learning theory.

The subcategories and terminologies used to explain the concepts are so wide, deep, and broad that they will not be discussed in fine detail for the purposes of this book. Instead, we will give you a whistle-stop tour of the main ideas behind these learning theories. The notion of experiential learning (learning by reflecting on experience) and different learning styles will also be considered to give you essential background knowledge before we outline some guidance for organizing teaching.

Behavioural learning theory

According to Jarvis et al. (2003), the behavioural learning theory has been the most influential approach to learning in the past century and forms a basis for education, as it arose from the functional and scientific fields. Here, the aim is to reduce knowledge and skills into small measurable outcomes. Behavioural theorists allude to earlier definitions of learning as being more or less any permanent change of behaviour resulting from experience.

The behavioural theory tends to refer mainly to the stimulus–response relationship of a human or animal with their environment. Behavioural approaches concentrate mainly on the development of behaviours (usually observable and therefore outward) as opposed to internal thought processes. This is the strength of behaviourism, but it is also its weakness, as it tends to reduce human learning to sets of behaviour without much thinking. The theory is based on the stimulus–response principle, whereby the resulting response is reinforced (strengthened) by reward or punished (weakened) by aversive methods. Jensen (2000) describes behaviourism as a rule-based approach that manipulates learners and the environment to such an extent that they have no voice or choice in the process. This may be correct, but such rewards and punishments do help to shape responses and can lead to ways of motivating students. For example, consider Maslow's (1954) hierarchy of needs (Figure 6.1): once one stage is satisfied,

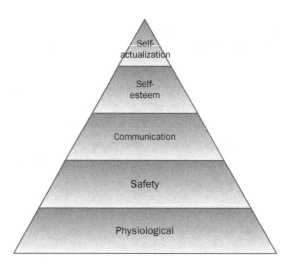

Figure 6.1 Maslow's hierarchy of needs

we can move to the next stage. The need to move to this next stage is a motivating factor for the learner and the rewards and punishments help to shape the way in which the learner gets there. Quinn and Hughes (2007) offer some criticisms of Maslow's hierarchy of needs, such as that there is evidence of people reaching the higher stages while having deficits in the lower stages and that it does not quite explain why people engage in activities that might not be related to any biological or intellectual deficits. However, it is important to note that, in assisting learners, the nurse needs to be aware of how to maintain motivation by increasing rewards and reducing punishments. In this way, the learner is accepting of the methods chosen to learn. If a student is punished or sanctioned, then they are less likely to take the same risk in learning again.

Classical conditioning

The first aspect of behavioural theory that we consider here is classical conditioning. According to Jarvis et al. (2003), classical conditioning arose from the work of Pavlov, famous for his work in noticing the changes in how dogs salivated in response to differing stimuli with or without the presence of food, and later work by John B. Watson applying similar mechanisms (associating aversive experiences to specific stimuli) to human subjects, particularly the infamous 'Little Albert' experiments. In these experiments, a young child (Albert) was given a cuddly toy and also subjected to a loud, startling noise at the same time, which eventually led to the child becoming fearful of the cuddly toy alone. To conduct such experiments in the modern age would be ethically very questionable, but from these research studies it has become understood and accepted that the basic element of learning is association—that is, association between the stimulus and the response (Figure 6.2). The response of the subject is the behaviour to which the whole theory relates. In nursing terms, the stimulus is the trigger or situation with

$$Stimulus \Longleftarrow Association \Longrightarrow Response$$

Figure 6.2 Association between stimulus and response

which the nurse is presented and the response is their resulting behaviour. So a facilitator needs to understand the necessary stimuli and expected behaviours in specific nursing situations: for example, a student may need to learn the correct response when presented with stimuli such as a chart highlighting a rise in a patient's temperature.

Operant conditioning

Operant conditioning (so-called because it relates to 'operations' in the environment) was developed by B. F. Skinner and built on the work of the classical conditioning researchers and also on the work of Thorndike (Jarvis et al., 2003). Thorndike noticed that behaviours of animals that were, at first, random (law of effect) became strengthened when repeated and rewarded with food (law of exercise). Skinner's work introduced similar aspects, but recognized the power of the reward or the punishment in shaping behaviour. The rewards act as a *reinforcer* to certain behaviours. For example, if a reward is given to a person immediately after the desired behaviour, the person is more likely to exhibit that behaviour again. The reward therefore acts as a positive reinforcer of the behaviour. If it is desired to reduce or extinguish certain behaviour, then instead of a reward, an aversive experience, or a *punisher*, would be given *immediately* after the behaviour, with a view to decreasing the frequency, intensity, or severity of the behaviour.

Behaviours can also be strengthened or reinforced by other means: for example, if a person is experiencing something that they feel is aversive to them, they may develop a behaviour to escape that experience. Therefore, the removal of the aversive experience should strengthen certain escaping/avoidance-type behaviours. Nothing is being given after the behaviour to reward it; instead what *is* happening is the punisher is given before the actual behaviour and the behaviour is intended to stop this: for example, if we are too hot, then we would remove a layer of clothing to cool down. This is known as 'negative reinforcement' because the stimulus is actually removed and the behaviour is still strengthened. So we learn to remove layers of clothing if we are too hot in future. The removal of the aversive stimulus (in this case, heat) is rewarding.

Basically, the association now occurs not only between the stimulus and the response, but by the association between the response and the further external response that provides reward or punishment. This is illustrated in Figure 6.3 and Table 6.1.

It has been suggested above that reward or punishment is totally controlled by external means, but this is not entirely accurate. Rewards or reinforcers can be either **intrinsic** or **extrinsic**, and many things in life can be used as reinforcers. Intrinsic reinforcers coming from within the person, such as feelings of satisfaction and self-competence,

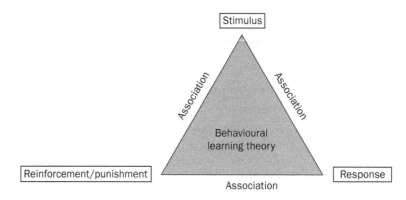

Figure 6.3 Operant conditioning

and extrinsic factors coming from the environment, such as praise, pay, privileges and good grades.

Applying operant conditioning in practice

In order to apply operant conditioning to your practice as a newly qualified nurse, you need to consider how to provide reinforcement to the learners with whom you may be involved, which should be appropriate to the level they are at in Maslow's hierarchy of needs. As far as possible, the reinforcers should be positive and rewarding in order to encourage the student. It could be safely assumed that the students' physiological and safety needs are met, so they are more likely to be motivated by social praise, which should reward their need of communication and self-esteem, thus encouraging them to develop the behaviour further. Reprimands for doing the wrong thing are punishers, and although effective in the short term, can be damaging to relationships and reduce the students' willingness to participate in learning experiences. They are likely to limit further communication and damage self-esteem unless communicated in a professional, constructive, and kind manner. Rather than telling a student that they are doing something wrong (an example would be saying something like 'No, No, that is totally wrong!'), phrase your response in a constructive way by saying something like 'You need to do it this way', or 'You need to improve that technique', and then tell them how to do it. Once they do something approximating what you want, give them the reward.

Table 6.1 Operant conditioning

	Rewarding experience	Aversive experience
PRESENTED	Positive reinforcement (strengthens behaviour it follows)	Punishment (weakens behaviour it follows)
REMOVED	Punishment (response cost: weakens behaviour it follows)	Negative reinforcement (strengthens behaviour of escaping)

Theory into action

Think of the learning experiences that you have had during your nurse education. What kinds of rewards were you given by those teaching you in practice? How did you feel when you were rewarded or punished?

As you approach your final-year placements, it is increasing likely that you will be asked to undertake some teaching for junior students or care assistants. Consider the positive rewards that you could give and try some out in practice.

Shaping

An important aspect in behavioural approaches is the reduction of behaviours into smaller components that can be achieved easily, then subtly developed into more complex skills. This is known as 'shaping'—whereby understanding and skill are developed in a gradual process (Entwistle & Peterson, 2004). By reinforcing the student on completion of the skill or being able to demonstrate some knowledge, they can then be moved on to the next level. Shaping is important when a student is not able to meet a learning outcome. The skill should be broken down so that they can therefore achieve an easier step (leading them to be able to be reinforced), which is then developed into more complex stages, step by step.

Social learning theory

Another learning theory is that of social learning theory or role modelling, based on the observations of Albert Bandura. The basic principle is that learners will imitate the behaviours of others. If these are then reinforced, then such behaviours will be strengthened. This theory is based around research that involved observations of how children responded after seeing others behave in certain ways before them, concluding that they were quite likely to copy or mimic behaviours of adults that they had witnessed. Jarvis et al. (2003) suggest that Bandura's work highlights that learning occurs as a mutual proactive process whereby the individual 'acts back' towards the environment and its influences. Therefore it is important, as a nurse, to demonstrate exactly the types of skill and ability that you wish your learners to develop, as they will imitate you. The more the behaviour is witnessed, the more likely this will then be repeated by the learner. It is important that these behaviours are not just modelled in a teaching/learning situation, but that they are also practised continually, because the more the learner witnesses a correct behaviour, the more that behaviour can be modelled. If the learner is only exposed to correct techniques while being taught, but then witnesses different behaviours occurring more frequently in the everyday world of practice, they will probably adopt the latter approach. This is the notion of taking 'short cuts', or not 'practising what is being preached', but copying what are the most prevalent behaviours.

....

⊖ Theory into action

Think of some of the mentors with whom you have worked. What kind of role models were they in relation to being consistent with what they taught you and how they practised? Consider those you thought to be the best in teaching you and the methods they used to model the practices for you.

In your final-year placements, try to be increasingly aware of how you behave and ask your mentor for feedback on your own role modelling.

....

Cognitive learning theory

Cognitive learning theory is important to understand as it provides a deeper explanation of how people learn and understand, and it includes the internal mental processes of the learner as a fundamental basis. This theory answers the criticisms aimed at behavioural learning theory, which considers learning as simply being programmed responses to external stimuli. This is because cognitive theory includes the learner's ability to discriminate, generalize, and transfer skills, knowledge, and understanding to new or different situations. According to Burke et al. (2005), this is the ability to transfer knowledge learned during instruction to different situations. The different situations are usually the real-world domain in which the skill is practised. Therefore cognitive learning theory includes the notion of thinking between the stimulus and the response (Figure 6.4). In order to do this, it recognizes the role of perception, memory, and information-processing as internal mechanisms. Therefore, to assist students, we need to understand how thinking and learning occurs as opposed to straightforward behavioural aspects, and how to develop these.

A main proponent of cognitive learning theory is Bloom, who developed a taxonomy (or classification) of educational objectives related to cognitive learning (Quinn & Hughes, 2007). Bloom suggested that a skill consists of:

- a psychomotor component (the actual hand–eye coordination and behavioural motor/physical dexterity necessary);
- an affective component (the attitude and application required to carry it out effectively);
- a cognitive component (the level of understanding about the task that is required).

Stimulus ⟺ Association + thinking ⟺ Response ⟺ Reinforcement

Figure 6.4 Cognitive learning theory (unlike that shown in Figure 6.2, this theory includes the notion of thinking between the stimulus and the response)

For example, if you consider learning a clinical skill such as taking a blood pressure, there is first the 'hands on' element of learning how to operate the equipment; second, one learns when the skill is relevant and appropriate to carry out on a patient; and third, a student must understand the anatomy and physiology of the cardiovascular system. Bloom developed this taxonomy to represent the sequential and deepening levels of cognition.

1 **Knowledge**

This is knowing straightforward facts about the subject/issue being considered.

2 **Understanding/comprehension**

This is knowing how the subject/issue works or what its utility is.

3 **Application**

This is the ability to put the subject/issue into practice in the real world or to be able to explain its uses.

4 **Analysis**

This is the ability to break the subject/issue down into its component parts.

5 **Synthesis**

This is the ability to transfer the understanding about the issue and come up with new ideas of how it can be used.

6 **Evaluation**

This is the ability to place a value on all aspects involved in the issue as they are applied to different situations. Evaluation utilizes judgement based on the evidence provided in previous levels.

The lower levels (1 and 2) suggest that the learning is achieved by reception or rote (when we learn something by repetition, 'parrot fashion' such as learning 'times tables' off by heart in maths). This may be an important way to learn, but is very superficial. The methods employed can be used to convey information itself, but the learner may have very little understanding about it.

The latter stages in the taxonomy (3, 4, 5, and 6) show how the individual can develop higher-order thinking skills so that the knowledge provided now has meaning. At these stages, the learner is more likely to be discovering the knowledge, understanding, application, and value from the learning themselves, and involves a move from superficial understanding to deeper understanding. This notion of 'surface learning' (superficial repetition of knowledge) to 'deep learning' is discussed by Marton and Saljo (1976).

- -

➡ Theory into action

Consider a topic or skill that you have recently learnt at university or on placement. If you had to teach this skill to someone else, how would you break the teaching session into sections applying Bloom's taxonomy above?

- -

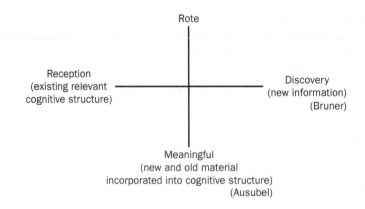

Figure 6.5 Methods of learning (adapted from Quinn & Hughes, 2007)

The concept of 'meaningful learning' as opposed to 'rote learning' was discussed by Ausubel (1968), who suggested that using the students' previous knowledge as a starting point is important, as otherwise they will not be able to make the links between new knowledge being presented and what they already know and understand. Bruner (1960) suggested the notion of 'discovery learning' as opposed to reception learning. This concept states that the nature of learning is more valuable to the individual if they find things out for themselves, which leads to deeper learning (Figure 6.5).

The notion of moving to deeper levels of learning by making associations between the student's prior knowledge ands experiences, and building on this cognitive learning, requires a number of considerations. According to Hartley (1998) these are as follows.

- **Well-organized and well-structured instruction**
  The instruction should be in incremental stages, so that each stage is achieved before moving on to more complex aspects.
- **Attending to the perceptual features of the task**
  Individuals perceive things differently, so it is necessary to check out the understanding of the learner in relation to the concepts being focused upon.
- **The importance of prior knowledge**
  An idea of the starting point of the learner's understanding is essential in order for them to be able to incorporate new knowledge and skills.
- **Awareness of individual differences**
  Individuals have different preferences for types of learning and instructional approaches, so using a variety of approaches at different stages is important.
- **The importance of feedback**
  Feedback is as important as new knowledge so that the student can ascertain where they are in relation to the task being learned.

These aspects relate very closely to the theory proposed by Piaget, that a learner 'assimilates' information by processing it against prior held knowledge and that prior beliefs can 'accommodate' the new knowledge into a whole new set of understandings and behaviours. Piaget had an influential role in the sphere of theory related to children's cognitive development, as did Vygotsky, who suggested that it is not only the individual child's potential that is important in learning, but also the opportunities, environments, and socialization that can enrich their learning. This he called the 'zone of proximal development' (Jarvis et al., 2003), which means that an individual can have a certain capacity, but that this can be hindered in poor or lacking social and learning environments.

 Thinking about

Think of some of the aspects that you have learned throughout your nurse education. How were these knowledge and skills developed? What kinds of explanations were you given that helped your understanding and what approaches hindered your understanding?

Brain-based learning

Another factor related to improving the cognitive abilities of individuals is brain-based learning. This means that, in order to best facilitate learning, we should not only look at the structure of learning, but also incorporate the physical and physiological understanding of how the brain works. Basically, brain-based learning requires us to ensure that all physical needs are met, such as those in Maslow's hierarchy of needs (water, food, air, safety, and shelter), or these will interfere with effective learning. So it is a matter of creating optimal physical conditions to ensure optimal cognitive functioning. There is a need to ensure that there is a balance between the amount of stimulation and relaxation offered to provide good learning experiences. Too much stimulation causes stress and a feeling of threat, so learning is reduced. Too much relaxation means there is very little change in environmental stimuli, which provides little opportunity to learn new things, (Jensen, 2000). Therefore the teacher needs to consider of a variety of activities and the time scale in which they are employed.

As human beings, we gather in information about the world around us through our senses. We also process our experiences of the world internally in a sensory way. So, for example, when remembering or imagining, we create sensory experiences internally. We process information in the following ways:

- visually;
- auditorily;
- kinaesthetically;
- olfactorily;
- gustatorily.

In other words, we see hear, feel, smell, and taste (O'Connor & Seymour, 1990). The activities that we provide in order for a learner to develop understanding of the situation need to incorporate differing aspects of these sensory processes. Individuals have preferences for certain sensory modes (the issue of preferences will be discussed later in this chapter). Therefore you might match your teaching approach with a student's preferred method of processing information—that is, visually, auditorily, kinaesthetically, and to a lesser extent olfactorily and gustatorily! However, as you cannot always easily find out individual preference in instructional situations, we have to go back to the notion of varying our activity to ensure that we do match it at least on some level.

Practical tip

The use of pictures, drawings, diagrams, or objects might satisfy those with a visual preference. Discussion, questions and answers, or reading some narrative about the topic might satisfy those with an auditory preference. Getting hands-on experience and being involved in completing tasks might satisfy those with a kinaesthetic preference, and so on. The use of all of these types of activity might produce a sensory-rich learning approach in which the learner can develop in relation to the aspect that they are learning.

 Thinking about

Think of the sensory mode from which you most prefer to learn: visual, auditory, or kinaesthetic. What kinds of activities appeal to that preference? For example, do you prefer to be shown things such as diagrams or pictures? Do you prefer to have discussions or questions and answers about topics? Do you prefer to have hands-on practical experiences? If you like all of these approaches, for which one do you have the strongest preference?

Multiple intelligences

Howard Gardner (1983) developed the concept of people having preferences for different modes in different situations and challenged the previously accepted concept that intelligence could only be measured in one way. He suggested that, because of these preferences for different sensory processes, individuals actually expressed their intelligence in different ways and therefore could be disadvantaged by the former established ways of assessing intelligence. He named these multiple intelligences. Basically, someone might not be able to solve problems using one processing approach, but may be able to do so if they use the approach that they prefer. These multiple intelligences or processing preferences are as follows.

- Visual/spatial
- Verbal/linguistic
- Logical/mathematical

- Bodily/kinaesthetic
- Musical/rhythmical
- Interpersonal
- Intrapersonal

The notion here is that, once again, a learner can be assisted to learn, by either matching their preferred approach or by using a variety of approaches to ensure that their preferred approach is at least not missed.

Practical tip

Following the above approach may not always be easy in busy clinical areas, so the aspect of getting to know the learner well is important. Then you can involve them in activities and situations in which they can best learn.

Experiential learning

An approach considered within the cognitive school that assists in the process of multiple intelligences mentioned above is experiential learning. This is a bridge between the theory of learning and the concept of preferences for learning styles. It is an approach discussed by Kolb (1976) based on previous work of Lewin, and also includes the concepts of assimilation and accommodation purported by Piaget. In the experiential learning cycle, the student goes through a number of stages in order to optimize the learning potential (Figure 6.6).

Kolb argues the importance of the person–environment interaction, and therefore the experiences that the learner has and the way in which they process the information. This is considered to be a cyclical process that has four stages (Boyatzis & Kolb, 1995).

- **Concrete experience**
  This is the actual event or activity. Being involved enables individuals to become immersed in actual clinical learning situations.

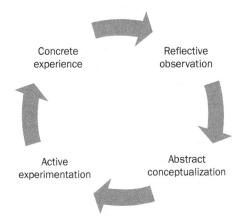

Figure 6.6 The cycle of experiential learning

- **Reflective observation**
  This occurs after the event, allowing the learner to reflect on their experiences from different perspectives.
- **Abstract conceptualization**
  This stage is used to develop explanations of what has happened, come up with new ideas, and begin to understand logical theoretical approaches to be applied in the situation in future.
- **Active experimentation**
  This is then used to test developing hypotheses as a problem-solving approach in practice.

Practical tip

When instructing a student, these phases are important.

1 Provide the student with the experience.
2 Follow this up with some time for discussion and reflection on the situation and gather information about it.
3 The next stage is to include some problem-solving exercises or question-and-answer sessions based on the theoretical knowledge necessary for the situation.
4 Finally, the student needs more supervised practice in the situation in order to establish the knowledge and skills needed in the specific context. In doing so, learning from experience should take place.

. . . .

Thinking about

Think of a skill that you learned in the clinical area. Reflect on this and identify the parts of the skill development that link to the stages above. What forms did these take?
Did you always go through the whole cycle or parts of it? Which parts of the cycle did you prefer?

. . . .

It is important to note in this theory that the concepts of concrete experience and abstract conceptualization are polar opposites. The same is true of reflective observation and active experimentation. Both have, on one side, some involvement in the practical arena and, on the other side, more internal or information-gathering and problem-solving processes. According to Bentham (2002), this relates to preference of perception (how information is taken in by the individual, such as a preference for concrete experience or abstract conceptualization) or a preference for processing (how information is internalized, either by active experimentation or reflective observation).

The theories of brain-based learning—multiple intelligences and experiential learning—provide an opportunity to further discuss the concept of learning style preferences. This is because they allude to individual preferences in cognitive style, sensory modality, and instructional approach.

Learning styles

As mentioned earlier, learning styles are preferences of students for a particular approach towards the subject matter to be learned. However, in a systematic review by Coffield et al. (2004), a number of issues were raised regarding the use of learning styles; the authors pointed out that care must be taken before applying the use of learning styles without carefully considering their validity and usefulness. The review showed that validity and reliability was questionable in a number of learning style theories and tools. The authors do point out, however, that it is accepted that the main value in understanding the concept of learning styles is for students/learners to be able to raise their awareness of their and others' learning styles as a self-awareness activity. It is beyond the remit of this chapter to discuss all learning-style theories and tools; instead, the learning styles proposed by Kolb (1976) and Honey and Mumford (1992) will be discussed here, as they are very commonly used in education.

Kolb

Kolb (1976) states that if individuals prefer certain types of learning at specific points, then they have particular learning styles (Figure 6.7) (Coffield et al., 2004).

- Between concrete experience and reflective observation, the learning style is known as being a **diverger**. This means that you may be imaginative and aware of meaning and values, and prefer observation to action.
- Between reflective observation and abstract conceptualization, the learning style is known as being an **assimilator**. This style suggests a preference for reasoning, having ideas, and logical problem-solving.

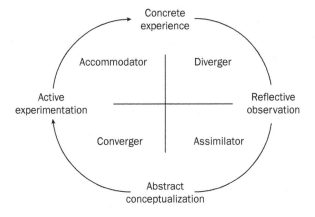

Figure 6.7 Learning styles (Kolb, 1976)

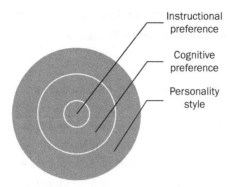

Figure 6.8 Curry's onion model (1983)

- Between abstract conceptualization and active experimentation, the learning style is known as being a **converger**. This style suggests being good at solving practical problems and making decisions.
- Between active experimentation and concrete experience, the learning style is known as being an **accommodator**. This style means that you are intuitive and can adapt to changing situations using trial and error.

Kolb devised a multi-item questionnaire known as the 'learning style inventory' (LSI) to ascertain an individual's preference for learning styles. This is an established and popular tool in education and other fields such as management, but questions have been raised about its validity (Coffield et al., 2004).

In 1983, Curry outlined the 'onion model' of learning styles. This model suggested that individuals have a personality style (which is fairly fixed and stable), a preference for the cognitive style (or sensory mode of learning, which is relatively fixed but can develop), or a preference for instructional method (which may be flexible). This can be seen in Figure 6.8.

By identifying students' preferences and matching the sensory mode, cognitive or instructional approach, optimal learning should be achieved. Ford and Chen (2001) suggest that there is some evidence supporting the notion that matching learning styles with teaching styles may be beneficial and has potential in enhancing student learning. Hallock et al. (2003) support this and suggest that research indicates that when individual's learning styles and the teaching approaches they are exposed to match, enhanced learning occurs. Kolb argues that mismatching of learning styles leads to ineffective learning or the learner not engaging in the learning process.

Honey and Mumford

Honey and Mumford (1992) accept Kolb's model, but disagree with the polar nature of the preferences and argue that each one has strengths of its own. This means that an individual can be an 'all-rounder', so they can learn in differing situations or just have a preference of one learning style, suggesting that that approach will provide the best learning experience for them. They accept the main premise of Kolb's styles, but have a different perspective from him. Honey and Mumford's styles (1992) are as follows.

- **Activists**

  This style relates to Kolb's concrete experience preference. Someone with this preference would prefer here-and-now activities and like to get involved in lots of new activities. However, they often get bored once into a project and look for new experiences.

- **Reflectors**

  This is similar to Kolb's reflective observation preference. Individuals with this preference like to gather information and ponder all perspectives before making decisions. They are likely to keep diaries and listen to all sides of a debate.

- **Theorists**

  This is similar to Kolb's abstract conceptualization preference. People with this preference like problem-solving and logical approaches based on evidence and knowledge.

- **Pragmatists**

  This is similar to Kolb's active experimentation. This is applying what is learned in practice. People with a preference for this style like to try things out in practice and experiment with new techniques and approaches.

Honey and Mumford suggest that different, less-established preferences of the individual can be developed by widening the repertoire of types of learning activity to which they are exposed. In a similar way to Kolb, they also designed a 'learning style questionnaire' (LSQ) to be used to ascertain individual strength of preference for each style.

Practical tip

In considering learning styles, the main premise is to understand that individuals all learn differently, so if only one approach is used, then some learning will not appear accessible to some students. Ideally, some form of assessment (or, indeed, the use of a formal tool such as the LSQ or LSI) to ascertain individual preferred styles should be completed so that the most appropriate type of instructional method that matches the style of the individual learner can be employed for effective learning to take place. Alternatively, in the absence of such knowledge or in dealing with larger groups of individuals, a variety of techniques need to be employed for learners to be able to take best advantage of the learning opportunities available.

....

Theory into action

From the descriptions of learning styles given above (Kolb, or Honey and Mumford), which would you prefer? What kinds of learning activities do you engage with most and which ones provide you with the most effective means of learning?

....

Humanistic learning theories

The final topic related to learning theories to be discussed here is that of humanistic learning theory, sometimes referred to as adult learning theory (Quinn & Hughes, 2007). This theory places the locus of control firmly with the learner. In behavioural learning theory, the locus of control is external in manipulating the environment and the reinforcers or punishers; in cognitive learning theory, it could be argued that it is shared between the person doing the teaching and the learner, as some more explorative approaches are used rather than straightforward stimulus–responses. Humanistic learning theory differs in that the principle suggests that the learner is the one that brings with them the motivation to learn; therefore the teacher needs to acts as a facilitator rather than instructor, or as is commonly stated ' a guide on the side as opposed to a sage on the stage'. Bentham (2002) suggests this main difference is because humanistic learning theory deals with the internal private mental world of individuals. It has as a fundamental principle consideration of the capacity for human growth and development and an individualistic approach (Miettinen, 2000).

The main theorists to consider within this field are Maslow (1954), Carl Rogers (1983), and Malcolm Knowles (1980). As mentioned earlier, Maslow's hierarchy of needs does form a basis for how individuals' learning can be reinforced by having their needs met. In the humanistic learning theory, the higher-level needs of communication, self-esteem, and self-actualization are the internal drivers and motivators for the individual to pursue learning, therefore suggesting that the individual comes with a desire and a preparedness to learn. Maslow's concept of self-actualization is considered to be a major motivator and driver for individuals wishing to experience new or further learning opportunities. Quinn and Hughes (2007) suggest that Maslow basically referred to self-actualization as the person becoming the best that they are able to become and is related to discovering their identity and purpose or destiny.

The formal type of education (which is usually applied to children) is known as 'pedagogy', which basically means the art and science of teaching children. According to Jarvis et al. (2003), Knowles (1980) had introduced the term 'andragogy', as he believed the art and science of teaching adults is different from the mechanisms required with children. (Note that the term 'pedagogy' is often used to describe teaching methods or strategies.)

Adults come with their own motivating factors, individual preferences, and aspirations. They are able to make their own decisions, so therefore, in respecting this, adult learners may enter into some form of agreement with the teacher as to how best to meet their own individual needs. Obviously, in nursing, some of these outcomes are set: for example, in the NMC (2010) standards of proficiency and the various learning outcomes incorporated into their nursing course. However, processes should be in place whereby the individual identifies and negotiates what and how they need to learn in order to achieve the outcomes. This is a basic tenet of adult learning and humanistic approaches.

Facilitating in adult learning

Rogers (1983) suggests that the instructional role is that of being a facilitator. Negotiations take place and the 'learning contract' is developed. A learning contract should include aspects such as the learning outcomes to be achieved, some sort of personal development plan that might identify the strengths, needs, and goals, a description of learning actions and the activities to be undertaken, and an agreement of the product and evidence to be produced to demonstrate achievement of the outcomes. In doing so, each individual learner may have very different approaches to achieving the outcomes, but the outcomes and therefore the standards still remain and quality is maintained. So the facilitator may take up a **coaching** role, giving advice and suggestions and acting as a support mechanism for the student when they are undertaking their learning journey.

In order to be successful in such a facilitator/coaching role, Rogers (1983) suggests that there is a fundamental requirement for the facilitator to embody unconditional positive regard incorporating trust, empathy, and genuineness. Unconditional positive regard is the polar opposite to aspects of behavioural learning theory, whereby conditions are firmly put in place before rewards and reinforcements, sanctions, or punishments are given. It means that there is a sense of acceptance and respect about the learner with no conditions on that acceptance. However, it is a mutual responsibility and the student should also therefore provide respect to the facilitator. Banning (2005) suggests that this is very much a move away from a didactic (authoritarian) role to one of empowering the student. However, in the current climate of targets and outcomes, sometimes there may be a pressure to return to more didactic methods to ensure that standards are met (Rolfe & Gardner, 2006).

The basis of ensuring good facilitation is the art of communicating well on an adult level with the learner. Outcomes need to be identified and, in nurse education, they are givens. In teaching junior nurses, you quickly need to establish trust. This means that you need to act as a role model without expecting them to do things that you would not be prepared to do yourself. It is important that you are aware of current evidence-based practices in order to deliver appropriate, relevant, and best advice to the students. This should not be too difficult, as such practices also reflect the more current empowering approaches advocated in healthcare environments (Akerjordet & Severinsson, 2008).

....

💡 Thinking about

Think of the mentors with whom you have worked. What steps did they take to gain your trust? How did they negotiate your planned learning experiences in order to meet your course requirements? What were your experiences of unconditional positive regard?

....

Teaching approaches

This section will discuss teaching approaches that can be utilized in practice by newly qualified nurses. Teaching methods, as discussed earlier in the chapter, are sometimes be referred to as 'pedagogy' (Jarvis, 2002).

Plan

The starting point is planning. As mentioned above, some situations may be spontaneous, as they occur in practice, so there may not be enough time to plan thoroughly. For all other situations, some time must be spent on thinking about the instruction or formally planning it. This would usually include some consideration of detail of the students involved, the learning outcomes to be achieved, teacher activity, student activity, times and venues, methods of assessment, and methods of evaluation (Quinn & Hughes, 2007).

Structure

Howard (2009) suggests that the structure of the session needs careful thought, but can follow a simple format, as suggested in the old adage of 'tell, tell, and tell'. Basically, tell them what you will tell them, tell them, and then tell them what you have told them. In other words, provide an 'introduction' outlining what will occur in the session and stating the learning objectives. The next aspect is 'development', in which these aspects are fully explored. Finally, there is the 'conclusion', in which the content discussed is summarized as a conclusion. This structure should be used in any form of teaching approach.

Muijs and Reynolds (2005) suggest that teaching approaches fall into three distinct types, into which most strategies can be classified.

- **Direct instruction**
  This is where the authority lies with the teacher and includes information giving and demonstrations.
- **Interactive teaching**
  Here, students are encouraged to participate and provide answers or raise questions in more discursive forums or seminars or coaching approaches.
- **Constructivist teaching**
  This relates to problem-based approaches, in which there is some responsibility on behalf of the student to undertake some exploration and information gathering in order to solve a 'real-world' problem.

Methods

In direct instruction, you may be utilizing more didactic approaches. In the practice setting, this may be along the lines of a short presentation to a small group of individuals.

A mini-lecture (in similar ways to a large-scale lecture) is an efficient way of sharing information quickly (Quinn & Hughes, 2007). Care must be taken in using technology to present the information, such as PowerPoint or flip charts. Just as with learning environments, visual aids should be neat, tidy, uncluttered, and spacious. The information should be kept to a minimum and the points explained. Further detail can be developed through questioning or by providing supporting materials such as handouts. Non-verbal and verbal aspects need to be carefully orchestrated to create engagement with you as a presenter and to emphasize relevant or important points. It is also important for managing the students and any disruptions that may occur (Race, 2001).

Another form of direct instruction is by providing a demonstration. This might be in the practice area or in a lab or simulation area. Simulated learning involves imitating some facet of life, such as the use of equipment, including mannequins or actors who take on roles of patients (Quinn & Hughes, 2007).

Demonstration

A demonstration is described by Quinn and Hughes (2007) as a visualized explanation of facts or principles. The number of students observing such a demonstration needs to be carefully considered, as the presence of too many students will restrict the effectiveness of what can be observed, or what can be asked about the procedure. Once again, all equipment should be prepared and be in working order, and all resources needed be at hand. Howard (2009) highlights the importance of breaking a skill into smaller achievable stages and steps when demonstrating techniques. It is also best to have students behind you when observing the situation as they would face it rather than observing it in mirror-image view. Explain the procedure beforehand, demonstrate it, and then take feedback and answer questions. As Race and Brown (2005) suggest, you need to become an 'expert witness' and used to answering questions.

Small group interactive teaching

Demonstrations could also be considered to be interactive teaching. However, in the main, these are more likely to be small individual or group sessions, such as seminars or tutorials. According to Jarvis (2002), these methods align with the student-centred humanistic approaches that have developed over the past 30 years. In small groups, reflective approaches that perhaps follow the experiential learning cycle of Kolb (1976) can be used as a basis of discussion. Advanced organizers—(information given out prior to sessions (Ausubel, 1968)—are also used so that there is a defined focus for any prearranged sessions. Small group teaching might include role play, discussions, setting up of debates or microteaching (Quinn and Hughes, 2007). The skills of questioning need developing as well as the ability to 'scaffold' learning, which means developing a basic understanding, then releasing and discussing increasingly complex aspects of the area under study.

Problem-based learning

Constructivist teaching basically means providing the student with problems, or exercises, in which they need to seek out information in order to answer them. These can be resource-based exercises, in which learning materials such as workbooks, or online and computer-based learning opportunities, are developed and utilized (Howard, 2009). Once again, the skill as a facilitator is needed as opposed to being an instructor. Problem-based learning (PBL) is such an approach. It is a method that aims to help students to utilize fact-finding skills and apply them to contextually based scenarios that truly reflect the areas, situations, and people in which and with whom they will be practising. Wilkie (2000) points out that PBL is presented in the context that students are likely to encounter the situation in real life. PBL is described by Cooke and Moyle (2002) as a situation in which real clinical situations are used to develop learning and clinical reasoning responses in students. It is based on the delivery of a trigger or scenario reflecting real-world problems. There is a period of group facilitation to highlight information inherent in the situation, to develop hypotheses, and to identify gaps in knowledge. Following this, there is a period of self-directed study, during which students appraise evidence and return to the group to provide answers or solutions to the problem at hand.

Simply put, PBL is an approach that reflects a structure whereby students are directed around a problem and need some self-discipline to find the solution. Muijs and Reynolds (2005) suggest that any such approach follows a basis of a start phase in which the problem is given, an exploration phase in which the problem is analysed and information gathered, a reflection phase in which the information is shared and reconstructed in light of the problem, and finally an application and discussion phase, in which the problem is solved and the learning gained is extrapolated and identified.

Having discussed learning theories and some teaching approaches in detail to understand how to facilitate learning, we now move onto the next domain in the NMC (2008b) standards related to learning and assessment.

Assessment and accountability

As a qualified nurse, you may find yourself involved informally or formally in the assessment of student nurses. The role of mentor is one that you may find appealing once you have settled into your role as a qualified nurse. A nurse can become a mentor when they have completed at least one year post-registration and successfully achieved all outcomes required in the NMC standards for that stage. They can then enter a local register and be identified as a mentor, with a specific role in supporting and assessing student nurses.

As a newly qualified nurse, although not a mentor, you may be expected to participate in some assessments in the practice area by observing and giving feedback on a student's progress to the mentor. This section is intended to give you an overview of assessments, what they are for, how they can be guaranteed to be useful, how you can provide constructive feedback on a learner's performance, and how you can use a range of assessment methods to ensure that a learner meets their learning outcomes.

Rowntree (1987) suggested an assessment has five main aims:

- to provide a basis for job selection;
- to maintain standards;
- to motivate learners;
- to inform learners of their progress;
- to inform teachers (and, in this case, mentors/supervisors) about their performance.

As a newly qualified nurse, you may get the opportunity to be involved in some selection interviews, but it is the last four aims of assessment that are most important for you. The mentor/supervisor's responsibilities are related to assisting in the development and progress of the learner and in making sure that standards are met. Race and Brown (2005) suggest that the purpose of assessment is for students to be able to set their sights high and be able to achieve their intended outcomes. It is up to the person doing the assessment to communicate what the 'goalposts' are, and to help the learner to understand the nature of how they will be assessed and on what they will be assessed.

Assessment is the process of measuring and interpreting how students have responded to their instruction in relation to given required outcomes (Curzon, 2003). Quinn and Hughes (2007) suggest that assessment serves the purpose of providing valuable feedback to the student on their performance, development, and progress, and whether learning has taken place. Ultimately, it leads to a judgement as to whether they can be worthy of a publicly recognized award and right to practice. According to Wellard et al. (2007), nursing knowledge and skill is complex in nature; and they argue that assessment activities can be instruments of power (barriers to be overcome). We can all appreciate that students are inclined to want to learn more about passing assessments than learning about nursing!

Authentic assessment

Nursing involves knowledge, skills, and attitudes; therefore, an assessment method should be employed as to how these might be demonstrated to meet specific criteria. This calls for the need for *authentic assessment* approaches.

Cumming and Maxwell (1999) argued that assessment needs to be 'authentic' because of the need in measuring the learning outcomes required, and to ensure quality and standards in meeting the outcomes. The validity also needs to be inherent in the assessment in order to ensure contextual meaning so that the student finds motivation to be involved and pass the assessment not only for passing's sake, but also because the assessment leads to their actual development about the nursing knowledge and skills being focused upon.

Bathmaker (2003) argues that assessment is important to show that nursing students are conforming to standards to make decisions about the fitness of the individual for purpose.

Teaching and assessment

Muijs and Reynolds (2005) suggest that assessment takes up one-third of a teacher/mentor's time. This shows how interlinked teaching and assessment are: they could be considered within the same continuum of learning, and there could not be learning without both instruction and assessment. Barton (2009, in Hinchliff, 2009) suggests that a mentorship approach uses tools for assessment that includes teaching and support aspects, and that can be used for examination of performance. Muijs and Reynolds (2005) state that there are two important types of assessment.

- **Formative**: this is where information is gathered in an ongoing manner and the student is provided with feedback about how they are performing. It can still be a formal process. This type of assessment has being found to have a positive effect on achievement.
- **Summative**: this is where final judgements on the student's performance against specified criteria are made. This type of assessment is used as the quality control mechanism and to ensure that appropriate standards are met.

....

⊙ Theory into action

Reflect on your nursing course and your experiences of assessment in practice. What types of assessment have been used in order for competencies to be passed in your portfolio? From the methods used by the mentors whom you had, what were the most beneficial approaches used to provide formative feedback?

....

Key points

As a newly qualified nurse, you may not immediately find yourself in the situation of summatively assessing students, but you may very well be providing formative feedback on performance to some students informally or providing testimonies for them as evidence that they may use in a more summative situation with their mentor. You may also be reporting on the student's performance to the mentor.

How to provide feedback

When providing feedback on students, it is important that the mechanisms of judgement making are understood. Assessment can be judged by the performance of the learner compared with others, known as 'norm referencing', or they can be judged by their performance against given criteria, known as 'criterion referencing'. The latter is often used as a basis in nursing and higher education in order that the learners demonstrate that they meet the minimum standards required (knowledge of content and demonstration of skills).

Norm referencing

Barton (2009) suggests that norm referencing is often useful as a guide within formative feedback, as the individual can have their performance compared with their peers; any deficiencies are highlighted, therefore providing an opportunity to identify needs and actions to be taken to improve performance. Norm referencing can often highlight the expectations related to levels of performance: for example, more would be expected of a third-year nurse than a first-year nurse in relation to certain activities (this may also be reflected in the expectations within the criteria).

Criterion referencing

Criterion reference is really a final form of evaluation of performance and although it can be used as a basis for formative feedback, it is more closely related to summative assessment. This is because the knowledge, skills, and competence of the learner must be accounted for against statutory requirements. The development of assessment criteria is important to create reliability in the assessment process. This is almost the same as producing a checklist of aspects that can be ticked off on completion, or a set of behaviours describing how well someone has completed the task. The criteria are important, as ideally what is wanted is that at least two or more assessors can arrive at the same decision in light of the facts observed. This is known as inter-rater reliability.

An example of criterion referencing taken from the NMC (2010) standards of proficiency is:

> Nurses must communicate safely and effectively with individuals and groups of all ages, using a variety of complex skills and interventions including communication technologies.

This is a set standard, but it can be seen that problems with interpretation may still arise, as criteria will still need to be established for determining terms such as 'effectively', and there is a need for clearer definition of what 'complex skills' are and how they can be identified and measured. A good assessor will explore such criteria with the learner, identifying, negotiating, and agreeing on the terms and how they are demonstrated in the real-world context. For example, while working with people with learning disabilities in the community, you might discuss with a student specialist approaches to communicating, such as using sign language or a communication board, for those with limited communication abilities.

Hence, getting to know the student, identifying clear outcomes, providing supportive instruction, stating the method of assessment, and then making unambiguous decisions on the performance of the outcome is an important and continuous process. As Hartley (1998) points out, in order to help the student to meet their outcomes, we need to understand different methods of assessment and clarify our intentions.

⊖ Theory into action

Look back over your nursing practice portfolio. Identify the factors involved that were related to formative assessment. How were these structured and what processes occurred? In what way were the summative elements approached differently? Identify aspects that were norm-referenced and those that were criterion-referenced.

Points to consider

In your portfolio, there will be some proficiencies or competencies that you are required to pass. These might be considered as criterion assessments. Feedback whereby you are compared with your peers or others, perhaps with feedback such as 'you performed at a higher standard than expected for your stage of training', might be considered norm referencing.

Ensuring consistency between learning and assessment

The concept of 'constructive alignment' becomes important here and is a major factor to be considered in making the best of the learning experiences for the individual. Entwistle and Peterson (2004) suggest that this is a systematic approach to ensure that learning situations have strong links between the aims, mode of instruction, and assessment of learning. It is based on the work of Biggs (1999), who argues that there needs to be clarity and consistency between the learning outcomes that are set, the teaching methods employed for the student to learn them, and the way in which they are assessed. If learning is constructively aligned, then there is maximum consistency and the learner can make the most of the developmental opportunity.

Learning outcomes

Setting a learning outcome is the first stage in ensuring alignment in learning. According to Race (2001), learning outcomes should be more than official statements in course documents—they should underpin all teaching and learning situations. Therefore setting clearly identifiable learning outcomes can be done in a discussion with a student or more formally written into their assessment documentation. The outcomes should include the person completing the outcome (the learner, the student, you, etc.) and what they need to do (*will administer an intramuscular injection, will record a clients' history, will complete a behavioural assessment*), when they will do it (*at the end of the session, by the end of today, by the end of the placement*), and the degree of success needed to complete it (*successfully, independently, under supervision, etc.*).

The following are some examples of learning outcomes.

- 'You will administer an intramuscular injection by the end of today under supervision.'
- 'The learner will record a client's history by the end of this week independently.'
- 'The student will complete a behavioural assessment of a client by a [specific date (e.g. 1 January)] independently.'

Sometimes, more formal learning outcomes are written, with a stem statement such as:

- 'By the end of this teaching session (module, course, etc.), the student will be able to demonstrate . . . '

Following the stem statement, the actual required behaviour/activity/skill of the student is included, using such verbs as described in Bloom's taxonomy earlier.

1 'By the end of this teaching session (module, course, etc.), the student will be able to demonstrate **knowledge** of the principles of anatomy and physiology.'
2 'By the end of this teaching session (module, course, etc.), the student will be able to demonstrate an **understanding** of the principles of anatomy and physiology.'
3 'By the end of this teaching session (module, course, etc.), the student will be able to demonstrate **application** of the principles of anatomy and physiology.'
4 'By the end of this teaching session (module, course, etc.), the student will be able to demonstrate **evaluation** of the principles of anatomy and physiology.'

In each of the above cases, deeper levels of learning need to be demonstrated. Therefore the way in which these outcomes are tested would need to be different.

1 A simple multiple-choice test might be used to examine their knowledge.
2 A deeper question requiring some explanation in the answer (written or verbal) might be used.

3 An observed structured clinical examination (OSCE), which involves the direct observation of clinical skills assessed using a checklist (Jones et al., 2010), might be used to ascertain how skilled they are at applying their knowledge by working with a patient (usually simulated in exam conditions, but can be in real-world context).

4 Some problem-solving or research answering a specific assignment might be used to probe the depth of their knowledge of how principles are transferable across different fields, perhaps even followed up by some oral questioning or *viva voce* (live voice) examination.

It is apparent that some aspects are harder to articulate into learning outcomes than others as they are open to interpretation. It is best to identify in advance what would be required by the learner to specifically demonstrate these in practice.

Race and Brown (2005) stress the importance of feedback and suggest that students be encouraged to get involved in self-assessment. Feedback should, in the main, highlight the positive aspects of the work and turn any negative aspects into a positive by telling the learner what it is they need to do to improve in order to address their deficiencies.

Assessment in practice

Throughout a nursing course, students will have been exposed to a variety of assessment methods in their formal educational setting. These may include seen and unseen timed examinations, production of assignments and essays, OSCEs, and individual or group presentations, and they will be judged on their academic qualities as well as the knowledge and understanding of relevant content (Merricks, 2002). Students will come into the clinical area with specific sets of competencies that are expected to be demonstrated. In order to satisfy the NMC (2010) standards of proficiency, they will have to be assessed and signed off by appropriately qualified personnel. Quinn and Hughes (2007) suggest that assessment in the workplace may revolve around how the student constructs their personal practice portfolio, which may include reflective diaries as well as the competencies needed to be achieved. The main method of assessing a student's progress is by observing them in practice as they complete their required skills and tasks.

Observation

It is important that an effort is made in the relationship-building aspect, as being observed can be quite unnerving for the student. The observations may be rated against a checklist developed to identify the stages of the task and the criteria against which the student is been judged. Observations could be made in close proximity or in a more 'long-arm' fashion. However, a mentor cannot sign off a competence for a student if they have not actually observed it themselves or have not been provided with reliable testimony of observations from other recognized assessors/mentors.

A checklist for assessment

Overall, it is important that assessment:

- is valid, reliable, consistent, fair, and honest;
- has closely aligned learning outcomes, teaching activities, and methods of assessment;
- includes the student being given appropriate feedback that is commensurate to their performance and supportive of their further development.

....

Theory into action

Think of how you have been assessed in practice. How were the assessments set up? How were the observations conducted? How were you provided with feedback? What techniques were used to put you at ease?

....

Evaluation of learning

The NMC (2008b) states that the domain of evaluation of learning relates to the evaluation of learning in practical settings and how students relate their experiences. It is linked closely once again with the concept of constructive alignment of teaching and learning activities, methods of assessment, and feedback. In fact, this could be considered feedback on the whole learning process.

By evaluating students' experiences, further lessons may be learned and changes incorporated to improve future learning situations (Quinn & Hughes, 2007). According to the NMC (2008b), this is about ensuring that the learning environments are suitable and appropriate for student nurses to be learning optimal practice knowledge, skills, and attitudes related to the role of the nurse. Young and Maxwell (2007) state that evaluation can be:

- formal or informal;
- systemic or episodic;
- formative or summative.

Howard (2009) suggests that evaluation is important to improve outcomes, teaching processes, learning achievement, and ultimately patient/client care. They argue there are two major functions, as follows.

- To evaluate factual/physical aspects linked to learning outcomes, all of which are easily measurable (Has learning occurred?)
- To evaluate systems and processes that support and contribute to the fixed components of the course (Are the mechanisms working in an appropriately supportive way?)

Most nursing courses have formal ways of evaluating students' experiences throughout their education. These might be on a modular level or at course level. There are also mechanisms to explore their learning experiences while in practice. There might be tripartite meetings between the student, their personal tutor, and their mentor/supervisor in the clinical area. Evaluation may be required as a part of their formal portfolio documentation, and they may need to complete this as part of their mandatory requirements.

If an evaluation is completed formally, then there is usually some sort of questionnaire or instrument designed for the purpose. Most of these are answered anonymously, but it can also be transparent who filled a questionnaire, if necessary. Race (2001) suggests that involving students in self-assessment and peer assessment can help them to build confidence in their own abilities and in providing evaluative information. This increases their confidence and they can draw up the agendas for what is to be evaluated.

Key points

As a newly qualified nurse, you may not be called on very early in your career to be involved in devising formal evaluations. However, you may work with learners of whom there is a need for informal evaluation.

As discussed above, the main evaluative questions quite simply are as follows.

- **What have you learned?**
  This can be expanded to assess whether or not the student has learned aspects that reflect their intended learning outcomes and wider learning opportunities.
- **What has helped/hindered your learning experience(s)?**
  This can be expanded to include the student's thoughts and feelings related to environmental factors, the teaching and learning activities, and supportive mechanisms that they have experienced.
- **What could be done to further improve the learning experience for future students?**

It is important to let the person know that their views are valid and that they are been listened to. However, it is also important not to change approaches immediately (unless there is something remarkably obvious that needs to be changed), as evaluations tell you how an individual perceives a situation, and because individuals perceive situations differently, change should only be considered if there are consistent evaluative comments requiring some need for change or improvement. Evaluation is important and should not be treated as just an end-stage process (Howard, 2009).

Creating an environment for learning

It is recognized that the real world of nursing takes place in practice and that student nurses need to learn there. This provides the learner with opportunities to learn through observation or involvement, but care needs to be taken that they are not placed in situations that are too stressful or threatening. Likewise, the main intention of any clinical area is to provide care for the clients or patients who are catered for in either generic or specialist ways. Therefore student nurses will find themselves in situations in which they require formal learning that is not university or classroom-based, such as a busy hospital acute setting using highly specialized approaches or working in the community with nurses who visit and look after people in their own homes.

When providing learning opportunities for individuals, care needs to be taken to make sure that the physical, psychological, and social factors are addressed adequately (Bentham, 2002; Muijs & Reynolds, 2005). The student should have had adequate breaks and the instruction given in short spells to aid attention to the task. The environment should be appropriately heated and ventilated, with enough light and heat to function in. Noise should be kept to a minimum and any potential distractions should be addressed beforehand (Jensen, 2000). It is also important to maintain the balance between stimulation and relaxation so as to not create stress while heightening motivation.

Resources should be prepared and available before the instruction is given. Scheduled or timetabled use of rooms is advisable, but sometimes the learning experience may present itself spontaneously. Communication with other members of staff is important as they also will need to know when the instruction is occurring.

As mentioned earlier, the aspects related to the context of practice, evidence-based practice, and leadership are covered in other chapters in this book. In this setting, the three concepts combined basically mean that it is your responsibility to keep up to date in your practice using appropriate evidence to support this. In order to create effective learning for students, these practices should be role-modelled and opportunities taken to develop such practices in the work areas, and to disseminate the knowledge, skills, and attitudes related to them to others.

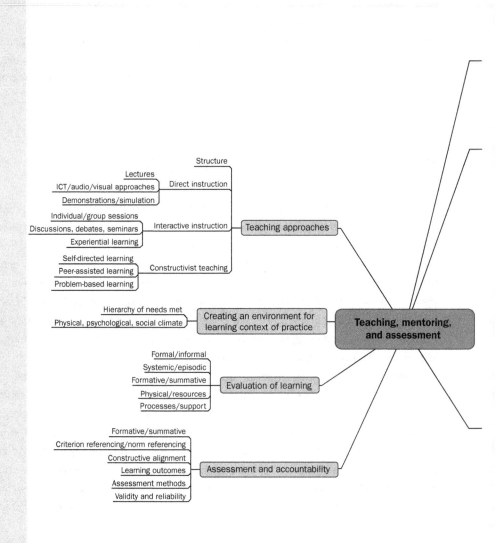

Figure 6.9

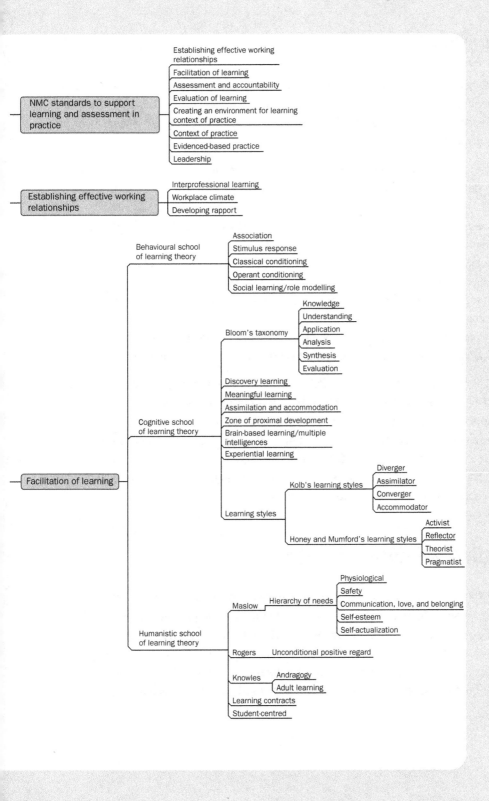

Summary

Newly qualified nurses have a crucial role to play in the practice-based education of student nurses, junior staff, and often other health professionals. It is important that, alongside being a good role model, that practice-based teaching and assessment follows these golden rules.

- Get to know your students and their course requirements.
- Understand the principles of learning and teaching.
- Set appropriate learning outcomes.
- Create environments that are physically, psychologically, and socially conducive for learning.
- Design relevant teaching and learning activities to optimize students' learning experiences.
- Use a range of assessment methods to ensure that students meet the learning outcomes.
- Provide constructive feedback on performance, including clarity on how to improve.
- Evaluate all aspects of the mentoring/supervising/ teaching experiences.

This chapter has looked at the NMC (2008b) standards in relation to supporting learning and assessment in practice. We have discussed learning theories and how these should shape our approaches to facilitating learning for students. The nature of assessment was discussed, as well as how to develop effective learning environments and teaching methods in a practice setting.

In this chapter, we have looked at several teaching, mentoring, and assessment approaches, which are summarized in Figure 6.9.

Online Resource Centre

 This textbook is accompanied by an Online Resource Centre that provides interactive learning resources and tools to help you to prepare for the transition from student to fully qualified member of staff. After you have completed each chapter and whenever you see this icon, please go to the ORC at your earliest convenience. If you have not done so already, save the ORC web address into your favourites: **http://www.oxfordtextbooks.co.uk/orc/burton**

References

Akerjordet K & Severinsson E (2008) Emotionally intelligent nurse leadership: a literature review study. *Journal of Nursing Management*, **16**: 565–77.

Ausubel DP (1968) *Educational Psychology: A Cognitive View*. Holt, Rhinehart and Winston, New York.

Banning M (2005) Approaches to teaching: current opinions and related research. *Nurse Education Today*, **25**: 502–8.

Barton D (2009) How to assess teaching and learning. In: SM Hinchliff (ed) *The Practitioner as Teacher*, 4th edn. Elsevier, Philadelphia, PA.

Bathmaker A (2003) The expansion of higher education: a consideration of control and funding. In: S Bartlett & D Burton (eds) *Education Studies: Essential Issues*. Sage, London.

Bentham S (2002) *Psychology and Education*. Routledge, East Sussex.

Biggs J (1999) What the student does: teaching for enhanced learning. *Higher Education Research & Development*, **18**(1): 57–75.

Boyatzis E & Kolb DA (1995) From learning styles to learning skills: the executive skills profile. *Journal of Managerial Psychology*, **10**(5): 3–17.

Bruner JS (1960) *The Process of Education*. Harvard University Press, Cambridge, MA.

Burke V, Jones I & Doherty M (2005) Analysing student perceptions of transferable skills via undergraduate degree programmes. *Active Learning in Higher Education*, **6**(2): 132–44.

Cable S (2002) The context: why the current interest? In: S Glen & T Leiba (eds) *Multi-professional Learning for Nurses: Breaking the Boundaries*. Palgrave, Hampshire.

Coffield F, Moseley D, Hall E & Ecclestone K (2004) *Should We be Using Learning Styles? What Research has to Say to Practice*. Learning & Skills Research Centre, London.

Cooke M & Moyle K (2002) Students' evaluation of problem-based learning. *Nurse Education Today*, **22**: 330–9.

Cumming JJ & Maxwell GS (1999) Contextualising authentic assessment. *Assessment in Education: Principles, Policy & Practice*, **6**(2): 177–94.

Curry L (1983) *Learning Styles in Continuing Medical Education*. Canadian Medical Association, Ottawa, ON.

Curzon LB (2003) *Teaching in Further Education: An Outline of Principles and Practice*, 6th edn. Continuum, London.

Entwistle N & Peterson E (2004) Conceptions of learning and knowledge in higher education: relationships with study behaviour and influences of learning environments. *International Journal of Educational Research*, **41**(6): 407–28.

Ford N & Chen SY (2001) Matching/mismatching revisited: an empirical study of learning and teaching styles. *British Journal of Educational Technology*, **32**(1): 5–22.

Gardner H (1983) *Frames of Mind: The Theory of Multiple Intelligences*. Basic Books, New York.

Hallock D, Satava D & LeSage T (2003) An exploratory investigation of the potential relationship between student learning styles, course grade, cumulative grade point average and selected demographics in on-line undergraduate business courses. *Management Research News*, **26**(1): 21–8.

Hartley J (1998) *Learning and Studying: A Research Perspective*. Routledge, London.

Honey P & Mumford A (1992) *The Manual of Learning Styles*, 3rd edn. Peter Honey, Berkshire.

Howard S (2009) How to make your teaching effective. In: SM Hinchliff (ed) *The Practitioner as Teacher*, 4th edn. Elsevier, Philadelphia.

Jarvis P (2002) Teaching styles and teaching methods. In: P Jarvis (ed) *The Theory and Practice Of Teaching*. Kogan Page, London.

Jarvis P, Holford J & Griffin C (2003) *The Theory and Practice of Learning*, 2nd edn. Kogan Page, London.

Jensen E (2000) *Brain-based Learning: The New Science of Teaching and Training*, revised edn. The Brain Store, San Diego.

Jones A, Pegram A & Fordham-Clarke C (2010) Developing and examining an objective structured clinical examination. *Nurse Education Today*, **30**(2): 137–41.

Knowles MS (1980) *The Modern Practice of Adult Education: From Pedagogy to Andragogy*. Prentice Hall, Englewood Cliffs, NY.

Kolb DA (1976) *Learning Style Inventory. Technical Manual*. Mcber and Co, Boston, MA.

Marton F & Säljö R (1976) On qualitative differences in learning I: outcome and process. *British Journal of Educational Psychology*, **46**: 4–11.

Maslow A (1954) *Motivation and Personality*. Harper and Row, New York.

Merricks L (2002) Assessment in post-compulsory education. In: P Jarvis (ed) *The Theory and Practice Of Teaching*. Kogan Page, London.

Miettinen R (2000) The concept of experiential learning and John Dewey's theory of reflective thought and action. *International Journal of Lifelong Education*, **19**(1): 54–72.

Muijs D & Reynolds D (2005) *Effective Teaching: Evidence and Practice*, 2nd edn. Sage, London.

Nursing and Midwifery Council (2008a) *The Code: Standards of Conduct, Performance and Ethics for Nurses and Midwives*. NMC, London.

Nursing and Midwifery Council (2008b) *Standards to Support Learning and Assessment in Practice*, 2nd edn. NMC, London.

Nursing and Midwifery Council (2010) *Standards for Proficiency for Pre-registration Nursing Education*. NMC, London.

O'Connor J & Seymour J (1990) *Introducing NLP: Psychological Skills for Understanding and Influencing People*. Aquarian Press, London.

Quinn FM & Hughes S (2007) *Quinn's Principles and Practice of Nurse Education*, 5th edn. Stanley Thornes Publishers, Cheltenham.

Race P (2001) *The Lecturer's Toolkit: A Practical Guide to Learning, Teaching and Assessment*, 2nd edn. Kogan Page, London.

Race P & Brown S (2005) *500 Tips for Teachers*, 2nd edn. Routledge, Oxon.

Rogers CR (1983) *Freedom to Learn for the 80s*. Charles Merrill, Columbus, OH.

Rolfe G & Gardner L (2006) 'Do not ask who I am . . . ': confession, emancipation and (self) management through reflection. *Journal of Nursing Management*, **14**: 593–600.

Rowntree D (1987) *Assessing Students: How Shall we Know Them?* Harper & Row, London.

Scott SD (2008) 'New Professionalism': shifting relationships between nursing education and nursing practice. *Nurse Education Today*, **28**: 240–5.

Young LE & Maxwell B (2007) Student-centred teaching in nursing: from rote to active learning. In: LE Young & BL Patterson (eds) *Teaching Nursing: Developing a Student-centered Learning Environment*. Lippincott, Williams and Wilkins, Philadelphia, PA.

Wellard SJ, Bethune E & Heggen K (2007) Assessment of learning in contemporary nurse education: do we need standardised examination for nurse registration? *Nurse Education Today*, **27**(1): 68–72.

Wilkie K (2000) The nature of problem-based learning. In: S Glen & K Wilkie (eds) *Problem-based Learning in Nursing: A New Model for a New Context?* Palgrave, Hampshire.

7

Being in charge: leadership and management

Rob Burton

The aims of this chapter are to:

➜ explore issues of transition to the role of newly qualified nurse and being in charge;

➜ explore theories of leadership;

➜ explore theories of management;

➜ outline strategies to help a newly qualified nurse to be in charge.

The transition to the role of newly qualified nurse

One of the first things that you will need to get used to as a newly qualified nurse is *being in charge*. This may mean being in charge of the care of a single client, or group of clients, as well as being in charge of the whole care environment, including all staff and other multidisciplinary team members. In order to do this, you will not only need to understand the care needs of the clients, but also to understand and be able to demonstrate skills of leadership and management. It is recognized that you should have a period of **preceptorship** and supervision on qualifying, but there may be times at which you do have to lead or manage teams during this period.

What does 'being in charge' mean? And what does it take to make the transition from being a student nurse to finding that you are the one who is responsible for yourself and the welfare of the patients, staff, visitors, and anyone else in the care environment? The focus of this chapter is on what you need to know and what you might need to do when you are leading and managing in a care setting for the first time.

We will discuss the concepts of leadership and management, and how to apply them in a new role and be able to feel confident and competent to do so. By identifying the different concepts and looking at how they can be applied, you should be able to analyse workplace situations and decide on the best leadership/management approach. Aspects of being in charge that tend to be common and generic in all settings are:

- the delegation of tasks within the team;
- dealing with staff issues;
- solving problems arising from unexpected circumstances.

Key points

The **Nursing and Midwifery Council** (NMC, 2010) identifies that one of the standards of **proficiency** for entry to the register as a qualified nurse is to respond to planned and uncertain situations, managing themselves and others effectively. The nurse should demonstrate the development of further management and leadership skills during their preceptorship and beyond.

Therefore, in the final year of training, you need to take as many opportunities to be in charge of a shift (under supervision) in your **field of practice** as possible to help you to achieve this.

Scenarios 7.1 and 7.2 describe typical situations in which you may find yourself as a newly qualified nurse, whether in a busy hospital ward setting or in a community nursing team or community home setting. There are common experiences that need the person dealing with them to show leadership qualities and to manage the situation.

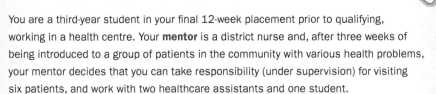

Scenario 7.1

You are a third-year student in your final 12-week placement prior to qualifying, working in a health centre. Your **mentor** is a district nurse and, after three weeks of being introduced to a group of patients in the community with various health problems, your mentor decides that you can take responsibility (under supervision) for visiting six patients, and work with two healthcare assistants and one student.

What would your priorities be in this situation? What would you need to consider?

Points to consider

In a situation such as Scenario 7.1, you would have to concentrate on the skills identified within the NMC (2010) standards of proficiency domains of professional values, communication, leadership, and teamwork. Some of these aspects have also been discussed in earlier chapters and include ensuring that the environment for the care management is safe for clients and staff, and making decisions related to managing risk. You would need to clearly communicate with the other staff members 'allocated to you', as well as with other members of the interdisciplinary team involved in care. It is your responsibility to ensure that these communications take place and your responsibility to delegate duties to others. It is here where your leadership qualities are tested. The principles of delegation are also discussed in Chapter 3, but it is clear that delegation requires leadership qualities and skills. For example, you will have the responsibility for recording and managing the information related to your clients and communicating this to colleagues, thereby demonstrating some management skills.

You will also have to manage your time and the time of those allocated to you to ensure that the care priorities are met equitably and competently among your clients. As the NMC (2010) states, nurses should be able to demonstrate proficiency in public protection, maintaining safe environments, and ensuring quality assurance, as well as delegating duties to others, while ensuring that they have adequate supervision. Scenario 7.2 will require all of these aspects to be demonstrated.

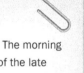

Scenario 7.2

You take a phone call as you commence the late shift on a busy care area. The morning staff are completing their duties for the day, and there is another member of the late shift just arriving. The environment is bustling with activity. You listen to the other person on the end of the phone; it is the nurse manager who was supposed to be in charge of the area for the late shift. They tell you that they are unable to come in on duty as there has been an emergency with their young daughter.

As a student nurse, you would probably have had a qualified nurse with you on duty to whom you could turn for advice, or deal with the matter themselves. Therefore, you could have looked behind or over your shoulder and confidently handed the issue on to them to deal with. But, now, you are qualified and currently the most senior member of staff on duty for the late shift. There is no one else for you to hand the matter to: you are the one who has to deal with this situation.

For a newly qualified nurse, this can be a stark realization. The healthcare assistants are looking towards you now with an expectation that you should do something about this. Your leadership abilities are now open to scrutiny.

A nurse in the situation described in Scenario 7.2 would have little choice but to take on a leadership role, even if that were to meant taking action by informing more senior staff of the situation. However, in some services such as small care homes or in primary healthcare settings, there might not be anyone more senior to whom to immediately turn. This may seem daunting at first, yet dealing with such issues is part and parcel of the responsibilities of newly qualified nurses and, rest assured, becomes easier to deal with, as practice helps you to recognize that there are standard approaches to many of these situations.

Definitions of leadership and management

We now look at the terms 'leadership' and 'management' in more detail to demystify them and to help you to recognize that there are structures and approaches that can be utilized to deal with potentially difficult events that occur on a daily basis. The terms need to be closely scrutinized because they are different concepts that can often be confused and misinterpreted as having the same meaning. Armstrong and Stephens (2005) suggest that management is about getting things done, and leadership is how things get done through people. There is clearly some overlapping of certain aspects of the two, so are they separate concepts? Can you be a leader without being a manager and can you be a manager without being a leader? Armstrong and Stephens (2005) provide further clarification, stating that:

> Management is concerned with achieving results by effectively obtaining, deploying, utilising and controlling all the resources required, namely people, money, facilities, plant and equipment, information and knowledge. Leadership focuses on the most important resource, people. It is the process of developing and communicating a vision for the future, motivating people and gaining their commitment and engagement.
>
> ARMSTRONG AND STEPHENS (2005: 5)

Emerging from the above statement, it can be seen that there are elements of responsibility related to **tasks** and **outcomes** and also elements related to **dealing with** and being a **role model** to the people in the service.

....

➡ Theory into action

In Scenario 7.2, how would you describe the role and responsibilities of the nurse taking the call? What are the leadership and management aspects, as outlined in the above definition of Armstrong and Stephens (2005)?

....

Although there is some overlap in both concepts, they clearly also have different properties and dynamics (see Figure 7.1).

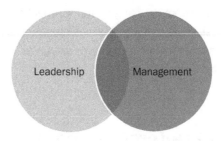

Figure 7.1 The overlap between leadership and management

Leadership

'Leadership' derives from an old English word *læden* (of Germanic origin), which means 'show the way' and 'be ahead of' (Chantrell, 2004: 297). 'To lead' can be defined in the following ways (*Collins English Dictionary*, 2010):

- to control or direct (a group of people); to be the person who makes decisions that other people choose to follow or obey;
- to show the way to (someone or something that follows), especially by going first;
- to guide;
- to cause to act, think, feel think, or behave in a certain way;
- to initiate the action of something;
- to influence;
- to be in front, be first, or be winning;
- to be the first, or foremost;
- as the position or the function of someone who is a leader.

This dictionary definition gives us a broad overview of leadership behaviours. The nurse in Scenario 7.2 has to make decisions, initiate actions, show the way, and influence and direct others. In taking the call, the nurse is also in the position of acting as leader with a function to fulfil, whether by choice or purely by circumstance. However, the definitions above may not capture the complexity involved, as leadership involves further elements related to a leader, such as being charismatic and inspirational, considerate, stimulating, and challenging (Thomas, 2006).

Leadership is concerned with leading and therefore, by implication, causing others to follow. It is important to recognize what role you are taking on in terms of leadership or 'followership' at any given time. Bartram and Casimir (2007) state that trust in the leader plays an important part in such a relationship. This trust can be fostered by:

- demonstrating competence;
- fair treatment of followers;
- showing genuine concern for the welfare of those being led.

Scenario 7.2 shows just how those words could apply to a newly qualified nurse. Even though there is a current requirement for newly qualified staff to have a period of preceptorship (NMC, 2006), unforeseen circumstances can still occur. This means that the practicalities of preceptorship are not always so easy and there may not always be others to whom to turn. The newly qualified nurse then needs to act in order to meet the needs of those in their care, the staff, and others working and visiting the environment.

In a study by Jackson (2005), 'doing something well' was a major factor in newly qualified nurses gaining job satisfaction. Another major factor was 'getting the work done', which included organizing and prioritizing. Indeed, in Scenario 7.2, the nurse taking the call would certainly need to organize something, even if this is purely ensuring that the information reaches more senior staff.

Jackson (2005) points out that co-workers are important as a source of reward in nursing. You need to gain respect through your actions, as other members of staff will be observing how you react and the decisions you make. If you can deal with such an issue fairly and confidently, you will be held in high esteem. Goleman et al. (2002) suggest that the leader in any group is the one to whom others look in order to provide assurance, clarity, or to do the job. The saying 'lead, follow, or get out of the way' could be seen as a useful piece of advice here. However, in situations such as that in Scenario 7.2, there is little scope for the nurse to be a follower or to get out of the way.

⮕ Theory into action

What skills do people in leading roles need? What actions do you think the nurse taking the call in Scenario 7.2 could take? What actions have you observed being taken by nurses in this kind of situation?

Peck (2006) suggests that a crucial element is the relationship between the 'leader' and the 'followers'. Akerjordet and Severinsson (2008) illustrate this point in discussing **emotional intelligence (EI)** as an important aspect of leadership. They suggest that EI is a set of skills that enable the leader to identify, process, and manage emotions by being knowledgeable, approachable, and supportive. A range of good leadership characteristics is given in Box 7.1.

Box 7.1 Some leadership characteristics

- Developing relationships
- Creating trust
- Fair treatment
- Maintaining team dynamics
- Providing assurance and clarity
- Doing the job
- Identifying and managing emotions
- Being knowledgeable
- Being approachable and supportive

These characteristics are translated into standards of proficiency by the NMC (2010), which include providing rationales of care, **interprofessional teamworking**, and delegation of duties where appropriate, as well as ensuring that nursing outcomes and interventions are clearly documented.

➡ Theory into action

Think of some of the people with whom you have worked in nursing in the past to the current day and reflect on the actions that they might have taken that correspond with those characteristics outlined above. If you came across anyone with these characteristics in a leadership role, what was the outcome of their actions? What are the opposite characteristics and potential outcomes?

You may have worked with qualified staff who appear to make the shift run smoothly and efficiently. You may find that those who do this more successfully are also those who develop and maintain good relationships with clients, staff, and interdisciplinary team members. They are people who are seen to make decisions rather than agonize over them (no matter how unpopular the decisions may be), but, most importantly, they demonstrate that they can show the way and are prepared to be involved in some of the tasks that they would expect other team members to complete. If these aspects are demonstrated, the person can create an aura of trustworthiness and reliability. The phrase 'leading from the front' can be taken literally!

Management

The origin of the word 'management' comes from the Latin *manus* for hand and was originally expanded to mean how to *handle* a situation, related particularly to managing a horse (Chantrell, 2004). This was then extended to controlling/handling other types of situation and person. According to Tyler (2004), the management process is related to the linking of the activities of people within an organization and the organization's goals. The central focus of management could be considered as being related to control and coordination. These are important factors to be considered while caring for patients or service users in health and social care settings. Even on a day-to-day, shift-to-shift basis, many aspects of coordination are needed to ensure the smooth running of any service to ensure best outcomes for all.

Clegg et al. (2005) suggest that management was historically a concern for rulers such as the monarchy, lords, and religious orders. Through the Industrial Revolution, military development, and beyond, these notions have evolved into systems of control within organizations as they developed. The latter therefore required aspects of control related to surveillance and drill in order to ensure that tasks and duties required by organizations were satisfactorily completed. The definitions below give an indication of how management is viewed in the modern world (*Collins English Dictionary*, 2010):

- the technique, practice, or science of managing or controlling;
- the skilful or resourceful use of materials, time, etc.;
- to be in charge of; to administer;
- to succeed in being able to do something;
- to exercise control or domination over;
- to wield or handle a weapon.

The last bullet point is interesting, as managers can be seen to have the power to *wield* rewards or punishments, emphasizing the notion of power and authority within a management position. These definitions thus suggest that the role of a manager is one that brings with it authority and power in relation to rewards and sanctions.

....

➔ Theory into action

In considering the types of health or social care services in which a newly qualified nurse might find themselves, who might hold such managerial positions? What are their responsibilities in relation to the service provided? How is their control exercised?

....

Leadership and management: the theory

It is now necessary to look at the theory underpinning the practice of leadership and management with a view to analysing how these can be applied in the role of the qualified nurse. There are many differing theories with confusing titles and definitions that overlap as regards the aspects they describe. Some of the key theories will be discussed below, bearing in mind that this is not an exhaustive list. The concept of leadership theories will be explored first.

Leadership theories

According to Pointer (2006: 128), leadership is:

A process through which an individual attempts to intentionally influence human systems in order to accomplish a goal.

From this definition, it is implied that leadership resides with a person rather than a position. Therefore, the theories that encompass leadership theory tend to allude to aspects related to individuals and their personalities, behaviours, and styles. Personality, or trait, theories will be considered first.

Trait theory

Handy (1999) suggests that trait theory implies that the individual is more important than the situation. Trait theory, or 'great man' theory, is based on the assumption that leaders have particular recognizable traits or characteristics. Most early studies focused on historical leaders to determine the characteristics considered necessary to be a leader (Marquis & Huston, 2009). They focused on people such as military, religious, or political leaders. Many traits such as age, gender, weight, height, and ethnicity were thought to make these 'leaders' stand out (Clegg et al., 2005). Other aspects highlighted have been being tall, male, white, well educated, and wealthy, but these can be deemed to be dependent on social norms and cultures that drive the social settings, which is a weakness in this theory.

Some other traits identified are honesty, integrity, being able to inspire followers, and charisma. Handy (1999) also suggests that further common traits in leaders include intelligence, initiative, self-assurance, and the **helicopter factor**, which is the ability to rise above situations and see what solutions are needed by being able to appreciate all of the factors involved. Davison and Peck (2005) argue that the focus on traits shifted as leadership began to be applied to wider areas such as education, sport, and community development.

Digman (1990), Keller (1999), Judge and Bono (2000), and Gregoire (2004) further discuss trait theory in terms of what is described as the 'five factor', or the 'big five', model of categorizing leadership traits (see Box 7.2).

Box 7.2 The 'big five' model of categorizing leadership traits

- **Surgency/extraversion**

  This is related to the energy with which a leader demonstrates their enthusiasm and positive emotions and beliefs towards a task. This could also be considered as a drive and willingness to be at the front.

- **Conscientiousness**

  This is related to being focused on the job in hand. Achievement and dependability are inherent traits.

- **Agreeableness**

  This is an ability to relate to others, providing trust, warmth, and kindness.

- **Adjustment**

  This is the ability to deal with issues in a rational manner without becoming anxious or emotionally distracted.

- **Intelligence**

  This is related to openness to experiences, creativity, and imagination, and being perceptive and thoughtful.

Thinking about

Think of someone with whom you have worked who you consider an effective leader.

1   Which of the traits in Box 7.2 did they have and how were they demonstrated?
2   Is there anyone who you have considered to be a poor leader?
3   What were their traits? How did they compare and contrast with those of the effective leader?
4   What traits do you feel you have that might highlight your leadership potential?

The big five *traits* might be better described as *behaviours* or *habits*. This is because individuals may not be able to do anything about their height, weight, gender, age, or attractiveness (traits sometimes associated with leaders), although they could further develop skills and abilities that may improve their leadership qualities. Abilities such as conscientiousness, reliability, agreeableness, being able to communicate well, developing problem-solving strategic skills, and intelligence can all be worked on and developed (Keller, 1999).

Handy (1999) points out that the notion of trait theory has been criticized because it is hard to define a discrete set of traits that apply to all leaders. The traits that were initially identified were becoming more numerous and differentiating as professions and industry grew, which effectively led to questions being raised as to its subsequent acceptance as a theory. This diversity began to show that leaders can come from a variety of backgrounds with a variety of different characteristics. According to Peck (2006), trait theory still persists to an extent when leaders are 'head hunted' to turn around 'failing' organizations.

Stephen Covey (1989), in his book *The 7 Habits of Highly Effective People*, suggests that there is a **character ethic** and a **personality ethic** that defines individuals in relation to interpersonal and leadership situations. The 'character ethic' includes integrity, humility, patience, industry, and justice, to name but a few. The 'personality ethic' differs in that it focuses on public images, attitudes, and skills that are related to processes of human interaction. Basically, this concept is related to promoting positive imagery and developing and maintaining public relations. It could be argued that the character ethic is based on **intrapersonal behaviours** and the personality ethic is based on **interpersonal behaviours**. Covey suggests that the character ethic is a primary driver in leadership and the personality ethic secondary. Therefore habits or behaviours that develop the character ethic help to develop both. Covey describes habits as internalized principles and patterns of behaviour. These include:

- **knowledge**—of what to do and why to do it;
- **skills**—how to do it;
- **desire**—wanting to do it.

By utilizing these habits, individuals can move through a continuum from *dependence* to *independence* to *interdependence* in achieving goals.

Thinking about

What 'habits' have you noticed in some of the people whom you considered to be leaders in care areas? What behaviours would you class under character ethic and which would you classify under personality ethic?

What habits do you feel you have that can be linked to these classifications?

Armstrong and Stephens (2005) suggest that leadership skills develop as a result of experiences that form the individual. We can see that this is a move away from traits and personality into behaviours and attitudes. They suggest that true leadership occurs when individuals can find meaning from negative situations and trying circumstances. Scenario 7.3 is a statement from a newly qualified nurse. She clearly shows how, when faced with responsibility, she had to quickly move towards a position of independence.

Scenario 7.3

When I qualified I went to work in a group home (registered nursing) for seven adults with learning disabilities and complex needs. Once there, I was often the shift leader and found that most of the challenging issues that I faced were related to managing the shift team. As the only qualified nurse on shift, delegation of duties was to unqualified staff, many of whom had worked within the home and/or company for several years. I had to overcome a significant age difference in conjunction with my newly qualified status – 'proving my worth' was my most difficult task.

NEWLY QUALIFIED RNLD

In 'proving her worth', the nurse in Scenario 7.3 demonstrated her ability to deal with others and get them on her side, demonstrating a move towards interdependence. This is a situation in which most newly qualified nurses will find themselves. Those seen to lead from the front, making confident, efficient decisions that are effectively communicated, will gain the trust of fellow staff members. This requirement is highlighted by the NMC (2010) when it requires nurses to demonstrate effective interprofessional working while respecting the contributions from all team members.

 Theory into action

Reflect on Scenario 7.3 and highlight the issues relating to dependence, independence, and interdependence. What type of knowledge would help the nurse? What types of skill might she need? What might create the desire for her to succeed?

So far, leadership has been discussed as a range of attributes inherent in the person, as aspects related to character or personality, habits, and behaviours. It is now necessary to consider aspects related to leadership styles.

Leadership style theory

According to Sellgren et al. (2006), leadership styles are related to behaviours that build on leadership dimensions of task and interpersonal relationships. Style theory is different to trait theory, as it proposes that there can be differences in the ways in which leadership is approached. Clegg et al. (2005) suggest that the behaviours of a leader can be observable. They suggest that you either act like a leader or you don't. Different actions of leadership relate to different styles of leadership.

Marquis and Huston (2009) state that a major contribution to leadership style theory was made by Kurt Lewin, who identified three major styles of leadership: **authoritarian**; **democratic**; and **laissez-faire**.

- **The authoritarian style** is characterized by a downward flow of information, control, coercion, commands, decision-making, and giving of rewards or sanctions.
- **The democratic style** is characterized by two-way communication, encouraging the sharing of ideas and decision-making, and the use of constructive criticism.
- **The laissez-faire style** allows individuals to be empowered to complete the tasks. The work is delegated and the member is trusted to carry it out successfully. Communication flows up, down, and across the members of the team; little direction is given and criticism is withheld.

Barr and Dowding (2008) suggest that these styles reflect the power in the relationship between leader and followers. In a workplace, there are a range of differing situations. Some of these situations need more direction from the leader than others. In a health setting in which there might be an acute situation such as dealing with people with traumatic physiological needs or where patients might be displaying aggressive/violent behaviours, there is a need for powerful direction from the leader. Therefore the authoritarian style of leadership would be recommended.

Decisions need to be made quickly and each team member needs to know or be told exactly what their roles and responsibilities are. In this situation, it could be argued that the team is dependent on the leader and looks for direction from them. Barr and Dowding (2008) point out that effective communication from the leader is important in such scenarios. There is no room for ambiguity when instructions and directions are being given. There is not enough time for questioning or discussing options, so clear decision-making is necessary. The communication should be clear and effective. Good communication is also the basis for the other styles.

A democratic approach might be useful within nursing when working practices are being reviewed or developments considered. Marquis and Huston (2009) suggest that this style is effective in longer-term situations. It is useful as a method for empowering members of the team and valuing their contribution; however, it can be less effective than the authoritarian style due to the time it takes to coordinate ideas and opinions. The danger is that some decisions may be a compromise to suit all. This could be related to Covey's independent concept. Here, the team members are allowed to express their own views to the leader for consideration.

The laissez-faire style of leadership requires the person leading to hand over power in the situation to those considered as subordinates or followers. The team is left to manage the situation itself. Tasks are delegated with the confidence that those carrying them out have the abilities to complete them effectively. These aspects of different styles for different situations will be discussed in the section on contingency and situational leadership theory. Basically, it could be argued that this style may be demonstrated when staff nurses are delegated to lead teams in a clinical environment in the absence of more senior staff. This requires trust in the abilities of the person left in charge, and relates very much to Covey's interdependence concept. It is important to remember that ultimate accountability should lie with the person who makes the decision to delegate to a junior worker, although the latter will still have their own professional accountability to consider (NMC, 2008).

The style theory represents two different interpretations of leadership that you may need to consider: **fixed** and **flexible**. The 'fixed' interpretation would align to the trait or behavioural characteristics of the person, suggesting that they always operate in that style. This may or may not be successful. It may also affect their popularity in the team, as it could lead to admiration, antipathy, or even fear of the person. They may be effective, but at the cost of their relationship with the team. Alternatively, they could be popular because of their style, but be ineffective as a leader.

The alternative 'flexible' interpretation suggests that, as a leader, you should be able to adjust to the circumstances faced and utilize whichever style is recognized as being most effective in that particular kind of situation. This fits a behavioural model and focuses on adaptability of the person.

....

💡 Thinking about

Think of some of the people with whom you have experienced working who have been designated or described as leaders.

Identify characteristics of those who you believe had leadership styles that were authoritarian, democratic, or *laissez faire*.

Identify times and situations that you recognize as requiring the different style(s) to be adopted.

Which style do you associate most with yourself?

What situations have you been in during your course that demonstrates the necessity of using different styles?

....

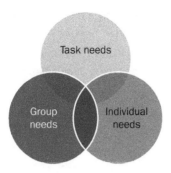

Figure 7.2 Adair's effective leadership considerations

In developing an understanding of style theory, it is important to recognize that the style depends on the interrelationship between a number of factors including:

- the person considered to be the leader;
- the individuals considered as followers or subordinate/teamworkers;
- the purpose or task/outcomes needed.

This is similar to Adair's (1988) model of the interrelationship between the **task**, the needs of the **individual**, and the needs of the **group**. The leader needs to assess these needs and maintain the balance or development of each (Figure 7.2.)

There are some important historical authors with ideas related to style theory. Blake and Moulton (1964) suggested the importance of **concern for production** and the **concern for people**. McGregor (1960) suggests that there are two types of subordinate worker who need different approaches from the leader. This is his famous **theory X** and **theory Y**. Basically, theory X represents workers who are unmotivated mainly due to tasks that are unfulfilling, therefore requiring the leader to be directive and instructional, with a need to provide extrinsic rewards in order to encourage participation. Theory Y represents a workplace in which the workers enjoy going to work and the rewards are intrinsic.

The process of leadership, therefore, becomes quite complex when considering styles. You need to understand the work environment, the outcomes required, and the tasks used as a vehicle for this. Individuals need to be understood, as well as the dynamics of an effective working group or team. The context is important as you need to be able to adapt styles that fit the situation, ranging from being authoritative to democratic, or laissez-faire.

Contingency/situational theory

Blanchard and Spencer (2000) are considered to be major theorists in relation to the contingency theory, more popularly known as situational theory. They identify and develop the styles of leader mentioned above, such as authoritarian, democratic, and laissez-faire, and provide their own descriptions. Blanchard (2007) suggests that those who stick to one style exclusively are only a fraction of the leader they could be, particularly if they take up an extreme position or style. He suggests there are four styles of leader and that these should be utilized to recognize the requirements of the task in hand and the individuals that are being led. The styles are:

- directing;
- **coaching;**
- supporting;
- delegating.

Therefore, there is a formula for finding the right approach between meeting the supportive needs of the workers and the completing the task. The qualities of the followers need to be taken into account along with the level of skill they have plus their level of motivation. Therefore a balance is needed between the support and direction provided by the leader.

- Someone with a high level of motivation and a low level of skill will need directing.
- Someone with a low level of motivation and a low level of skill will need coaching.
- Someone with low level of motivation and a high level of skill will need supporting.
- Someone with a high level of motivation and a high level of skill will need delegating to.

This can be seen in Table 7.1.

....

➡ Theory into action

What would you need to do to find out about the level of motivation and skill in your fellow colleagues? Discuss with your mentor or preceptor what the best approaches to finding out such things are and how they take differing approaches in different situations.

....

The key point is that your leadership style should be flexibly adapted to meet the needs of the individual and the situation faced. These styles can also be applied in the completion of a task/skill or new project. In the early stages, there will need to be clear direction from the leader. This is followed by a period of coaching during which the skills of others are developed. The stage of supporting is then applied in terms of ensuring resources and skills are maintained. Finally, when the leader is confident that everything is in place, the followers can be entrusted to make independent decisions based on their level of skill and therefore have tasks or duties delegated to them. Delegation is highlighted by the NMC (2010) as a required standard of proficiency, so it is important to be aware of the right kind of situations in which to do so.

Table 7.1 Situational leadership

	Low direction	High direction
High support	*Follower behaviour*	*Follower behaviour*
	Low level of motivation	Low level of motivation
	High level of skill	Low level of skill
	Leader style	*Leader style*
	Supporting	**Coaching**
Low support	*Follower behaviour*	*Follower behaviour*
	High level of motivation	High level of motivation
	High level of skill	Low level of skill
	Leader style	*Leader style*
	Delegating	**Directing**

Thinking about

Think of a responsibility that you have had to undertake as part of a team at some point.
Identify the stages of the task at which the behaviours of directing, coaching, supporting, and delegating were applied.
What were the behaviours of the leader at these stages?
What worked well at each stage?

You may have been involved in developing a new method of reporting in the workplace or implementing a specific kind of care plan for a client, which needed to be communicated to the care staff to ensure its success, or you may have been involved in introducing and learning how to use a new piece of equipment. Goldblatt et al. (2008) suggested that nurses finding themselves as shift leaders often find tension between managing the present shift and focusing on ideas or aspects that extend beyond the boundaries of the specific day. The shift leader has many responsibilities and has a large degree of control. This means that they have to consider many factors.

A shift leader often finds themselves making decisions about delegation of duties as it is impossible to carry out all duties associated with successfully managing a shift alone. It can be seen with this example, therefore, that the notion of *situational* leadership is particularly important—especially depending on the skill levels of the supporting staff on a given shift. Some days, there might need to be more direction; others, more delegating.

Goldblatt's study also discusses the concept of the leader needing to be like an octopus, with one head and many arms. When delegation is used, you may have to relinquish some control to more junior staff, yet your eyes may then need to be turned to further developments, such as the support or coaching of other staff and the development/completion of further tasks.

....

⊖ Theory into action

Discuss with a qualified nurse the strategies that they have found most useful in dealing with balancing the management of patient care and the management of staff while in charge.
   How did they develop these strategies?

....

In answering the above question, it may be useful to think of it in terms of time and responsibility. Some aspects will be urgent, which need dealing with, and others, although important, may not be quite as pressing, but will still need to be dealt with in the long run. Goldblatt et al. (2008) proposed a model with aspects related to considerations of time and responsibility when considering the running of shifts (Table 7.2.)

....

⊖ Theory into action

Think of the differing kinds of situation in which you have observed qualified nurses over the course of a typical shift. What styles of leadership have you noticed them using in these situations? How effective were they for the situation at hand?

....

Transactional and transformational leadership theory

The concepts of transactional and transformational leadership could be considered an amalgam of all of the other theories. Judge and Bono (2000) highlight that these ideas were originally developed by Burns in around 1978, and Bass (1985). They suggest that transactional leadership is almost an authoritarian style whereby the leader establishes the outcomes required in the task and communicates this to the followers,

Table 7.2 Goldblatt's (2008) model of time versus responsibility

		Responsibility	
		Maximum control	**Releasing control**
Time perspective	**Present shift**	Presence	Instrumental support
		Supervision	Emotional support
			'Keeping the peace'
	Broader managerial focus	Information-gathering	Empowering
		Problem-solving	Enabling
		Learning	Team learning

or subordinates, and then monitors the performance during the delivery of these. This is very similar to McGregor's theory X.

According to Marquis and Huston (2009), the concept revolves around control in relation to 'day-to-day' operations and is closely associated with the role of the manager. Stordeur et al. (2001), however, suggested that this can create stress if the workplace is too control-oriented. Transformational leadership could be deemed to associate more with Goleman et al.'s (2002) notions of emotional intelligence and leadership, whereby a leader handles their own and the followers' emotions in a positive way. It is about empowerment, inspiring the workforce, and acting as a positive role model—perhaps almost like the coach in situational leadership.

Stanley (2008) argues that transformational leadership demonstrates the interdependence of leaders and followers. Sorensen et al. (2008) suggest that these transformational aspects are crucial in nursing leadership. Having a clinical focus is important, but nurses need to be able to develop strong interpersonal and social skills in order to meet the needs of the patients, families, public, and staff. They need to be able to enter into negotiations and make difficult decisions. Stordeur et al. (2001) found favourable responses from staff when faced with transformational leadership role models.

Hendry (2004) points out that there are four basic components suggested by Bass's original work.

- **Idealized influence**

  This aspect is related to the 'charisma' of the leader and the influencing factors that this brings in terms of admiration and respect from followers.
- **Inspirational motivation**

  This relates to how the leader models desired behaviours, therefore creating meaning and challenges for the followers.
- **Intellectual stimulation**

  This relates to how the leader engages the followers to be creative, and problem-solves in relation to the challenges presented in the workforce.
- **Individualized consideration**

  This relates to the ability of the leader to identify and show concern for the development of individual members of the team.

Laurent (2000) provides a good example in Scenario 7.4 of how these might apply in practice.

Scenario 7.4

A nurse has just completed a consecutive run of five night shifts. On coming on duty, the shift leader finds that the nurse has made a medication error, which fortunately has not resulted in any harm to a patient.

In a transactional leadership approach, the perception might be that this is a crisis situation and that the nurse needs some remedial intervention or sanction. Alternatively, a transformational leader would listen to the nurse and ascertain any developmental needs and education or skill development that they may need, and take steps to ensure that the nurse is supported with these.

Bartram and Casimir (2007) argue that trust is an essential part of transformational leadership. It requires that each party can depend on each other so that reciprocation will occur when necessary. This can be developed by the leader being competent and skilled so that their presence as a role model is accepted and utilized as a basic level or standard. Fair treatment and consideration of the followers' best interests are also important.

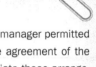

Scenario 7.5

A recurring issue in my workplace is debate about the duty rota. The manager permitted flexibility, so staff would often swap shifts (sometimes without the agreement of the person being swapped). As a shift leader I sometimes had to negotiate these arrangements between staff members.

STAFF NURSE

As mentioned above, a transactional leader might make a unilateral decision and state that person A or person B must do the shift. This might be a necessary tactic if all else fails. However, transformational leadership requires that the leader is empowering, fair, and considers individual needs. Therefore, it is necessary to gather the facts. In doing so, a mediator role can be adopted by the nurse in charge. The best result would be that the leader then presents the facts as they stand and checks that all parties understand and agree that this is a fair appraisal of the situation. The leader can then either leave the decision between the parties or enter negotiation in order to secure agreement, disagreement, or agreement on difference (De Bono, 2004).

However, the leader also needs to explain the constraints and provide boundaries on what must be achieved and by when. In doing this, the followers may find a solution themselves, thus transforming the working environment. The leader can still make the final decision (transactional leadership) if there is no satisfactory result, yet by taking a transformational approach, this should lead to decisions that eventually are advantageous for all.

Baillie (1999) suggested that newly qualified staff nurses found it difficult to adjust to this role. They needed to maintain trust with the workforce while ensuring that all work was completed satisfactorily. This might therefore mean that, sometimes, the nurse would complete a number of tasks themselves in order to make sure that this happens.

Therefore gaining trust while leading the workforce can be a delicate balance and quite a challenge. This is applicable to newly qualified nurses from all fields of practice. However, as Anderson and Kiger found in 2008, opportunity to develop such skills was beneficial for final-year student nurses. By being given the relevant opportunity, they found themselves developing confidence, professionalism, and the ability to manage care.

Theory into action

Seek out with your mentor or preceptor some opportunities (under supervision) to manage individual shifts and to deal with issues such as delegation of tasks and dealing with rota changes. Reflect on these experiences, noting what types of challenge they present and the methods that are useful in dealing with them.

Management is a different concept from leadership as it relates to the role or position that is ascribed to a person. Shortell and Kaluzny (2006) suggest that leadership is one role of a manager and suggests that a leader can be a manager performing the leadership requirements. Therefore not all leaders are managers, but all managers perhaps need to be leaders. They do suggest that people are placed in managerial positions that have associated expectations or managerial roles.

Therefore these aspects can be considered in light of a care environment in which nurses might be part of the workforce. What roles do staff have that require a leadership element? Think of roles of staff from lower bandings to those with higher bandings. In the NHS, a newly qualified nurse is likely to be at band 5, so may have some supervisory, planning, and organizing responsibility for those from lower bands and students.

Theory into action

Seek out the band descriptions from *Agenda for Change* (Department of Health 2004), and look at the expectations and responsibilities from band 5 and those below it. (Alternatively, seek out the job descriptions in the care area in which you are currently working.) Make a note of the requirements that relate to having responsibility for the supervision and management of those on lower scales.

What kinds of decisions are made at each level? For example, a support worker may have to make very small decisions in providing care to individuals while following prescribed plans of care. These may also need to be communicated to a shift leader. A shift leader may have to decide which staff to delegate certain duties to, and to decide which tasks gain priority. They also need to be able to report to senior staff about day-to-day issues affecting the running of the care environment, thereby contributing to larger-scale change processes.

The senior staff may not have much direct care responsibilities (although in some smaller units this may have to be inevitable), but they need to maintain the integrity of the service and have wider responsibilities, including the service users or patients, staff environment, and others involved. They will have to report these aspects at an organizational level. Therefore it can be seen that, at all levels, the leader has to make specific decisions while providing broader information in an upwards direction from which more senior staff can make decisions about the level below.

Egan (1993), in looking at the nature of organizations, suggests that they need to consider three main aspects: **organizational processes**; **change**; and what he describes as the **shadow side of the organization**—for example, culture, politics, and social systems. The first aspect of organizational processes requires management principles in which he places leadership in the sixth position of flowing through:

- strategy;
- operations;
- structure;
- human resources;
- management;
- leadership.

Armstrong and Stephens (2005: 13) suggest that a leader should **define the task**, **achieve the task**, and **maintain effective relationships**.

We would suggest therefore, in accommodating the theories already discussed, that the key elements in leadership in creating small-level or grand-level change are:

- know where you want to go (goal/outcome);
- decide when and how you are going to get there (strategy formulation);
- communicate this vision to others (communication);
- fill others with enthusiasm for this vision (motivation);
- cause the first steps to happen/take the first steps (action).

In order to demonstrate that leadership qualities lie with the person, their behaviours, and abilities in getting things done, one needs to quite simply look at ordinary life experiences: leadership qualities can be seen in all arenas of life, such as the familial, social, or work.

....

➡ Theory into action

Think of a non-work-based instance in which people willingly followed you. This does not need to be a huge or important event: in fact, it is better if it is something small—for example setting up a get-together with friends, going on an outing, or going on holiday.

Now answer the following questions.

- What did you want to achieve? (**Goal/outcome**)
- What factors influenced your decision about how and when you would do this? (**Strategy formulation**)
- How did you let the other people involved know about it? (**Communication**)
- How did you convince the others to join you in this? (**Motivation**)
- What were the first steps that you took? (**Action**)

....

Here is an example—using organizing a family get-together as a basis.

- What did you want to achieve? (**Goal/outcome**)
  - To host a family party
- What factors influenced your decision about how and when you would do this? (**Strategy formulation**)
  - My house was not big enough to accommodate all of the people I wanted to be there.
  - It had to be on or near the date of the birthday.
- How did you let the other people involved know about it? (**Communication**)
  - Telephone conversations and text messages
- How did you convince the others to join you in this? (**Motivation**)
  - Floated the idea past everyone first – provided them with the reasons.
  - Told them that I would organize it and that all they would need to do would be to turn up.
- What were the first steps that you took? (**Action**)
  - The first move made was to book the table at the restaurant.

Take some time now to compare your answers with the example and, in particular, to think about the elements required in your leadership approach. In the example, the following aspects mentioned earlier were important.

- **Goal/outcome**
  The time was right and there was an internal drive and will to do it. A goal was clearly identified early in the process.
- **Strategy**
  The practical elements needed to make the idea happen were carefully considered, weighed up, and a decision made as to what was considered to be the best way of achieving the vision.
- **Communication**
  The fastest possible method of communication was used, the first choice being telephone, rather than text messaging, letters or emails based on a need to gauge how people were feeling about the idea and to hear how they sounded taking their tone of voice into consideration. The personal touch adds more weight.

- **Motivation**

  The first step in motivating others was to communicate my reasons, but retaining awareness that my reasons might not be attractive to others. It was important then to listen very carefully both verbally and non-verbally to the responses and to realize that although others may share the desire for it to happen, they did not have enough enthusiasm to undertake the entire organization required. Identifying that I would contribute to the solution was a motivating factor, as the others knew that I was willing to participate in completing the task and the obstacle was removed.

- **Action**

  Although only one very small step was taken—it only consisted of one short telephone call—it represented for the others involved that the event was really going to happen.

To see how these aspects can be applied to a broader situation, let us return to Scenario 7.2, in which you take a call informing you that the senior nurse will not be turning up for the late shift and consider what you need to do.

- **Goal/outcome**

  The goal is clear: the care area needs to be run in such a way that minimum standards are met, all individuals in the environment are safe, and optimum achievement occurs within the constraints given. You now have the perfect opportunity to demonstrate your leadership skills and to demonstrate your ability to solve the problem in the fairest way possible. You will no doubt have a strong internal desire to ensure that your first experience of leadership is successful.

- **Strategy**

  You now need to assess the practicalities of what needs to happen and decide on what would constitute a successful shift. One of the very early decisions needing to be made is whether, and how, a replacement should be sought for the one missing member of the team. It may be that, in considering the tasks, the workload could be shared among the remaining staff. You may volunteer to provide cover for a short while until you (or someone senior) can organize someone else. You may have some identified people who can be contacted in such circumstances; there might be staff in nearby services who perhaps could be spared or moved, or you may need to contact outside agencies. In contacting senior staff, it is always best to have either completed these actions first, or if you need permission for further action (such as being allowed to provide overtime), to let them know of your intended actions and that you seek their approval.

- **Communication**

  All of the members of your team need to be made aware of the situation in the swiftest way possible and made aware of what you propose to do as a result.

You will be able to gauge their concerns from their verbal and non-verbal responses. Remember the staff nurse who felt that she had to prove her worth to junior staff: there is an expectation from junior staff for swift action. There is also a need to communicate with senior staff. However, this may need to be carefully judged. If there are actions that you can take to remedy the situation and report your actions to them rather than pass the problem directly to them without any thought or action, this will be much better received.

- **Motivation**

  Having listened to the concerns, you are now in a position to propose what you would like to do, giving your reasons and linking these to the concerns and reasons of the other staff. Any perceived obstacles to achieving the vision need to be identified and, if possible, removed at this point. You need to consider how you can maintain the morale of the staff in what could obviously be considered a negative situation in which some or all staff may have to do extra work.

- **Action**

  It is important that you do something that may be small, but which represents for others that you have been decisive and that you are working to resolve the situation. This could simply be to begin the telephoning process to attempt to replace the missing staff member. In the end, it does not matter if you succeed in this initial action; what is important is that you do something that all those involved regard as being important. Finally, you need to record your actions and decisions.

Important questions to assist decision-making

A simple way to find answers at each of the stages above is to ask yourself questions in order to seek out more detail, or find wider, more generalized, areas in which alternatives can be found. It is the process of analysing the situation into chunks of more easily understandable information, sometimes referred to as 'chunking up' or 'down chunking' (O'Connor & Seymour, 1990).

To chunk down in order to get the detail, you ask a question similar to 'What is an example of X?' (X is the situation or concept at which you are looking). This will provide more specific information related to it. In order to chunk up to find general or broader information, you ask the question: 'Of what is X an example?' In answering this type of question, you can gain the 'helicopter view' or wider perspective of the situation or concept. In other words, the answer provides us with generalizations in relation to the situation. Whether chunking up or chunking down, at each level, you can also ask: 'What is an alternative example?' This will give you more information or suggestions about what to base your decisions on.

So, from Scenario 7.2, 'What do I need to do to secure more staff?' is a chunking down process. The answer might provide a basis for actions to consider. In posing this type of question, the leader can ascertain the *specific aspects* required to gain a successful outcome. In other words, this helps you to identify choices for action in the situation. At each stage, more detail is provided.

Alternatively, the chunking-up process would warrant the question: 'What would securing more staff do?' The answer to this would perhaps highlight the *value of actions* to be taken. Securing more staff would ensure that the area is covered and that the care needs of all clients can be met.

⊖ Theory into action

Discuss with your mentor/preceptor similar types of decision that you have observed been taken by them while in charge. How did they set the goals? How did they work through the decisions?

This technique of chunking up or down can be used in each of the stages mentioned earlier (goal/outcome through to action) until you reach a point at which you know what is needed. By asking the alternative question, you may be able to offer solutions with which the other people involved will agree. Agreement can also be brokered using this technique by finding out the level at which your proposal or action is attractive to the followers, either by generalizing or specifying what is required.

You will be more successful in motivating the others if you make them aware that it is well-cared-for patients etc. that you are all working towards. The other staff members are likely to care very little about whether or not you succeed, but they certainly will want to feel that they have succeeded in their own right. Knowing that you and they are working towards the same end goal is a real motivating factor! In using these techniques, we can often find answers or alternatives to the challenges faced in day-to-day or longer-term situations. Remember—if you do not know what to do, you can always ask the question: 'Who could help me find out what to do?' It is important to note, however, that whatever actions you take must align with your employer's policies and procedures.

You should be prepared to be the one doing the extra work at times, as this shows that you are a willing role model and prepared to 'walk the talk' and take your share of the responsibility. However, you should not always be the one volunteering to work extra! Doing so at times will add to the sense of fairness needed when you request others to do the task.

Clinical leadership

This aspect of leadership has been left until last as it is really an approach that is about specialization and may not necessarily be something in which a newly qualified nurse will be involved, but it can be an aspiration for some. However, the NMC does require nurses to be proficient in creating and utilizing opportunities for promoting health and well-being. The leadership aspect revolves around the client/service user and not necessarily a team of staff in one care area.

Moving into clinical leadership roles is a developing area of opportunity for qualified nurses. Woodring (2004) describes this role as a leader in healthcare delivery systems across all care areas and not just in one area. The role requires accountability in meeting care outcomes by utilizing evidence-based care in designing packages of care with health professional teams in healthcare services. According to Stanley (2008), clinical leaders need to be approachable and open, good communicators, and role models who can demonstrate to others positive values and beliefs. They need to be visible, knowledgeable, and clinically competent. As they are not directly managing individual staff, they need to be able to make decisions and ensure that these are carried out across a number of teams.

It appears therefore that there are different ways in which to achieve leadership roles that do not necessarily require management positions and day-to-day authority for staff and teams. Harris (2004) suggests that these are ideal roles for those nurses who become proficient in a high level of practice and expertise. However, they have a crucial role across many teams, so they have to use leadership skills in order to be successful—particularly those related to situational leadership.

Both clinical leadership roles and management/leadership roles are available to all qualified nurses in their careers. However, there are different ways in which nurses exploit these opportunities. According to Bondas (2006), there are four main paths: the path of ideals; the path of chance; the career path; and the temporary path.

- **The path of ideals** involves the nurse making a conscious choice to become a leader, mainly because of their beliefs and values and wanting to create change.
- **The path of chance** is a passive route by which they became leaders, usually due to situations requiring them to step up to the role or others recommending it to them.
- **The career path** is one in which the nurse sets out a plan of how they want their career to develop based on ambition and perhaps influenced by salary and status.
- **The temporary path** is the path in which nurses usually take on the role in an 'acting up' capacity. This is almost a trial run at the role, in which the nurse can then decide whether or not to purse leadership roles.

....

➲ Theory into action

Seek out the opportunity to speak to a manager, a team leader, and if possible a clinical leader. Find out whether they consciously chose their career pathway or whether it happened by chance and circumstance. What are your aspirations in relation to leadership roles?

....

However future healthcare systems and the nursing profession are organized, there will always be a requirement for nurses to demonstrate leadership skills at all levels within it in order to create small-scale and large-scale changes that impact on the care of individuals. As mentioned earlier, although leadership and management can be considered different concepts, they are inextricably linked and the theories do overlap. It is now important to focus on some theories of management.

Theories of management

Armstrong and Stephens (2005) suggest that management is concerned with defining and achieving ends.

> Management is deciding what to do and then getting it done through the effective use of resources.
>
> ARMSTRONG AND STEPHENS (2005: 3)

This brings an added dimension for the qualified nurse than the previous discussions related to leadership. This added dimension is the fact that responsibility for the effective functioning of the healthcare setting (and, at higher levels, the organization) lies with the manager.

Handy (1999) argues that the role of a manager is similar to that of a general practitioner presented with a patient. The manager must identify symptoms, diagnose the cause, decide a strategy to deal with it, and commence the treatment. Pedler et al. (2007) also offer a similar process of diagnosis, goal-setting, action, and evaluation. Tyler (2004) suggests that there are three main aspects of a manager's role, as follows.

- **Interpersonal**
  The manager is a figurehead and organizational representative, leading staff and liaising with external parties.
- **Informational**
  Where there are responsibilities for monitoring information internally and externally and disseminating it as appropriate.
- **Decision making**
  The manager makes decisions on actions to create change, manage conflict, and allocates and negotiates resources.

Although it may be some years after qualifying before a nurse might take up a managerial position as described above, some of these factors may echo in their role of managing a shift in the healthcare setting. Endacott (1999) found that such a role included making important decisions about the running of the area and particular decisions about individuals' care. This involved:

- **presence;**
- **information-gathering;**

- **supportive involvement;**
- **direct involvement**.

Egan (1993) suggests that management has three desired outcomes, as follows.

- **Satisfied customers**
  In the case of the newly qualified nurse, this relates to experiences of patients/service users, and their relatives/friends/representatives. This is an area in which the qualified nurse is on the front line and the one in immediate contact, whereby the aims of the organization are ultimately achieved within the interactions with patients and families.
- **Committed and productive employees**
  The qualified nurse needs to maintain the effective functioning of the team when in charge of a care area. Although they may not ultimately be responsible for selecting the team members, they have a responsibility to deal with matters affecting the team's performance on a daily basis, and to report any strengths or deficiencies to senior staff.
- **Financial returns**
  It is not usually within the remit of the staff nurse to create profit for the healthcare organization (although this may be the case when working for some private healthcare providers). However, it is necessary that the qualified nurse ensures that the resources at their disposal are being used effectively, without waste, to ensure financial effectiveness that is balanced with meeting the needs of those in their care and the healthcare team.

Thinking about

The above principles can broadly be translated as managing *clients and relatives, staff,* and *resources*. Think of an average shift in an acute setting, a community residential or care home, or as part of a community team, and then make a list of the types of duty or responsibility with which you would generally need to deal if in charge, under the headings of clients, staff, and resources.

Even though it may be many years before you consider management positions or aspects, it is always beneficial to understand the principles involved and to be aware of the contributions that you can make. Using Egan's (1993) concepts of six master tasks from his book *Adding Value* as a basis, comprising a process through 'strategy', 'operations', 'structure', 'human resources', 'management and supervision', and through to 'leadership', some of the wider management theories will be discussed below.

Strategic management

Crossan (2003) suggested that strategic management is concerned with successful performance and is more than just decision-making planning in that it is also about developing the culture within the organization. Qualified staff may have to rise up the career ladder before being able to make fundamental decisions about the nature of the organization for which they work, but they can have a direct influence on the culture of the organization by the ways in which they perform their duties and act as role models. Crossan (2003) suggests that nurses do need to be more involved in making these factors apparent and therefore being involved in decision-making and suggesting ways in which services can move forward. However, nurses need support and skills development in order to be able to do this.

Gallo (2007) suggested a development ladder of four stages that a nurse may go through once qualified (Figure 7.3). As a newly qualified nurse, the main area of your influence is likely to be at stage 1 or 2 of the steps. However, with adequate training, expertise, and experience, the other steps can be achieved.

Armstrong and Stephens (2005) point out that strategic thinking is about the purpose, or at least the sense of purpose, of the organization. It is about defining modification and new directions as situations change. Therefore your contribution is important in at least informing the strategy: by highlighting what those necessary changes need to be on the front line and how current initiatives are currently operating. You may be nervous as a newly qualified nurse, but your opinions, if expressed appropriately, may

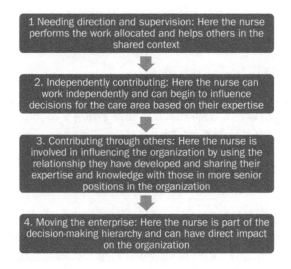

Figure 7.3 Four stages through which a nurse may go once qualified (reprinted from Gallo, 'The new nurse manager: A leadership development program paves the road to success', *Nurse Leader*, **5**:3 (28–32), 2007, with permission from Elsevier)

still have some weight. Some areas appreciate the benefits that a fresh pair of eyes can bring. Indeed, having just completed three years of education in a variety of settings, you may have the advantage of experiencing some useful approaches and initiatives that may not have been thought of by the staff in your current work or clinical placement. By sharing these, you can have an impact and contribute to the strategic development of the organization.

Bruce and Langdon (2000) suggest that a good strategist is a team player, stays calm, is a skilled communicator, can balance short-term and long-term needs, and sees problems as opportunities. They suggest that a process consisting of the stages **analyse–plan–implement** should be utilized. Here, any newly qualified nurse should be able to spot that the nursing process they use in caring for their patients (assess, plan, implement, evaluate) is very similar to this suggestion, if not an expanded version of it, which could be applied to strategic thinking in the work environment. In Egan's (2002) other major work, *The Skilled Helper*, he suggested that there is a need to identify the 'present state', the 'desired state', and the 'resources required' to get to the position of setting and meeting outcomes. This is another example of strategic thinking if applied to the work environment as a whole.

⊙ Theory into action

Think of a problematic work situation that you have encountered and use the process of analyse–plan–implement to suggest a new strategy towards it, while maintaining the same resources.

Operations management

According to Egan (1993), this aspect is related to the day-to-day running of services, with the main focus being on ensuring that satisfaction of the customer is achieved by delivery of a quality product. In the case of a qualified nurse, this means ensuring that clients' needs are met to as high a standard as possible. It is about turning the strategy into action at the point of delivery. However, the important aspects of operations management are keeping the client as the central focus and utilizing the best evidence to create efficient and valued care. Barr and Dowding (2008) point out that quality is basically being **effective** and **efficient**. So, for a qualified nurse delivering care, this means that there is a need to ensure that the care is provided to the highest possible standard, using resources in an efficient, cost-effective manner.

The qualified nurse is often the interface between the service and the clients. As well as their technical competence, a nurse needs to understand the importance of communication with patients, junior staff, other professionals, and senior staff within the organization. Iles (2005) suggests that this requires you to be able to secure agreement about what is to be achieved, ensure that you have the skills and resources to achieve it, and provide feedback at all stages of the interactions. This needs to operate in both upward and downward communication exchanges. In most cases, it is obvious that patients/service users need to have their needs met.

You need to communicate effectively to let service users know the steps that will be taken in moving towards this goal (as nothing can ever be fully guaranteed). This means highlighting what is realistic in the situation. In discussions with your senior managers, you need to inform them of the situation as it is at ground level, in order to request the appropriate resources and support needed to ensure optimum care delivery.

Structural management

Egan (1993) suggests that structural management relates to how work is divided throughout the organization, including information flow and decision-making processes. Anderson-Wallace (2005) argues that structural management tends to look at how hierarchies of authority and power are set up and highlights the roles and responsibilities associated with these. It is about how rules, processes, and procedures are decided on in the organization and how these are communicated throughout the workforce. It is about the division of labour and how this is managed.

As a newly qualified nurse, you might not be involved in the large-scale decision-making and organizing of the structural aspects of the service in which you work, but you will be involved in aspects on a micro level, such as being in charge of a team in the day-to-day running of the care area. In this role, you may have to decide on how workload and tasks are distributed among the staff team. These decisions may have to be taken on the actual day once all staff are assembled and the duties required are recognized, or it may be that there needs to be more mid- and longer-term planning in which you may become involved, such as the allocation of responsibilities.

An effective healthcare provider will need efficient communication systems at all levels. Heller (1998) argues that informal direct communication between workers is the most effective. Other communication technologies should be available when this direct contact is not possible. You need to communicate with the team under your supervision if in charge of a shift. This means that there is a need for a visible style of management in order to foster open communication, without being oppressive and reducing the **autonomy** of trusted workers where relevant.

Endacott (1999) suggested that the nurse did not always control the bedside work of other nurses, but did take up a role in which they intervened when their expertise or advice was needed. Their roles fell into the earlier mentioned categories of presence and being there, gathering information, supportive, and direct involvement in patient care.

Theory into action

Imagine that you are responsible for a group of six clients in a community nursing home. These are divided into separate areas in two groups of three. You are allocated one support worker to assist you. What steps could you consider to demonstrate effective communication, presence, information-gathering support, and involvement in care?

Here, you would have to provide the support worker with discrete instructions on what tasks are required, with which group of clients, and delegate some of these to them. You then need a mechanism for them to report back to you. You might seek their opinion on some approaches, but will still need to make appropriate decisions. You may organize some times when you are able to observe them in order to provide support and assistance where necessary. Most important is the notion that the support worker can access you if needed.

Another factor that impacts on structural management is the large-scale introduction of information technologies in healthcare environments as a way of improving communication systems. Wojner (2001) suggested that healthcare informatics systems were designed for healthcare practitioners to integrate interdisciplinary approaches via computer science in order to identify, collect, process, and manage data to support practice, education, and develop **evidence-based practices**.

Keen (2006), however, suggests that there is little evidence that this is as cost-effective as, or is the panacea that, it is purported to be. Often, the technology becomes a back-office function rather than is utilized in front-line clinical work. How many times have we heard that the paperwork, now transferred to computers, takes up too much of a nurse's time, removing them from opportunities to spend more time with clients and their families? Therefore, if a nurse is managing a shift, they not only have to consider the clients, their relatives, staff, and other professionals, but they also need to make sure that the technologies are being utilized properly.

In this case, training in the use of such technologies is important for the qualified nurse, and the supervision of others while under their management becomes a crucial role. It is important therefore that you use the hierarchical structures to ensure that information about the effectiveness of such systems is communicated to senior management personnel.

 Theory into action

Think of the practice settings in which you have been involved. What types of technological equipment and approaches did you experience? What were the benefits and disadvantages of these? Is there another technology that you use (such as a mobile phone with various applications) that you think would be useful in the workplace? How do you think you could introduce this to a working environment?

Tyler (2004) argues that it is important that there is alignment between the organization's emerging aims and priorities, the demands and possibilities of the roles and jobs within services, and the individual, with their abilities, hopes, and aspirations. In other words, there needs to be alignment of the individual, the job, and the organization.

Human resources (HR) management

According to Leatt et al. (2006), organizations such as those providing health care employ a wide range of individuals within the teams in their healthcare settings. Having the appropriate skills and knowledge to carry out the organization's goals is critical. Usually, HR management is deemed to be an organization-wide role, but Tyler (2004) points out that managers at all levels make HR decisions about the workforce that reports to them. As a newly qualified nurse, this term might appear daunting and outside your remit. However, you will be responsible for making or communicating decisions that may affect junior staff, whilst maintaining approaches that are relevant to meeting the goals of the organization. These may include decisions related to development and change, reducing costs, and maintaining standards and quality.

Osborne (1997) argued that it was important that nurses were involved in decision-making at a number of levels, particularly as close to the client as possible, and that this included decisions to be made within multidisciplinary teams. Iles (2005) argues that this can be difficult sometimes due to the nature of relationships between professionals. Members of groups considered to be lower status may sometimes find expressing their views and opinions difficult, particularly if doing so to those regarded as having a higher status.

In setting out a structure or management map, Phillips (2005) shows how a nurse operates within wider systems such as the individual teams, the service as a whole, and the organization. An adapted version of this can be seen in Figure 7.4, which shows

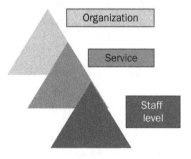

Figure 7.4 Nurses can contribute to decision-making

how nurses can contribute to decision-making at the organizational level above their current position, therefore showing how influence may filter upwards from ground level to senior executive positions.

Qualified nurses working in the staff team will contribute (with others at the same level) to discussions held at unit, and subsequently service, level. This may also include discussions related to the performance of, and needs of, junior staff. Those in senior management positions at service level will also then contribute (with others at the same level) to discussions at the organizational level. It is widely recognized that information can usually flow downwards in such a hierarchy, but you need to believe that these systems can also work effectively for you in creating change, by using it for disseminating information in an upwards direction too.

In order to have good HR management, certain considerations needed to be borne in mind. According to Barr and Dowding (2008: 179), these are:

- workforce planning;
- recruitment and selection of appropriate staff;
- induction, training, and development;
- performance management and appraisal;
- employer well-being and support;
- outsourcing.

Theory into action

To understand the above processes, it might be useful for you to consider them from your own experiences. Therefore, reflect for a few moments, then write a list of aspects that you have experienced or would expect in your own employment in relation to the above bullet points. For example, what were the recruitment processes? How were you inducted and how were your developmental needs identified? How has your performance been appraised?

Therefore, if, as a staff nurse, you are required to carry out specific tasks, you may need to alert senior staff to the amount and skill mix of staff needed to carry out such tasks. You may be required to train, teach, and educate others in the work environment. There will also be times when you need to alert staff to any deficiencies in their work (while remembering that it is also important to alert them to the positive aspects of their work).

Duty rotas

One of the aspects of which you may find yourself needing awareness is the organization, or more realistically, the *reorganization* of a duty rota. It is usually the responsibility of more senior staff to provide the rota for the service area. Thomas (2006) argues that such a rota should be completed in four-week to six-week periods to ensure minimum staffing levels and skill mix for each shift. This includes managing annual leave, study leave, and the involvement of agency staff where necessary. In relation to annual leave and study leave, these should have been agreed and planned as far in advance as possible, so should be recorded on the rota in the first instance. These are usually placed in a diary or request book and agreed by the manager of the service. This then needs to be followed by ensuring there is adequate senior or qualified cover as necessary and stated by the care manager in line with policy. Next, the numbers and skill mix of staff need to be met within the rota.

However, day-to-day occurrences happen such as sickness, or a sudden request for a change of shift, or changes in work demands, which may require the rota to be amended. Such amendments may have to be made by you if you are in charge of the shift, or if a manager delegates the task to you. If you are involved in developing or amending the rota, it is important to be as fair as possible in ensuring equality in shifts, meeting the needs of staff with family commitments and meeting requests of staff. Remember, if staff feel that they have been provided with a favour that suits them, then they should also be willing to return the favour at some point. What should not happen is that some people always get favourable shifts at the expense of others, without thorough negotiation. Staff who have been provided with favours in having their requests accepted should recognize that this will not always be the case and that they are expected to work the shifts prescribed to them within reason. In the authors' experience, completing a rota can appear to be an easy task on paper, but remember that we are dealing with people and that your decisions will need to be communicated clearly. The ability to show flexibility while meeting the requirements of the service is paramount.

Marquis and Huston (2009) highlight that staff shortages can occur on a day-to-day basis. The range of ways to deal with this are usually already decided at managerial level, but may include closed unit staffing, whereby staff from the area not on shift are contacted to cover. This is usually agreed by all of the team as a recognized approach. There may also be some scope for providing overtime. If this is necessary, it may be appropriate for you to contact the budget-holder before making any decisions to allow this. There is also the option of contacting agency or pool/bank staff to cover and, again, you may need to alert the budget-holder before sanctioning this. The important thing is to take action as soon as the staff shortage/difficulty becomes apparent.

Management and supervision

It can be seen in the above sections that there is a great deal of overlap in the concepts suggested by Egan (1993), as he states they are all in play at any one time, and each stage may have more importance at given times than others. However, each one is important before the next can be considered. So each level may have aspects of the previous stage, which is then built on. This brings us to management and supervision. The infrastructure and its rules have been set in place and it is now important that the workforce adheres to these in order to meet the strategic vision of the organization.

Systems of audit and discipline and reward therefore need to be put into place and utilized by the workforce. Marquis and Huston (2009) suggest that performance appraisal is an important managerial role. This requires the person identified as manager to objectively collect data through a formalized system, maintain the appropriate documentation, set goals and action plans, and establish mechanisms for review and feedback. According to Armstrong and Stephens (2005), further management roles and functions relate to health and safety, risk management, and policy development. It is about resolving unsatisfactory situations within the work environment, problem-solving, and decision-making.

Within this aspect of management, there might arise issues related to power and authority. This can occur due to a number of factors across physical, psychological, sociological, political, and emotional domains. These include factors such as age, gender, position experience, and skill. As a newly qualified nurse with responsibilities on a day-to-day basis for management of care areas, be that in hospital wards, clinics, residential and care homes, or as visiting community nurses, these aspects need to be addressed. Marquis and Huston (2009) suggest that although power usually comes with the position or status of the employee—in this case, the nurse—it can be gained by utilizing a number of skills, including:

- maintaining energy;
- demonstrating a positive professional persona in all situations;
- working hard and being seen to be doing so;
- knowing when to ask for help and from who;
- understanding the culture of the organization;
- continually developing skills and expertise;
- maintaining a broad vision;
- being flexible;
- demonstrating assertiveness (while avoiding aggressive and bullying tones);
- having a sense of humour;
- ensuring others are empowered.

In demonstrating these behaviours, power can be earned by gaining respect from colleagues and superiors. In doing so, value is added to the workplace, as teams will tend to be more cooperative.

Egan's final stage is that of pragmatic leadership, which has already been discussed in depth in this chapter. There needs to be leaders at all levels throughout the hierarchical structure of the organization to maintain the vision of the organization and to create change.

To summarize, management may not directly be the first remit of the newly qualified nurse and these concepts may be more applicable to organizational management—but they can still be considered in the day-to-day running of a care environment.

First, if you are in charge of a care area, you need to have in place a *strategy* for the day. There will be prescribed activities, duties related to individuals or the environment, that must occur on that day only and any other contingencies that may arise. Therefore, at the start of the day, the nurse needs to set out their strategy of how these would be best addressed and handled.

Second, in setting out the strategy, there is the need to fully understand the *operations* and maintaining of standards that is required. The nurse also needs to fully understand the *structural* nature of the organization and how this filters down to the day-to-day running. Therefore the nurse in charge will delegate tasks and duties to the workforce and issue commands on how to feedback on these to ensure everything is in order.

There are issues of *HR management*, such as ensuring that staff with the right skills are deployed to the right duties and that they are given feedback on their performance and assisted where necessary. The issue of *management and coordination* are therefore important throughout the day, and the nurse needs to understand what events are happening, including any that are unforeseen, and they then need to demonstrate flexibility and positive decision-making skills before reporting back on the day to senior staff.

⊖ Theory into action

Think of a nurse whom you know or of a time when you have been in charge of the care area for a day (or even longer). What considerations were made in relation to strategy, operations, structure, HR, management and supervision, and leadership?

Armstrong and Stephens (2005) point out that managers have to be leaders, but that leaders might not always be managers. Management is about making decisions to achieve results and leadership is about the relationships between people in order to ensure that change occurs, and results are achieved. Therefore theories of leadership such as trait, style, contingency/situational, transactional, and transformational, as well as clinical leadership have been discussed. It is necessary for nurses in the new healthcare systems to show leadership qualities. These skills will be needed on a day-to-day basis and in longer-term developmental scenarios.

The chapter has so far included discussion related to leadership and management. As a newly qualified nurse, it might seem that such large-scale organizational aspects of leadership and management may occur further on as your career develops; however, on a day-to-day basis, you may find yourself responsible for ensuring maximum achievement of care needs for their patients/service users, which includes awareness of all of the above theories and how they might be applied.

NMC standards of proficiency

As mentioned earlier in the chapter, nurses are required to demonstrate leadership and management roles in order to be able to register their nursing qualification with the NMC to enable them to practise as nurses (NMC, 2010). The standards are divided into four domains, as follows.

- Domain 1: Professional values
- Domain 2: Communication and interpersonal skills
- Domain 3: Nursing practice and decision-making
- Domain 4: Leadership, management, and teamwork

The standards of proficiency state that in order to provide care management and personal and professional development, nurses should expect to take on leadership roles within healthcare teams and to supervise and facilitate the work of others. These roles are important in order to establish and monitor safe delivery of care. These notions of delegation and working in harmony with other professions are emphasized by the NMC. This is strongly expressed throughout the NMC standards.

The Department of Health document *Modernising Nursing Careers* (DH, 2006) states that, due to the changing nature of health care, with a focus on health promotion, primary care, and community developments, nurses need to demonstrate effective leadership skills within their varying roles. Therefore one of the elements set out as a priority in the document is leadership management and supervision. Mooney (2007) found that newly qualified nurses expressed some anxiety with some of these roles, including dealing with other professionals. Gerrish (2000) also highlighted that newly qualified nurses were anxious about some of their managerial duties, such as delegating to others.

Collaborative working

Pedler et al. (2007) suggest that collaborative working in teams can be difficult when you might be in a position of having no formal authority over them, and your own professional team may have differing aims and agendas. These can be created because of a lack of clarity of roles and responsibilities. So the first lesson is to ensure that you make yourself clear. This means that clarity is necessary in the requests that you make, the information that you request or provide, and the instructions that you give.

Collaboration means sharing while maintaining your own boundaries. There are several mutual benefits of learning from sharing with other professionals. Heller (1998) suggests that taking steps such as socializing in a professional sense with other disciplines helps to show that you are willing to listen to them, and you can gain awareness of what and why they are carrying out certain tasks/approaches. However, there is also a need to utilize assertiveness skills to maintain your own authority in such arenas. This again boils down to clarity: creating clear goals/outcomes, clearly communicating these, and being clear about the potential consequences or benefits of the actions requested. Once again, making decisions and suggesting them to others is a good way of leading from the front. It shows that you can take initiative, which will instil trust from others. For example, you will need to have a working knowledge of the care environment, the patients/service users within it, and the planned events during your shifts. Griffiths and Hewison (2004) argue that it is important to understand the differing professional approaches so that you can organize for other disciplines, such as physiotherapists or occupational therapists, to visit at suitable times when patients/service users are not likely to be tired or involved in other activities.

Dealing with complaints

As well as having to deal with staff being late, other professionals, and delegating workloads, other aspects with which a newly qualified staff nurse needs to regularly contend include dealing with complaints or conflicts with staff. Sometimes, these may be linked, as according to Walshe and Smith (2006) the highest cause of complaint after poor practices are attitudes of staff, followed by poor written and oral communication.

In order to address such issues, Owen (2009) argues that focusing on people, being positive, and being professional are important. This means that you should be able to be aware of others, find solutions, and stay loyal to the core values of the profession and employers. All care services have a complaints procedure that states exactly the steps that should be taken.

The most important aspect is communication. Relatives may make a complaint because they believe that their loved one is not receiving the level of service that they would expect. Whether the complaint is valid or not, it does need to be seen to be dealt with. You may need to explain the circumstances of the situation, because an explanation may suffice in helping the relative to understand why certain things are happening. You should alert them to the procedure for dealing with complaints if they wish to continue their claim. The formal procedure may need to be invoked if your explanation does not satisfy their concern. It may be necessary to alert your immediate line manager or senior staff of the complaint and it most definitely needs to be recorded.

Dealing with conflict

You should be able to coach and influence, give constructive feedback, deal with conflict, and motivate others. Dealing with staff conflict may be a regular aspect of your role as a qualified nurse. This may be as simple as staff disagreeing with you or each other, or the wider members of the interdisciplinary team. The main thing is that this is dealt with quickly and professionally. A golden rule, which has been stressed in this chapter throughout, is to not ask staff to do something that you would not be prepared to do yourself or might have done yourself at some time. According to Dann (2008), conflicts with staff can build up over time or can happen spontaneously. The aim is to create a state of negotiation to resolve the problem. First, it is vital that such conflicts should not take place in front of patients or relatives or others. The parties should be politely asked to move to a private area in the work area. Barr and Dowding (2008) suggest that it is important to keep calm; Dann (2008) is in agreement with this. The next stage is to listen to get to the facts. This may mean having to listen to all parties before making any decisions. You need to show empathy, in as much as you must be willing to listen to their point of view before making a decision. De Bono (2004) argues that it is important to reach a situation in which there is clear agreement, clear disagreement, or an agreement to differ (in which case, you can secure agreement on what the difference is). You may have to assertively request that they put differences aside and continue in meeting the service goals in order to provide safe, secure care for patients/service users. You may have to separate them or reassign tasks. It cannot be stressed enough that clarity of goals and their communication are of the utmost importance.

Taking action is something that junior staff will associate with you and a way in which you can start developing respect as a leader in their eyes. If these informal mechanisms are unsuccessful, then you may need to refer to senior staff. Aspects related to accountability, maintaining standards, and ethical issues will be addressed elsewhere in this book, with suggested appropriate actions to take.

. . . .

💡 Thinking about

Think back to your nurse training. What were the positive methods that senior staff used in influencing you, coaching you, and giving constructive feedback? What were the best approaches that you observed in dealing with conflict?

. . . .

Summary

This chapter has looked at the major theories related to leadership such as trait, style, situational, transactional, and transformational. The important aspect to remember is that leadership is related to your people skills. It is about your ability to observe the situation, identify problems, and create solutions. It is about taking action, leading by being seen to be involved, and doing some of the tasks that you would expect others to do, as well as giving clear direction and instruction.

Theories of management have been discussed, demonstrating how the organizational goals are aligned and that strategies are put in place to maintain them. It is about formal mechanisms and infrastructure, and how these are maintained or developed. It is about the day-to-day running of services by following the policies and procedures set in place by employing organizations and professions. It is about formally dealing with people at all levels of an organization reporting up from the ground floor.

Overall, it is hoped that this chapter has shown that there is a great deal of overlap of concepts related to leadership and management. Management may be a role achieved by position, whereas leadership demonstrates interpersonal power and influence. Managers should, as far as possible, be leaders, but leaders do not necessarily have to be managers. As a newly qualified nurse, these aspects may be challenging, but by transferring skills gained in other areas of life, observing others, asking questions, and practising by getting involved, they are skills that can be developed and integrated as you progress in your career.

- **Leadership** is related to achieving goals through people. It is about dynamic relationships, goal-setting, strategy, and action.
- Leadership encompasses theories related to traits, styles, contingency, and situational flexibility.
- Clinical leadership relates to extending roles, developing approaches, and decision-making across nursing and interdisciplinary teams to achieve positive outcomes for patients/service users.
- **Management** is related to making sure that goals are achieved.
- It is related to developing organizational structures and systems to accomplish this.
- It encompasses managing resources effectively and supervising people effectively.

In this chapter, we have looked at:

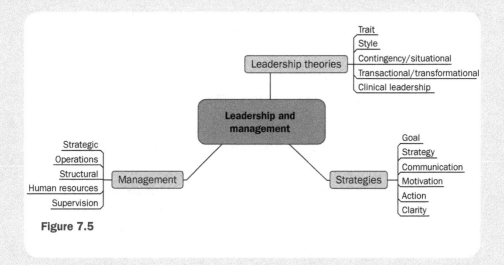

Figure 7.5

Online Resource Centre

 This textbook is accompanied by an Online Resource Centre that provides interactive learning resources and tools to help you to prepare for the transition from student to fully qualified member of staff. After you have completed each chapter and whenever you see this icon, please go to the ORC at your earliest convenience. If you have not done so already, save the ORC web address into your favourites: **http://www.oxfordtextbooks.co.uk/orc/burton**

References

Adair J (1988) *Effective Leadership*. Pan Books, London.

Akerjordet K & Severinsson E (2008) Emotionally intelligent nurse leadership: a literature review study. *Journal of Nursing Management,* **16**: 565–77.

Anderson EE & Kiger AM (2008) 'I felt like a real nurse': student nurses out on their own. *Nurse Education Today,* **28**: 443–9.

Anderson-Wallace M (2005) Working with structure. In: E Peck (ed) (2005) *Organisational Development in Healthcare*. Radcliffe Publishing, Oxon.

Armstrong M & Stephens T (2005) *A Handbook of Management and Leadership: A Guide to Managing for Results*. Kogan Page, London/Sterling, VA.

Baillie L (1999) Preparing adult branch students for their management role as staff nurses: an action research project. *Journal of Nursing Management,* **7**: 225–34.

Barr J & Dowding L (2008) *Leadership in Health Care*. Sage, London.

Bartram T & Casimir G (2007) The relationship between leadership and follower in-role performance and satisfaction with the leader: the mediating effects of empowerment and trust in the leader. *Leadership and Organization Development Journal*, **28**(1): 4–19.

Bass BM (1985) *Leadership and Performance Beyond Expectations.* Free Press, New York. In: TA Judge & JE Bono (2000) Five-factor model of personality and transformational leadership. *Journal of Applied Psychology,* **85**(5): 751–65.

Blake RR & Moulton JH (1964) *The Managerial Grid.* Gulf Publishing, Houston, TX. In: BL Marquis & CJ Huston (eds) (2009) *Leadership Roles and Management Functions in Nursing,* 6th edn. Wolters Kluwer & Lippincott, Williams & Wilkins, Philadelphia, PA.

Blanchard K (2007) *Leading at a Higher Level.* Prentice Hall, London.

Blanchard K & Spencer J (2000) *The One Minute Manager,* revised edn. Harper Collins, London.

Bondas T (2006) Paths to nursing leadership. *Journal of Nursing Management,* **14**: 332–9.

Bruce A & Langdon K (2000) *Project Management.* Dorling Kindersley, London.

Burns JM (1978) *Leadership.* Harper & Row, New York. In: TA Judge & JE Bono (2000) Five-factor model of personality and transformational leadership. *Journal of Applied Psychology,* **85**(5): 751–65.

Chantrell G (2004) *Oxford Dictionary of Word Histories.* Oxford University Press, Oxford.

Clegg S, Kornberger M & Pitsis T (2005) *Managing and Organizations: An Introduction to Theory and Practice.* Sage, London

Collins English Dictionary (2010) Harper Collins, Aylesbury.

Covey S (1989) *The 7 Habits of Highly Effective People.* Simon and Schuster, London.

Crossan F (2003) Strategic management and nurses: building foundations. *Journal of Nursing Management,* **11**: 331–5.

Dann J (2008) *Emotional Intelligence.* Hodder Education, London.

De Bono E (2004) *How to Have a Beautiful Mind.* Vermillion, London.

Department of Health (2004) *Agenda for Change: Final Agreement.* DH, London. Available at: **http://www.dh.gov.uk/en/Publicationsandstatistics/Publications/PublicationsPolicyAndGuidance/DH_4095943**

Department of Health (2006) *Modernising Nursing Careers: Setting the Direction.* DH, London.

Digman JM (1990) Personality structure: emergence of the five-factor model. *Annual Review of Psychology,* **41**(1): 417.

Egan G (1993) *Adding Value: A Systematic Guide to Business Driven Management and Leadership.* Jossey Bass, San Francisco, CA.

Egan G (2002) *The Skilled Helper: A Problem-management and Opportunity-development Approach to Helping,* 7th edn. Brooks Cole, Pacific Grove, CA.

Endacott R (1999) Roles of the allocated nurse and shift leader in the intensive care unit: findings of an ethnographic study. *Intensive and Critical Care Nursing,* **15**: 10–15.

Gallo K (2007) The new nurse manager: a leadership development program paves the road to success. *Nurse Leader,* **5**(4): 28–32.

Gerrish K (2000) Still fumbling along? A comparative study of the newly qualified nurse's perception of the transition from student to qualified nurse. *Journal of Advanced Nursing,* **32**(2): 473–80.

Goldblatt H, Granot M, Admi H & Drach-Zavary A (2008) The experience of being a shift leader in a hospital ward. *Journal of Advanced Nursing,* **63**(1): 45–53.

Goleman D, Boyatzis R & Mckee A (2002) *The New Leaders: Transforming the Art of Leadership into the Science of Results.* Time Warner, London.

Gregoire MB (2004) Leadership: reflections over the past 100 years. *Journal of the American Dietetic Association,* **104**(3): 395–403.

Griffiths M & Hewison A (2004) How to work with other professionals: multiprofessional and collaborative working. In: J Hyde & M Cook (eds) (2004) *Managing and Supporting People in Healthcare.* Bailliere Tindall, London.

Handy C (1999) *Understanding Organisations,* 4th edn. Penguin, London.

Harris S (2004) Clinical leadership. In: J Hyde & M Cook (eds) *Managing and Supporting People in Healthcare.* Bailliere Tindall, London.

Heller R (1998) *Managing Teams.* Dorling Kindersley, London.

Hendry B (2004) The human aspects of organisational change. In: J Hyde & M Cook (eds) *Managing and Supporting People in Healthcare.* Bailliere Tindall, London.

Iles V (2005) *Really Managing Health Care,* 2nd edn. Open University Press, Maidenhead.

Jackson C (2005) The experience of a good day: a phenomenological study to explain a good day as experienced by a newly qualified RN. *Accident and Emergency Nursing,* **13**: 110–21.

Judge TA & Bono JE (2000) Five-factor model of personality and transformational leadership. *Journal of Applied Psychology,* **85**(5): 751–65.

Keen J (2006) Information technology and information systems: so beguiling, so difficult. In: K Walshe & J Smith (eds) (2006) *Healthcare Management.* Open University Press, Maidenhead.

Keller T (1999) Images of the familiar: individual differences and implicit leadership theories. *Leadership Quarterly,* **10**(4): 589–607.

Laurent CL (2000) A nursing theory for nursing leadership. *Journal of Nursing Management,* **8**: 83–7.

Leatt P, Ross Baker G & Kimberley JR (2006) Organization design. In: SM Shortell & AD Kaluzny (eds) (2006) *Health Care Management: Organization Design and Behaviour,* 5th edn. Thomson Delmar Learning, New York.

Marquis BL & Huston CJ (2009) *Leadership Roles and Management Functions in Nursing,* 6th edn. Wolters Kluwer & Lippincott, Williams & Wilkins, Philadelphia, PA.

McGregor D (1960) *The Human Side of Enterprise.* McGraw-Hill, New York. In: BL Marquis & CJ Huston (eds) (2009) *Leadership Roles and Management Functions in Nursing,* 6th edn. Wolters Kluwer & Lippincott, Williams & Wilkins, Philadelphia, PA.

Mooney M (2007) Professional socialization: the key to survival as a newly qualified nurse. *International Journal of Nursing Practice,* **13**: 75–80.

Nursing And Midwifery Council (2006) *Preceptorship Guidelines.* NMC Circular 21/2006. NMC, London.

Nursing and Midwifery Council (2008) *The Code: Standards of Conduct, Performance and Ethics for Nurses and Midwives.* NMC, London.

Nursing and Midwifery Council (2010) *Standards for Proficiency for Pre-registration Nursing Education.* NMC, London.

O'Connor J & Seymour J (1990) *Introducing NLP: Psychological Skills for Understanding and Influencing People.* Aquarian Press, London.

Osborne SE (1997) Grasping the nettle: the involvement of the nurse in management decision making. *Journal of Advanced Nursing,* **25**: 871–2.

Owen J (2009) *How To Lead*, 2nd edn. Pearson Education, London.

Peck E (ed) (2005) *Organisational Development in Healthcare.* Radcliffe Publishing, Oxon.

Peck E (2006) Leadership and its development in healthcare. In: K Walshe & J Smith (eds) (2006) *Healthcare Management.* Open University Press, Maidenhead, 323–41.

Pedler M, Burgoyne J & Boydell T (2007) *A Manager's Guide to Self-development*, 5th edn. McGraw-Hill, London.

Phillips J (2005) Knowledge is power: using information management and leadership interventions to improve services to patients, clients and users. *Journal of Nursing Management,* **13**: 524–36.

Pointer DD (2006) Leadership a framework for thinking and acting. 125–47. In: SM Shortell & AD Kaluzny (eds) *Health Care Management: Organization Design and Behaviour*, 5th edn. Thomson Delmar Learning, New York.

Sellgren S, Ekval G & Tomson G (2006) Leadership styles in nursing management: preferred and perceived. *Journal of Nursing Management,* **14**: 348–55.

Shortell SM & Kaluzny AD (2006) *Health Care Management: Organization Design and Behaviour*, 5th edn. Thomson Delmar Learning, New York.

Sorensen R, Iedema R & Severinsson E (2008) Beyond profession: nursing leadership in contemporary health care. *Journal of Nursing Management,* **16**: 535–44.

Stanley D (2008) Congruent leadership: values in action. *Journal of Nursing Management,* **16**: 519–24.

Stordeur S, D'Hoore W & Vandenburghe C (2001) Leadership, organizational stress, and emotional exhaustion among hospital nursing staff. *Journal of Advanced Nursing,* **35**(4): 533–42.

Thomas J (2006) *Survival Guide for Ward Managers, Sisters and Charge Nurses.* Churchill Livingstone/Elsevier, Edinburgh/London.

Tyler S (2004) *The Manager's Good Study Guide.* Open University Press, Milton Keynes.

Walshe K & Smith J (2006) *Healthcare Management.* Open University Press, Maidenhead, Berkshire.

Wojner AW (2001) *Outcomes Management: Applications to Clinical Practice.* Mosby, St Louis, MI.

Woodring BC (2004) Clinical nurse leaders: new roles, new responsibilities, new preparation. *Journal for Specialists in Pediatric Nursing,* **9**(4): 129–34.

Getting the job that you want

Graham Ormrod

The aims of this chapter are to:

- ➔ offer strategies to assist you in finding and getting the job you want;
- ➔ help you to reflect on your strengths and areas of development;
- ➔ explore how best to prepare for interview;
- ➔ assist you to match your strengths with the person specification;
- ➔ offer insight into the interview procedures;
- ➔ promote strategies on coping with disappointment and how to get the next job.

Introduction

You have come to an absolutely crucial time in your career not only as a student, but also with regards to your future career generally. No doubt you will have thought about this moment since you started your nursing course and probably even further back than that. Starting and successfully completing your course will have been the first few steps in what will hopefully be a long, exciting, and fulfilling career.

You will probably have also been talking about job opportunities to your friends and colleagues more and more as the time for decision-making became closer and closer. Discussing your thoughts, plans, and aspirations with those whom you trust can be very positive; however, this can occasionally lead to *more* misunderstandings and confusion, and thereby raise, rather than reduce, anxiety at this already highly pressured time. Therefore be cautious!

In this chapter, we will explore various ways of ensuring that you show yourself in the best light, help to increase the likelihood of getting your ideal job, and generally do yourself justice. It is important to remember, however, that despite what you might now think, there will always be more than one job out there for you. You might presently think:

> 'This job on the paediatric intensive care at the local trust is the only job for me'

Or

> 'Working in the team with that community psychiatric nurse who was so supportive when I had my placement there is an absolute must!'

Considering very specifically the job that you would like is clearly an important step in actually getting it. However, the crucial stage here is consideration of *why* this particular job is so attractive. It is essential that, as far as is possible, the *reality* of the job is clear to you and that the reality meets both your current skills and expertise, and also your aspirations.

It is important to reduce the risk of becoming disheartened by putting 'all of your eggs in one basket'. One of the great things about nursing as a career is its variety—a variety that brings many different options and opportunities. Being able to recognize and grasp these opportunities, while matching them to your skills, experience, and aspirations, is a key part of finding a suitable and rewarding job.

So where might you start your career?

According to Hood (2010), every nurse has an established set of values—that is, values that they see as being important in their life. No two nurses share an identical set of values and selecting the ones that are the most important can be a difficult task. Nurses learn *professional* values as part of their socialization as a student, but some of these values can change over time. Hood (2010) suggests that certain areas of nursing *generally* cater to different sets of values. So nurses who value technologically complex skills tend to pursue what might be broadly viewed as critical care environments. Depending on the field the nurse is in, this environment can be found in intensive peri-operative areas, accident and emergency, or some areas caring for individuals with particularly complex challenging behaviours. Nurses who place greater value on long-term relationships may choose to explore career options in other areas, such as in caring for those with long-term conditions, school nursing, or caring for clients with learning disabilities in their own homes. While not claiming to fully capture the complexities of the personal and professional context, this type of initial approach and consideration might help to work out where you see yourself heading in your career—not least because, as Hood (2010) further asserts, unlike most other professions, nursing offers many career opportunities that fit with a nurse's *personal* values and allows them to develop a personal vision of their future.

So, once you have identified your future vision and identified your career direction, what strategies might you use to make this happen? If you speak to your **mentor**, personal tutor, or other colleagues, they may tell you that they didn't arrive at their current job along a carefully crafted and meticulously planned career path, but that they took advantage of interesting opportunities as their insight and particular interests became clearer. While it may be true that most careers don't necessarily follow exact and predictable paths, it is also true that opportunities don't simply appear out of thin air and there is a need to be proactive in exploring any possibilities.

A structured 'linear' career path, if such a thing exists, would follow a sequential series of carefully judged steps and may best suit the nurse who enjoys structure and meeting designated deadlines.

> 'In two years I will be a mentor, by five I will be a charge nurse and by ten years I will be working as a nurse specialist in palliative care.'

However, a lot of nurses have a fulfilling and enjoyable career following a far less 'linear' career path, relying more on unpredictable circumstances and key critical career incidents. Such paths are not totally random, however, and can still be formulated by considering particular and specific interests and relevant outside experiences, and then seizing the opportunities as they arise.

Nursing, and health care generally, changes all of the time and this is probably truer now than ever before. Exploring and recognizing the possibility of a less linear path in your career *may* increase the likelihood of taking opportunities creatively as they arise and perhaps encourage a more flexible approach in times of such change. However, it might conversely encourage a less focused approach to career development, leading to inertia and feelings of being 'left behind' *if* the individual nurse is not continually reflective of their current position and proactive in their exploration of career possibilities.

The term 'career mapping' can be used to denote the continuous process of career development. This is when any career changes unfold as the nurse engages in professional practice and lifelong learning, having identified their individual values, coupled with what Hood (2010: 566) calls an 'envisioning' of their nursing career. This overall vision, essentially picturing yourself in the future, creates a *blueprint* for personal action to make that envisioned future become reality.

Getting your ideal job can be very complicated. Some considerations are often called internal—that is, essentially about *you*—whereas others might be viewed as more *external*—for example, the current job market or the competition for the job that you want and so on.

One of the tools that can help clarify your thinking in relation to both internal and external issues of career planning is the **SWOT analysis** (Table 8.1). Much of the development of the SWOT analysis came from the area of sales and marketing, and in this context phrases such as internal (meaning the strengths and weaknesses of a particular organization) and external (the opportunities and threats from outside of the organization) might appear more appropriate and fitting. However, *the process can also be very useful* for an individual wishing to clarify their career planning.

Table 8.1 A partly completed example of a SWOT analysis

	Strengths	Weaknesses
I N T E R N A L	Current knowledge of specific clinical area from my placement	Newly qualified—therefore lack of experience
	Good teamworker	Need to stay in particular local area
	Enthusiastic and well motivated	First time had to apply for a job
	Chose the area for 'elective placement' so face known	Nervous of 'blowing own trumpet'
	Opportunities	**Threats**
E X T E R N A L	Recent investment in the service—so opportunities are available	Whole cohort looking for a job at same time
	Department are looking for newly qualified staff	More experienced competition
	Job is at local trust	Possibility of trust merger so may need to work cross-site

· ·

⊙ Theory into action

Complete a SWOT analysis similar to the example above. Be honest and realistic, but also as creative as you can, and avoid false modesty. Remember this is only an initial guide to where you might concentrate your thinking.

 You can print off a blank version of the SWOT analysis from the Online Resource Centre.

It is important to consider weaknesses as 'areas that could be further developed'; therefore this analysis will be not only a reflection of your current self, but also a record of your potential.

Try to put yourself inside a prospective employer's head, particularly as you consider your strong points. What might they be looking for?

If this is the first time that you have undertaken such an analysis, you may find it easier to start by simply listing key words. This can be developed further if necessary.

· ·

So what are you going to do with this information? You are going to use it to 'market' yourself! This can be a three-step process.

Determining your objectives

Your objectives might include:

- your ideal job;
- other jobs that you might consider;

- how you intend to make the transition from student to registered nurse;
- your two/five/ten-year career goal.

Developing a 'marketing' strategy

Think about the following.

- Which organizations or trusts might you 'target' to achieve your objectives?
- How will you discover what opportunities are available there?
- How will you then communicate your wishes to them?
- What help can I get to do this? What support network have I got? Could the university help? Could my mentor help?

Putting together an action plan

It is essential that the strategies are turned into actions.

- What do I need to do?
- When do I need to do it?
- What are the goals that I want to achieve?
- What are the specific timetables and deadlines?

Short-term career planning

The above processes allow you to focus more clearly on your realistic goals and objectives, which make it more likely that you will accomplish them. Your SWOT analysis may have highlighted barriers to your achieving these goals, such as lack of motivation or procrastination, or perhaps less personal barriers, such as family and peer pressure, or even financial considerations.

....

💡 Thinking about

Consider your current situation. What is it with which you are happiest? Now consider what would improve this situation in the future. What kind of activities do you particularly like? What kind of activities do you avoid?

Complete the table.

Key activities	
Activities I particularly enjoy	Activities I try to avoid

_____

_____

_____

_____

_____

Once you have made this list as comprehensively as possible, take a close look at your proposed career path and the job for which you thought you might apply

How does the list above match the key characteristics of your ideal job? Are there any surprises? Does your proposed job have more likes or dislikes?

Preparation: what type of job do you want and why?

_If_ you allow it to be, finding a job can be quite a traumatic and disheartening experience. To help to keep you focused and motivated during what can be quite a long and arduous process, it is important to consider who might be your support network. Who might be able to offer you advice and support?

 Theory into action

Write down whom you might include in your support network. How, specifically, might they be able to help?

As your nursing career progresses, you will undoubtedly develop a supportive professional network of colleagues and friends. This can facilitate learning by sharing best practice, discussing differences in practice, exploring current and future priorities and initiatives, and generally helping and encouraging you. Your support network may be less structured and less obvious at this stage in your career; however, there are still people who might support and advise you. One obvious person who might help you during this time is your personal tutor, who hopefully will be a trusted adviser who has seen you grow and develop professionally during the time on the course. Similarly, you will have mentors who have contributed to your growth and development as they have been assessing your practice.

Support networks outside of nursing, such as friends and family, appropriately utilized, might also be able to assist you in clarifying your thinking. Such 'critical friends' can often put into words more precisely the skills that you have, but might be quite reluctant to acknowledge as you generally struggle to 'blow your own trumpet'.

Key points

It is fair to say that just as nursing equips us with many transferable skills in other areas of life, the opposite is also true. This is important to remember when you are trying to sell yourself. So why include aspects of your 'personal' life in your application, curriculum vitae (CV), or even at interview?

- What might being involved in the local parent–teacher association say about your abilities and skills?
- What does the fact that you have completed the Duke of Edinburgh's Award say about your ability?
- Similarly, why might the fact that you like to go hill climbing in your spare time be of any interest to a prospective employer?

The above examples can be included in your application or discussed at interview as they offer evidence of skills that may be valuable to an employer. They may show that you are reliable, trustworthy, and committed. *Or* they may show you are self-reliant, a good time manager, and able to complete difficult tasks. *Or* they may even indicate that you have a well-rounded personality and have strategies outside of work that may help you to handle pressure and stress. *Or* all of the above!

Although you should include only *relevant* information, it is still possible to be quite creative by including information that makes you stand out from the crowd.

Finding the job

By now, you would have confirmed the type of work that you prefer and clarified the skills that you have to match the requirements of this role. So how can you find the jobs that are presently available? It is important that you know about the many resources available to locate employment opportunities.

- Each trust or employer will have an area accessible to employees and others where internal job openings are advertised. Do you know where this is in your current placement area? Ask your mentor for advice.
- Similarly, current vacancies will be available on the employer's website.
- There are also many websites available that allow you to search for specific jobs appropriate to newly qualified nurses. For example, in the UK:
  - **http://www.jobs.nhs.uk/**
  - **http://www.rcnbulletinjobs.co.uk/**
  - **http://www.staffnurse.com/**
- Some nursing journals also contain classified advertisements with available opportunities, such as *Nursing Times* (**http://nursingjobs.nursingtimes.net/**).

This website also offers an email service, through which you can receive email updates on all the suitable jobs.
- You may also find some jobs in your local paper.

The next difficult question: 'When should I apply?'

There is no absolutely correct answer to this, unfortunately—especially for student nurses coming to the end of their nursing course. The variables involved here are as follows.

- Is there a job available?
- Is it appropriate for a newly qualified staff nurse?
- When does the vacancy need filling?
- When can I start?

Because of all of these issues, it is important not to be too disappointed if you do choose to apply and you don't get invited for interview, or if you do receive an invitation for interview, but do not subsequently get appointed. Obviously, this may simply be because they need someone to start *now*. If you are unable to take up the opportunity for a few months, then you may be unsuccessful simply due to that fact.

Therefore, although it is true to say that there may never be agreement on when best to apply in these circumstances, it seems logical to say that more than a couple of months prior to the time at which you can officially start may inevitably lead to disappointment. Although *all* interview experience may be seen as useful in some way and part of a useful and ongoing learning process, even if, in real terms, you have no chance of being ultimately appointed, it is likely to irritate the interviewer if you have not been open and transparent about your position and ability to take up the opportunity. Discussing your specific situation openly and honestly with the contact person on the job advertisement may reduce your potential for disappointment and the likelihood of wasting their valuable time.

Remember that you may want the next job in that particular area and you don't want to be remembered as a time-waster.

So how can you increase your chances of getting an interview?

It is important to think of the interview as a wonderful opportunity and recognize that you are largely in control of the impression that the interviewer will form of you. Although many people might be critical of the whole interview process generally as a means of matching the right person with the right job, it is *not* purely chance if someone is successful at interview.

You will probably have heard people say, and may have also said yourself:

'How can they really know about me in such a short time?'

Or

'It is just whether your face fits or not, it isn't really about the individual person that's why it's so unfair.'

Or

'It is just about being in the right place at the right time.'

There *may* be some truth in these comments, but who knows? *However*, it is important to realize that the interview process is not simply determined by chance, and that you can have significant control and influence over the way in which the interview is conducted and more importantly over the outcome. We can be critical all we like, but interviews are not going to go away; indeed, employers spend a significant amount of time, effort, and money trying to ensure that they pick the right person for the job.

How can you improve your chances of success?

Key points

Remember that the best students don't necessarily get the job; the best prepared do.

The three main ways in which you can improve your chances are preparation, preparation, and preparation! For example, it is essential to keep up to date with what is happening in health care generally and especially in the specific area in which you are interested. If you don't, you could quite easily come unstuck at an interview when a question is asked that relates to current practice, policies, or new initiatives in that particular area. Knowledge and understanding of the current major issues will allow you to impress the interviewer with your insight and also your enthusiasm. It is undeniably impressive to an interviewer if a candidate is able to relate their knowledge of current issues to the specific job for which they are being interviewed.

Application form and/or CV

You never get a second chance to make a first impression. The unique personal profile on an application form or curriculum vitae (CV) tends to be the first thing the potential employer will read apart from the routine matters of name and contact details. Therefore, it is vital that you use this opportunity to work for you. The point of this section is to summarize, in no more than a few words, your major qualities and 'selling points'. The person reading this is not interested in what a wonderful person you are. They are, however, very interested in whether:

- you can do the job on offer;
- you have a real understanding of what the job entails;
- you have the appropriate experience and history;
- you will be able to do the job well;
- you will get on with the rest of the present team.

So it is important to concentrate on the benefits that you can bring and keep to the facts, avoiding overblown exaggeration and hype.

Key points

If you write your application form or CV as a 'solution to someone else's problem', it should make a favourable impression on the reader—that is, the person who needs that solution.

Unfortunately, this approach does mean that each job application is deserving of a very specific and individual approach, which can feel onerous and time-consuming. However, this time is definitely worth it: not only does it improve the impression that you are giving and the impact your application will make, but it also concentrates your mind on precisely why you are the right person for this *particular* job. There is no more certain way to lose a job than to speak of caring for patients undergoing surgery when the prospective employer is a charge nurse on a medical ward, for example.

Hopefully, your preparation, reflection, and the exercises that you have undertaken to clarify your thinking and understanding will have made you confident about what makes you stand out and right for the job. Let's be honest: if *you* don't know this by now, you cannot expect those reading your application form to invest significant effort in exploring and spotting it for you.

CV template

There are many different types of CV template available. Avoid gimmicks and unfamiliar formats as these can detract from, rather than enhance, the information included. The important thing is to make it easy for the reader to pick out the content that they are looking for so that the CV shows you in your best light as a prospective candidate (Box 8.1).

 You can print off a blank version from the Online Resource Centre.

Box 8.1 CV template

Name

Address (home and term)

Telephone (home and mobile)

Email

Personal profile

A succinct, approximately three-line sum-
mary of your unique selling points, which
will make you stand out from the crowd.

Education and qualifications

Date   University, Course, Qualification

                Subject

                Dissertation *(if relevant to job)*

Date   School/college

                A levels *(grades if good)*

Other qualifications

Date   School

                GCSE – number of subjects,

                including Maths and English

Work experience (most recent first)

Date   Trust, hospital or company

                    name, job title

                    Main responsibilities

Skills gained (communication, teamwork,
interpersonal, problem-solving)

Skills

For example, IT skills

Other relevant skills

Interests and activities

Only include these if they are focused and
relevant to the specific job for which you are
applying.

References

Usually at least two appropriate references
are required.

Application form, job description, and person specification

Each job advertisement will include both a job description and a person specification. It
may sound obvious, but these are very important documents! The job description will
include details such as job title, job location, and who the job holder is accountable for
and to, and so on. It will also include a job summary or job purpose. For example, this
section may include a paragraph similar to this:

> The post holder will participate in the delivery of high standards of care to chil-
> dren and their families. They will assess the care needs and develop, imple-
> ment, and evaluate programmes of individualized nursing care within a multi-
> professional setting, and work collaboratively and cooperatively with others to
> meet the needs of children and their families/carers.

The job description should then give more specific and crucial aspects of the job and
the role, including areas such as:

- clinical duties;
- management;
- professional/education;
- health and safety.

Studying the job description thoroughly will enable you to confirm both your interest in this particular job and also the appropriateness of your application.

While no two job descriptions will be identical, they generally tend to include certain information. Box 8.2 shows a fictitious example that could help you to assess your current position and focus your preparation.

Box 8.2 A sample job description

Title: Qualified Nurse
Grade: Band 5
Reports to: Charge Nurse
Accountable to: Charge Nurse
Job summary: To be responsible for the assessment, planning, implementation and evaluation of evidence-based individualized programmes of care. The post-holder will also assist in the management and organization of nursing work in the ward/department.

Key responsibilities:

1 **Clinical/professional**

   1.1 To work within the code of professional practice, and within policies, procedures, and guidelines of the department.

   1.2 To ensure that high standards of nursing care are maintained and act when standards are not being maintained.

   1.3 To participate in the assessing, planning, implementation, and evaluation of individualized programmes of care.

   1.3 To recognize changes in clients' conditions that require the intervention of others and refer on as appropriate.

2 **Management/operational**

   2.1 To support the Charge Nurse in risk assessment and minimization.

   2.2 To manage verbal complaints, inform the Charge Nurse, and refer on when unable to resolve.

   2.3 To participate in the investigation of incidents/complaints as required.

   2.4 To establish and maintain effective communication within the multidisciplinary team.

   2.5 Have an awareness of team members' skills/capabilities and be able to delegate tasks appropriately.

   2.6 Act as an innovative and enthusiastic role model, providing leadership, guidance, and advice to staff on operational and professional issues.

3 **Education/training**

   3.1 To support the Charge Nurse in providing a suitable and effective learning environment for students.

   3.2 To take responsibility for own continuing professional development and performance.

   3.3 To support the development of other team members.

4 **Quality/research**

   4.1 Monitor and ensure that standards of care are maintained and that policies/procedures and protocols are adhered to.

   4.2 Ensure own practice is evidence-based.

   4.3 Contribute to and participate in programmes of audit, including utilization of results in practice.

   4.4 Support the Charge Nurse in aspects of patient and public involvement.

   4.5 Actively participate in benchmarking clinical practice along with other areas.

The person specification

The other key document is the person specification. Again, it is essential that you study this carefully to see what characteristics are either essential for the job or merely desirable. Table 8.2 shows a specimen person specification that includes some of the generic points often included in such documents. The main thing to recognize is the fundamental rationale behind such documents. They exist to help to ensure that the *right* candidates are placed in the *right* jobs. They are also incredibly helpful for you to clarify the role you are applying for, prepare appropriately, ensure that you meet the essential requirements, and ultimately ensure that you stand a good chance of being successful in your application.

The person specification has four main aspects, as follows.

1 The specific requirements of the post
2 The qualities, experience, and skills that the candidate *must* have to be even considered for further discussion at interview
3 The qualities, experience, and skills that the employer would *prefer* the candidate to have before they invite them for further discussion at interview

Table 8.2 Example of an NHS foundation trust person specification for a qualified nurse—Band 5

Requirements	Essential	Desirable	How identified
Qualifications	First-level registration		Application form Portfolio
Experience		Experience working in specialty	Application form Portfolio
Training	Willingness to take responsibility for own continuing professional development	Insight into issues of recruitment and selection	Interview
Special knowledge/ expertise	Knowledge of nursing conditions and treatments relating to specialty Knowledge of local and national initiatives	Venepuncture Knowledge of specific drug therapy related to specialty	Portfolio Interview
Disposition: adjustment, attitude, commitment	Approachable and supportive to support staff Positive attitude Ability to prioritize workload of self and others Flexible and adaptable Good interpersonal and communication skills		Interview
Practical/ intellectual skills	Ability to motivate staff Excellent written and verbal communication skills	IT skills	Application Interview
Attendance record	Ability to maintain a satisfactory level of attendance		References

4 The way in which these qualities and skills are to be identified: application form, portfolio, reference, or interview?

⊙ Theory into action

By using the example in Table 8.2 or a real person specification, work through each of the items in it, and note down a personal example that shows that your experience, skills, or personality fits closely with what is required.

Consider and write down how you would provide appropriate evidence that you fit these requirements.

Write your answers in proper sentences and say them out *aloud*.

How comfortable does it feel to say the words?

Imagine saying them for the first time in the stressful environment of an interview. The more you are able to rehearse, the more comfortable you should feel at the real interview.

Clearly, you must provide proof that you have all of the characteristics marked as essential if you are to be successful in the interview. If this proof is to be identified at the point of application, it is essential that you include such evidence/proof in your application form. If you do not include it, you will most likely fall at the first shortlisting hurdle. If you are not experienced enough for a job, then you might think 'fair enough', but imagine the greater disappointment of not being invited for interview simply because you had omitted to highlight your experience comprehensively, perhaps on the assumption that you might be offered the opportunity to further explore this at interview.

The person specification helps you either to confirm or discover what is really wanted for the role, allowing you to match your experience and skills to indicate to your prospective employer that you could do the job. So, if you lack some *essential* experience or skill, then considering that job application may be a waste of time; however, one area of weakness in the *desirable* column may not be devastating if you can 'wow' them on all of the others. Including examples of how quickly you have learned things in the past may offer reassurance that although you might not be as experienced as other applicants, you would be worth investing in (or taking a risk on!) because of all of the other excellent attributes that you would bring to the team.

If the job is not for a newly qualified staff nurse, there is little that you can do about that: this is simply not the job for you at this particular time. *However*, the effort you put in, and the preparation and thought invested in the application procedure, will certainly help when the right opportunity does come along. It is important not to *waste* valuable time, mindful of the effort and commitment that it takes to get a job—but continually considering your strong points and areas that you might need to develop may mean that you are ready when the next job comes along.

And, of course, the next job could always just be your ideal job!

Professional portfolios

As you can see from the above person specification, evidence of suitability is often provided by means of your professional portfolio. A key requirement of professional practice according to the UK's **Nursing and Midwifery Council** (NMC) is the continued development of specialist knowledge and competence to address new and ever-changing demands of the complexities of modern professional practice. This requires you to demonstrate responsibility for your own learning through the development of a portfolio of learning and practice, and to be able to recognize when further learning and development may be required. Your professional portfolio is an opportunity to showcase the professional skills and accomplishments that have been generated as part of your completion of your nursing course. Maintaining a professional portfolio is in the spirit of lifelong learning and reflective practice, and it is also habit-forming.

Even though an impressive and appropriately focused portfolio may not get you the job, it may well be the 'casting vote' if you are competing with other students for a particular job. There are no hard-and-fast rules as regards what a good portfolio should contain, but do make sure that the priority of the portfolio—that is, the key documents included—are related to the specific job for which you have applied and emphasize your suitability to take on this new exciting role.

Some other application tips

- Increasingly, applications are completed 'online' and if they do not offer the provision of spellcheck, take special care to verify that all of the information that you are providing has no spelling or punctuation errors.
- Consider sending a cover letter if possible. This can not only provide a general introduction and shed positive light on your personality, but also give you opportunity to include positive aspects about yourself that might not be appropriate to put in the job application itself.
- Always ensure that you give appropriate references. It will probably be expected that one reference/final summary is from your university. If you choose not to utilize your university reference, this will inevitably raise questions in the mind of the employer.
- Any further referees need to be chosen carefully. You need to know that they will be supportive and positive, and have insight into the requirements of the job being applied for to enable them to tailor their reference accordingly.
- Remember that you are applying for a professional post and the references need to reflect that. Your choice of referee may be a 'friend', but be aware that they are offering the reference in their professional capacity and not in their

capacity as a friend, and that this professional insight must be the main thrust of the reference.

- Remember also that it is common courtesy to inform a person before you use their name as a reference. You are risking the possibility of a less favourable reference if the request for a reference is a surprise to the referee!

Pre-interview

Consider ringing the contact person to confirm receipt of your application and discuss the key aspects of the job, as this shows interest and commitment. Imagine the scene during the shortlisting process: 'Well, this person never even bothered to contact me.' Obviously, *not* a good start! It is, however, essential to treat this step as an integral part of the application process and therefore to rehearse it carefully. It is also important to ring at the most appropriate time to catch the person at their best time, when they are most able to speak to you. This also indicates an appreciation of the circumstances of the ward, department, or work environment generally.

Your phone call may lead to an informal visit. If it does, again treat this as seriously as any part of the recruitment process. If the person interviewing is unable to speak to you, they may ask a trusted colleague to do so. However, rest assured that the interviewer is very likely to subsequently ask them their opinion and first impressions of you as a potential colleague. You may also want to consider a 'ghost visit' to the area. This means visiting unannounced as perhaps a member of the public would. What are your impressions of the place? Does it feel like somewhere that you might be happy to work? If there are staff there, do they look professional and supportive? If there are clients there, do they look content and supported? Although it would be rash to make a decision based solely on such a visit, it might be part of your overall decision-making process.

Word of warning: you are visiting an environment in which confidentiality is paramount and you are simply visiting the open access and public areas to gain a *flavour* of the environment. This is not a covert spying mission, and if you treat it as such, be prepared to be escorted from the premises by security and wave goodbye to any chance of employment.

....

➔ Theory into action

Many universities and placement providers give final-year students the opportunity to undertake practice job interviews. These can be very helpful, because you can receive some objective feedback in advance of a real interview.

If you do not have an opportunity to participate in these, do practise answering interview questions with a friend or by yourself so that you have rehearsed what you are going to say.

....

The interview

So the letter arrives inviting you for interview. How do you feel? Elated or full of trepidation? Enthusiastic or terrified? These emotions are totally understandable, but wasn't this why you applied for the job in the first place? It is perfectly normal to worry that you may go through all of the stress and anxiety of preparation for nothing. Coping with this anxiety is important, as interviewers can often detect it—and it inevitably affects your performance in a negative way. Try to think of your application as you doing someone a favour by being the person that they need to do the job.

The people who interview you are likely to be complete strangers, unless you are applying for a job in an organization in which you have already worked or have been a student. Interviews are just a common-sense way for people to find out about each other and ask each other questions. So, as well as the employer interviewing you, you also have the chance to make your own decisions about the employer, the job on offer, and the type of work environment, ward, or department, and so on.

Interviews are like examinations at the end of a course of study. You know that you have done well so far on the course and you know in advance roughly what areas the questions are going to cover. In the same way, you know that you have done well in the selection process up to this point or you would not have been invited for the interview. You also know in advance roughly what will be covered in the questions to be asked, because you have studied the details relating to the job. Similarly, most of the talking in the interview will be done by you and therefore you can have a fair measure of control over where the interview is going.

Of course, you cannot set the questions yourself, but you can calculate fairly accurately what subject areas will be covered and plan your answers accordingly. The only reason why you have been invited for interview is because the employer wants to find out more about you. You are not invited to be tricked, but to find out exactly who you are and how you would deal with certain situations likely to crop up in your job.

Key points

Remember employers are interested in three main areas:

- your qualifications and skills;
- your experience and work background;
- your personality and character.

The most important of these is personality and character, because skills can be taught and experience gained on the job.

Ten questions you might be asked

Note: these are in no particular order.

1 Why do you want this particular job?
2 What do you think your key strengths are?
3 What do you see as the major difference between your role as a student and as a qualified nurse?
4 What would you do if you were asked to do something that was beyond your level of competence?
5 What do you like least about nursing?
6 What would you expect from me as your charge nurse?
7 What would you do if you were to witness poor practice by a colleague?
8 What part of being a student did you find most difficult?
9 Caring for patients can be quite stressful. How do you manage stress?
10 What are you most proud of in your career so far?
11 How would you redesign a teddy bear?

Question 11 is a rogue! However, it indicates that you need to always be prepared for a question totally out of the blue. This might appear a little underhand, but may be used to see how you react. Remember that the employer wants a person to fill the post, so being purposefully obtuse and confusing is not the norm. Frightening tales of mind games being played by interviewers are usually simply rumours or urban myths . . . Although you never know!

Creating the best impression

It cannot be emphasized enough that first impressions are very important and that even though you will not get the job on image alone, it definitely helps. The impression that we give is based on so much more than just the words we speak. This first impression is based on appearance and behaviour generally, including clothing, posture, body language, and facial expressions.

Evidence seems to indicate that, with regards to first impressions, there is a '93 per cent rule'. What this means is:

- 55 per cent of the impression that we get is from appearance and body language;
  - 38 per cent is from the way in which a person speaks, including the way in which the voice is used, clarity of speech, and accent;
- *only 7 per cent is from the actual words that we say.*

This powerful realization is compounded by the fact that we are also highly affected by our visual impressions of others, particularly where quick decisions have to be made. Decisions with regards to a person's aptitude, friendliness, social status, education, politics, and even religion or sexuality have been shown to be made within the first one to two minutes of initial meeting. Some evidence indicates that these impressions are made even more quickly, in some respects even within seconds, and we underestimate this at our peril. The secret of success is in understanding how other people perceive you and using this information to your advantage by making sure that the impression you create works in your favour.

Some people may view the above observation cynically as another example of the inappropriateness of interviews as a fair and equal process. However, this is not about pretending to be someone else or putting on an act, but more about enhancing your strong points and minimizing your weaker ones. Your appearance is the most important aspect of the first impression that you create.

- A smart appearance shows that you have taken trouble over the way in which you want to come across and your choice of clothes indicates your attitude to yourself and to other people.
- Therefore it is probably best not to go to an interview in your uniform, as you may have thought of doing.
- Similarly, it is advisable to avoid wearing too much perfume and smoking, as this may trigger some allergies in the interviewer, and the smell of smoke not only emphasizes the habit, but also creates a very negative impression for some people—something that you most definitely do not want to do.
- It is advisable to arrive five to ten minutes before the scheduled time, as this gives time to relax and calmly consider your thoughts—you wish! Hopefully, you have also been able to visit the venue for the interview previously to give you one fewer thing to worry about and to work out the practicalities of getting there on the day. This preparation, along with arriving in good time, reduces anxiety. Arriving just prior to the scheduled time indicates appropriate self-confidence without putting undue extra pressure on the interviewer if you arrive too early.
- Whilst you are waiting, try to look relaxed, but 'busy': read a professional journal, or your set of potential questions, or your CV. If the interviewer accompanies the previous candidate to the waiting area, they will therefore be given a positive first impression.
- It is imperative that you bring *all* of your certificates and records as asked for in your interview confirmation letter. These may need to be photocopied and if you fail to bring them as requested, it gives a less-than-favourable impression with regards to your organization, preparedness, and even your ability to follow instructions. All of this might lose you crucial 'points' in the inevitably competitive job hunt.

When it is your turn, start off on a positive note by greeting the interviewer with direct eye contact and a firm handshake, and enter the interview room smiling naturally at all of the interviewers present. This approach indicates not only confidence and assertive-ness, but also a friendly and interested approach.

Sit well back in the chair *when invited to do so* and lean forward slightly giving the impression of just the right amount of keenness and interest. This position should also be comfortable, thus avoiding having to change your position too frequently, thereby distracting the listener from what you are saying. Equally distracting can be lots of hand movements, so you may want to consider clasping your hands lightly in your lap or rest-ing them on the arms of the chair. While gestures undoubtedly add variety to speech, too much gesturing can also imply anxiety and tension.

Practising interview techniques definitely brings rewards and instils confidence, so even though it might sound slightly bizarre to say 'practise sitting in a chair properly', give it a go. Hopefully, you will reap the rewards and you can then recount your funny and slightly embarrassing story to your new colleagues once you have been offered the job!

As mentioned above, you will be doing most of the talking in the interview and there-fore you might consider rehearsing some answers as well. It is very likely, for example, that you will be asked what you consider to be your strengths. Remember that you may not be asked in *exactly* those terms, but it is probably safe to assume that the under-pinning reason for asking at least one question will be to further explore your strengths and qualities. Therefore, as you already can take a good guess that this is going to be asked in some guise or other, it is a good idea to rehearse the aspects that will be inevi-tably included in your answer.

According to the person specification above, for example, you 'know' that you are going to be asked a question that is related to your 'ability to prioritize the workload of self and others'. Therefore an answer to such questions can, to an extent, be consid-ered and rehearsed. It is also effective to rehearse your answer *aloud*. Your answer may include comments such as:

> In my final placement I was lucky enough to be given the responsibility for the holistic care of a group of clients supported by my mentor. This included the appropriate delegation of aspects of care to a support worker. I found this experience very rewarding and confirmed to myself that I was able to ensure high-quality care by prioritizing not only my own workload but also the workload of others.

While this in no way attempts to be an ideal answer, it indicates certain areas that you might consider. If so, *literally* saying those or similar words for the very first time to complete strangers (or some might argue more stressfully to the charge nurse from the very placement you are describing!) when you are anxious, 'on show', and your mouth is a little dry, is not ideal. Therefore some level of rehearsal *may* help.

The STAR approach (Situation – *Task* – Action – *Result*)

The **STAR approach** is a technique that is sometimes used by interviewers to gather information about your capabilities and thereby your suitability for the job. It attempts to predict your future performance based on the past. An insight into this technique may help you to prepare prior to the interview.

Situation

You will be expected to present a recent challenge and situation in which you found yourself. These may be explicit, such as: 'Have you ever been in a clinical situation in which you were asked to do something you were unsure about? What did you do?' Or they may be less explicit and start: 'What would you do if . . .?'

Both of these examples offer you a chance to show evidence of how you would deal with situations you may come across in the job.

Task

What did you have to achieve in this situation? If, in all of your answers, the task as you broadly describe it was the maintenance of safe and quality care, you will not go far wrong. The interviewer wants someone *appropriately* confident, but *not* overly so. They want you to be an integral part of a functioning and supportive team, able to safety deliver high-quality care, but also mindful of your accountability and relative inexperience.

Action

What did you do and why? Where there alternatives and if so why did you reject them? If you are being interviewed by the charge nurse, for example, they will want to be reassured that you would be safe and competent, working in the best interest of the client at all times, especially in the change nurse's absence.

Results

What was the outcome? What did you learn from this experience and how might you use this learning in the future?

How to answer: some golden rules

- Always be honest. Perceptions of dishonesty or 'being economical with the truth' are bound to worry the interviewer, not least as it casts a doubt on *all* of your answers. Remember also that the NMC Code (2008) says: 'Be open and honest, act with integrity and uphold the reputation of your profession.'

- Always describe things in positive terms. If you are asked concerning a difficult or negative experience in your training, discuss this in terms of how you used the situation to learn and develop, and how you turned it into a more positive experience. If you speak of previous situations negatively, the interviewer will inevitably think that you will be likely to speak negatively of them or their team in the future. Anyone who creates a negative attitude will *always* be overlooked in preference to the positive and keen candidate. Moreover, nothing attracts people like enthusiasm, and working with someone who is positive and keen is exactly what an employer wants.
- Some experts advise that you should generally limit your answers to three statements, with each aspect sharing something about yourself. Such targeted and focused answers show that you are able to be thorough, succinct, and clear in your communication—an important part of your role as a qualified nurse.
- If you have been unable to show your knowledge during the course of the interview, this could be offered at the end of the interview. For example, 'I am aware of the importance of X new policy and if I were successful, I would be very keen to contribute to the team implementing that change', or 'I would be very excited by the opportunity to being part of this thrilling new initiative'.

At the end of the interview

It is advisable to have a couple of questions ready, as you will invariably be asked if you have any. This can cause anxiety in students applying for their first job, not least with regards to which questions to ask. The main rule is: only ask a question if it is necessary and appropriate rather than simply because you feel you ought to ask one.

Questions about training opportunities or the chance to take on greater responsibilities in the future show keenness and may indicate plans to stay in the job, whereas purposefully difficult, 'smart', or obtuse questions are a sure way *not* to get the job. It is interesting to consider that some interviewers may be slightly anxious themselves when conducting interviews and an interviewee who increases that anxiety is likely to be looked on unfavourably.

Avoid questions about holidays, uniforms, or any such practical questions. You can discuss those issues thoroughly after you have been offered the job. However, like many other aspects of the recruitment process, there are no absolute rights and wrongs in this. While admittedly you do not want to ask a question that might be difficult for your interviewer to answer and make them feel foolish, an insightful, articulate question may help you to stand out and indicates an interest and focus on the job. So the advice here is to go prepared with a question, but do not feel that you need to ask it if the circumstances do not feel necessary.

Finally, always thank the interviewers for their time and attention, and smile again before you leave on the same positive note. You may also consider writing a thank you letter as soon as possible after the interview, as this shows appreciation and highlights courtesy as a personal strength. You never know what the future might hold, and if you are not successful this time, you may be keen to be in a good position the next time an opportunity arises—especially if this was your 'dream job'.

Post-interview: What do I do now? How can I get the next one?

You need to develop strategies to support you through the potential ups and downs of the job-hunting roller coaster. It is quite easy, and to an extent inevitable, to feel that all of the hard work and commitment you have put in to achieving your qualification and registration is in itself deserving of a suitable job in the area in which you really want to work. Unfortunately, unless you are very lucky, it is likely that you are going to have to learn to cope with rejections.

This is why a personal support network is so important to help you to deal with and learn from the experience.

First of all, it is important *not* to take this rejection personally. Any job opportunity is likely to have attracted a number of applications and this is especially true at the end of your course, as many students are in exactly the same boat. You can improve your odds of getting a job by:

- getting feedback as soon as possible;
- reflecting on the feedback as objectively as possible (not easy especially immediately after the event);
- being very selective and applying only for jobs for which you are a very good match;
- using the techniques highlighted in the chapter that will give you that hidden advantage;
- being professional at each stage in the process;
- avoiding getting into a vicious spiral of an 'all or nothing' mentality whereby this feels as if the only appropriate job has now gone;
- getting the disappointment out of your system as soon as possible to ensure that you are in the best frame of mind to make the most of the next opportunity that comes along.

Summary

Being successful in applying for a job is far from simply good luck. There are genuine and *relatively* easy steps than can be taken to improve your chances. Some of the steps, both positive and negative, are reiterated in Table 8.3.

Table 8.3 Improving your chances for getting a job: common mistakes and reasons why applicants are successful

Some common mistakes	Some reasons for success
Lack of specific and focused preparation	Flexibility and caring and helpful attitude
Not answering the question fully or properly, e.g. answers too short or full of waffle	Positive attitude, especially in the face of challenges
Not showing any enthusiasm for the job	Enjoying working in a team
Not being clear about skills and abilities, i.e. too vague or too modest	Looking smart
Using jargon	Evidence of continual learning
Not showing full consideration of all aspects of the job, e.g. indicating a dislike for some key aspect of the role	Ability to handle change
Having an untidy appearance or too relaxed an attitude	Punctuality
Panicking	Ability to offer examples to highlight claims
	Use of endorsement of others, e.g. 'My mentor said . . .'
	Giving specific examples to show competence, adaptability, and expertise

Planning your career and making career decisions is clearly an important aspect of your life, but it essential that this is put into true perspective. Do not put so much pressure on yourself that it stops you from making any real choices, decisions, or plans, and *never* turn down an interview just because you are scared. Like someone once famously said: feel the fear and do it anyway.

In this chapter, we have looked at:

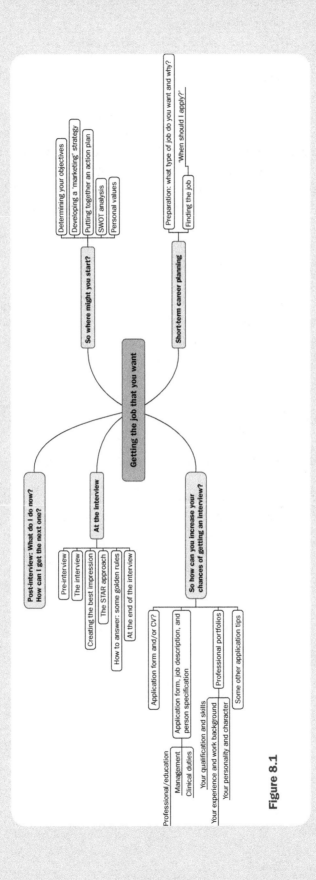

Figure 8.1

Online Resource Centre

 This textbook is accompanied by an Online Resource Centre that provides interactive learning resources and tools to help you to prepare for the transition from student to fully qualified member of staff. After you have completed each chapter and whenever you see this icon, please go to the ORC at your earliest convenience. If you have not done so already, save the ORC web address into your favourites: **http://www.oxfordtextbooks.co.uk/orc/burton**

References

Hood LJ (2010) *Leddy & Pepper's Conceptual Bases of Professional Nursing*, 7th edn. Lippincott, Williams & Wilkins, Philadelphia, PA.

Nursing and Midwifery Council (2008b) *The Code: Standards of Conduct, Performance and Ethics for Nurses and Midwives.* NMC, London.

Further reading

Eggert M (2003) *Perfect Interview: All You Need to Get it Right First Time*, 2nd edn. Random House, London.

Perkins G (2007) *Killer CVs & Hidden Approaches*, 3rd edn. Pearson Education, Edinburgh.

Yate MJ (2002) *Great Answers to Tough Interview Questions*, 5th edn. Kogan Page, London.

Preparation for personal and professional development

Val Ely and Rob Burton

The aims of this chapter are to:

- ➲ define and explore the concept of preceptorship to provide you with strategies to both seek and undertake preceptorship successfully following your qualification and registration as a nurse;

- ➲ define preceptorship, mentorship, and continuing professional development (CPD) in terms of determining their relationship to your professional role;

- ➲ define and explore the concept of CPD to ensure that you become a successful lifelong learner, in both your personal and professional practice, capable of planning your future career development;

- ➲ identify how preceptorship and CPD both form parts of the Nursing and Midwifery Council (NMC) emerging vision for revalidation;

- ➲ describe how CPD can assist you in your career development as envisaged in *Modernising Nursing Careers* (Department of Health, 2006) and (DH, 2010);

- ➲ explain how credit gained from formally accredited CPD activity can contribute to your future academic qualifications;

- ➲ highlight some strategies useful for your personal and professional development planning and life **coaching**.

Introduction

This chapter will examine the issues of personal and professional development from the point of qualification, initial registration, and beyond. The Chief Nursing Officer for England has recognized that the transition from student nurse to registered nurse is a 'challenging time for new nurses' (Department of Health, 2009: 4). **Preceptorship** is the key vehicle to help newly qualified and registered nurses to deal with this transition phase.

Preceptorship follows **mentorship** experienced by the student nurse during their pre-registration nursing education. As will be seen in this chapter, the elements of preceptorship include the individual newly registered nurse taking responsibility for their own personal and professional development and then embarking on a process of life-long learning. This, from the outset, makes the connection from pre-registration nursing education and training to 'lifelong learning', which is referred to by regulatory bodies as **continuing professional development (CPD)**, or as it can also be referred to in the nursing and health professional context, **learning beyond registration (LBR)**. However, a further link exists as the **Nursing and Midwifery Council** (NMC, 2010) has determined that preceptorship and CPD are crucial elements to its emerging policy on the **revalidation** process as does the Department of Health (2006, 2010) in terms of career development within *Modernising Nursing Careers* (**MNC**).

Therefore, to assist those nurses nearing registration or those who are newly registered, this chapter explores personal and professional development in the context of preceptorship, mentorship, and CPD. We will also discuss some personal and professional development planning approaches related to coaching and goal-setting, which you may use during your career beyond initial registration.

Definition of preceptorship

....

 Thinking about

As you approach qualification as a nurse, note down how you would define the term 'preceptorship'.

....

The Department of Health (2009) reviewed many definitions of the term 'preceptorship' when developing its preceptorship framework. Key definitions include:

> A foundation period [of preceptorship] for nurses at the start of their careers which will help them begin the journey from novice to expert.
> DH (2008A: 19)

> A period [of preceptorship] to guide and support all newly qualified nurses to make the transition from student to develop their practice further.
> NMC (2006: 1)

However, for the purposes of this chapter, our preferred definition of preceptorship for the Department of Health (2009: 11) framework is:

> A period of transition for the newly registered nurse during which time he or she will be supported by a preceptor, to develop their confidence as an autonomous professional, refine skills, values and behaviours and to continue on their journey of life-long learning.

 Thinking about

Now that you have read the above definitions, which definition do you prefer in terms of your aspirations for your impending period of preceptorship? It will be useful to write down your own definition of this term so that you can negotiate your learning needs and styles when your period of preceptorship begins.

Preceptorship in nursing

The current NMC preceptorship guidelines were published in 2006. These guidelines strongly recommend a period of preceptorship, on entering registered practice for the first time, entering a new part of the NMC register, or for those prepared as nurses abroad. This guidance addresses the role of the newly registered nurse, often referred to as the **preceptee**, and the member of staff who supports them during this period, the **preceptor**, the one-year recommended length for the period of preceptorship and the preparation requirements for preceptors. More recently, the NMC has commissioned research into its preceptorship policy, which demonstrates that this will be a constantly developing and changing approach in your nursing career; you will need to keep up to date with any changes as they occur in future, as you may be delivering preceptorship to others.

To confirm its commitment to preceptorship, indicated in **MNC** (DH, 2006) and underlined by the Department of Health (2008a), in 2008–09, the Department provided funding to strategic health authorities to support this initiative. As pre-registration nursing education moves to degree-level education, the Department (2009) asserts that support for a different type of preceptorship will be needed to enable the professional development of newly registered and graduate nurses.

So preceptorship is confirmed as an important activity in which you will be involved immediately following your qualification and registration as a nurse. In addition, as a 'preceptor' of the future, you are likely to provide preceptorship to many other newly registered colleagues.

Benefits of preceptorship in nursing

The Department of Health (2009) has outlined the benefits of preceptorship to:

- patients/clients;
- the newly registered nurse (preceptee);
- their employer;
- the preceptor;
- the nursing profession.

Ultimately, the goal of preceptorship is the provision of safe and effective nursing care to patients/clients by the newly registered, but still accountable, nurse. In keeping with the purpose of this book, it is worth taking this opportunity to focus on its key benefits for the newly registered nurse.

 Thinking about

Thinking ahead to your role as a qualified nurse, how would preceptorship benefit you both personally and professionally?

Threaded through the list of benefits identified by the Department (2009) are issues important for personal and professional development. The newly registered nurse can expect preceptorship to:

- result in respect and feeling valued by both team colleagues and their organization as a whole;
- ensure competence in their field of employed practice, resulting in greater confidence and as such linking with the principles of *Confidence in Caring* (DH, 2008b);
- increase their job satisfaction and organizational pride, as the preceptee is much more likely to understand both their team and their organization's corporate strategy and objectives;
- enable the preceptee to apply to their **field of practice** their understandings of the legal, ethical, professional, and regulatory body requirements gained from pre-registration nursing education;
- foster a personal responsibility for maintaining and developing knowledge and competence;
- grasp the evidence base and apply it to their new area of practice;
- identify and address their learning needs through onward CPD;
- result in accelerated progression through two pay increments for those organizations operating *Agenda for Change* (DH, 2004a).

In keeping with this, the Department (2009) recommends that the means of recording preceptorship should be congruent with the NHS Knowledge and Skills Framework (KSF) (DH, 2004b), your appraisal process, regulatory body CPD principles, and future NMC revalidation requirements. These will all be discussed in this chapter.

⊖ **Theory into action**

> Refer to your list above. Are there any similarities or differences to the benefits of preceptorship identified by the DH (2009)? If so, it might be helpful to amend your list so that you can share with your preceptor from the outset how you hope preceptorship can benefit you.

Implementing preceptorship

The Department of Health (2009) believes that its work with key stakeholders thus far has provided tentative indications that good preceptorship comprises two key elements. However, it acknowledges that these indications are yet untested. Nevertheless, the two key elements of good preceptorship seem to be a combination of:

- core theoretically based learning activities, whether taught, blended, or distance learning;
- supervision/guided reflection on practice.

The Department (2009) further suggests that the **core theoretically based learning activities** provided should be between four and six days in length, with the **supervised/ guided reflection of practice** taking around 18 hours to undertake.

⊖ **Theory into action**

> Does four/six days of core theoretically based learning activities and 18 hours of supervised/guided reflection of practice seem appropriate for you to meet your preceptorship needs? If not, consider how you will justify needing more or less than these suggested time periods. The following discussion may help you to decide.

According to the Department (2009: 18), the suggested learning methods for its recommended key preceptorship elements include:

- organizationally based preceptorship, e.g.:
  - ○ action learning sets;
  - ○ self-directed learning;

- o clinical practice focus days;
- o reflective practice;
- o shadowing;
- o one-to-one support (in person or remotely/electronically);
- preceptorship facilitated in partnership with universities that is delivered through an academically accredited programme—work-based learning, e.g. portfolio-building;
- web-based/blended learning programmes, e.g.:
  - o 'Flying Start England' (**http://www.flyingstartengland.nhs.uk/**);
  - o 'Flying Start Scotland (**http://www.flyingstart.scot.nhs.uk/**);
- attitudinal and behavioural-based learning, e.g. through role modelling.

⊖ Theory into action

What learning methods would you prefer to use? Does this help you to identify the learning activities and time that you will need for your period of preceptorship?

As we move from examining preceptorship towards exploring CPD, we will see how similar learning opportunities and strategies are available for personal and professional development. Thus good preceptorship is vital for establishing a pattern of successful lifelong learning and CPD.

The relationship between preceptorship, mentorship, and CPD

As a newly qualified and registered nurse, you will have experienced **mentorship** throughout your pre-registration nursing education. The NMC (2008a: 1) stipulates that:

> Students on NMC approved pre-registration nursing education programmes, leading to registration on the nurses' part of the register must be supported and assessed by mentors.

Furthermore, if you have undertaken your pre-registration nursing education after September 2007, you will have had a **sign-off mentor**. The NMC (2008a) states that the sign-off mentor, who has fulfilled additional criteria in their mentor training, must make the final assessment of a student's practice to ensure that the required proficiencies for entry to the NMC register have been achieved.

An immediate difference between preceptorship and mentorship seems to be clearly visible. As we have read in this chapter, preceptorship is only 'strongly recommended' by the NMC—that is, it is not compulsory. Mentorship, on the other hand, is a compulsory NMC requirement within pre-registration nursing education programmes. However, the likelihood is that all employers will require their newly registered and appointed staff to undergo the preceptorship process despite it not being made compulsory by the NMC.

Preceptorship, mentorship, and CPD are closely linked, as we will discuss in this chapter. To become a mentor, the NMC (2008a) requires that nurses have developed their own knowledge, skills, and competence beyond that determined at the point of initial registration. The vehicle for achieving this will first be preceptorship and then CPD. Equally, to become a preceptor and/or mentor, you will undertake a course to prepare you for this role. This will be part of your CPD, so again a link is established between preceptorship, mentorship, and CPD. The course will be accredited if provided by a university, so you may be able to count this towards a higher academic award. More discussion with examples will be provided on CPD and academic accreditation later in this chapter. Finally, as preceptors, mentors, and indeed NMC registrants, nurses must keep their knowledge and competence up to date. This is required by the NMC (2008b) Code, thus establishing once again the relationship between preceptorship, mentorship, and CPD.

Definition of the term 'continuing professional development' in nursing

As with preceptorship, there are a number of ways of defining CPD within the differing professional contexts to which the term applies. However, the Department of Health (2003) asserts that CPD encompasses a:

> wide range of learning activities through which professionals maintain and develop throughout their career to ensure that they retain their capacity to practise safely, effectively and legally within their evolving scope of practice.
>
> DH (2003: 9)

CPD requirements in nursing: current post-registration education and practice (Prep) requirements

The NMC stipulates its current CPD requirements for nurses within *The Prep Handbook* (NMC, 2008c), which comprises two standards.

The Prep CPD standard

The NMC (2008c: 11) states that the Prep CPD standard is about CPD of registered nurses. To meet it, nurses must:

- undertake at least 35 hours of learning activity relevant to their practice every three years;
- maintain a personal professional profile of their learning activity;
- comply with any requests to audit how they have met these requirements.

Given the variety of nursing practices, the NMC has no requirements regarding compulsory courses, nor does it accredit courses as being approved for CPD purposes.

The Prep practice standard

In order to meet the Prep practice standard, nurses must have undertaken a set amount of registered practice in their capacity as a nurse. This set amount comprises 450 hours at any point over a three-year period. However, as this standard is beyond the scope of this chapter, no further discussion will be included on this practice standard. Re-registration with the NMC requires compliance with the NMC Prep CPD standard discussed above.

....

 Theory into action

> Visit **http://www.nmc-uk.org**, and navigate to and read the current *Prep Handbook*.

....

Recording your Prep CPD

In terms of recording CPD in a personal professional profile, the NMC (2008c) recommends a format as shown in Box 9.1. It is important to understand that this is only a suggested template and that individuals are free to design and use their own approach. It is probably sensible, though, to include the recording prompts recommended by the NMC as a minimum dataset in any other format that a nurse may choose for their personal professional profile. The important point here is to record each of your learning activities; the format chosen for your record is of less importance. Some learning activities may be sensibly documented in one record. The NMC (2008c) suggests that a series of workshops attended could be an example of an instance in which it may be better to combine such learning activities into one record.

Box 9.1 The NMC suggested template for recording evidence of CPD learning in a personal professional portfolio, with advice for those preparing this document

Prep (CPD) period (the three-year registration period to which this learning applies)

From: *To:*

In this part of the document, recording the re-registration period in question might not be as relevant since the NMC has changed the three-year cycle of re-registration to an annual process. Nevertheless, recording the date of your personal professional profile entry is important.

Workplace – Where were you working when the learning activity took place?

Name of organization:

Enter the name of the organization at the time you were actually employed.

Brief description of your work/role

This part of the document deals effectively with your practice as a nurse in terms of your employment. This section may also be synonymous with your cv, but perhaps your personal professional profile allows more space to record your respective practice posts and employers. The NMC (2008c: 14) has provided examples of the work or role, which include the following:

1 If you are working with people in your care

2 If you are working in healthcare education

3 If you are working in healthcare research

4 If you are working in the management or administration of health care

5 If you are working in areas not directly related to health care such as consultancy

6 If you are not working, for example due to maternity leave, long-term ill health, carer's leave, or if you are retired

It is recommended that you include a brief description of your work role, but, for expediency, a written job description could be included in your personal professional profile instead. Certainly for those employed in the NHS, *Agenda for Change* has ensured that everyone has a job description for each role (DH, 2004a). Other employers mostly provide job descriptions too and generic documents could be personalized to reflect the actual role undertaken in more detail.

Nature of the learning activity

Date:

The date of the learning activity.

Briefly describe the learning activity: for example, reading a relevant clinical article, attending a course, observing practice, reading latest NMC guidance, discussing with a colleague a relevant clinical article.

State how many hours this took:

This section allows for factual information to be recorded about the learning experience itself including the activity type, date, and hours of learning undertaken.

Box 9.1 (continued)

Description of learning activity (of what did it consist?)

Describe what the learning activity consisted of – include for example: why you decided to do the learning activity or how the opportunity came about; where, when, and how you did the learning activity; the type of learning activity; and what you expected to gain from it.

This part of the document allows you to provide details of the learning activity, but this advice suggests many more types of CPD learning activity that you might undertake. Other CPD activities could include those suggested by the **Health Professions Council** (**HPC**) on its website for its registrants, as given below.

Work-based learning
- Learning by doing
- Case studies
- Reflective practice
- **Clinical audit**
- Coaching from others
- Discussions with colleagues
- Peer review
- Gaining, and learning from, experience
- Involvement in the wider work of employer (e.g. being a representative on a committee)
- Work shadowing
- Secondments
- Job rotation
- Journal club
- In-service training
- Supervising staff or students
- Visiting other departments and reporting back
- Expanding your role
- Analysing significant events
- Filling in self-assessment questionnaires
- Project work or project management
- Evidence of learning activities undertaken as part of your progression on the KSF (DH, 2004b)

Professional activity
- Involvement in a professional body
- Membership of a specialist interest group
- Lecturing or teaching
- Mentoring
- Being an examiner
- Being a tutor
- Branch meetings
- Organizing journal clubs or other specialist groups
- Maintaining or developing specialist skills
- Being an expert witness
- Membership of other professional bodies or groups
- Giving presentations at conferences
- Organizing accredited courses
- Supervising research
- Being a national assessor
- Being promoted

Formal/educational
- Courses
- Further education
- Research
- Attending conferences
- Writing articles or papers
- Going to seminars
- Distance learning

Box 9.1 (continued)

- Courses accredited by a professional body
- Planning or running a course

Self-directed learning

- Reading journals/articles
- Reviewing books or articles
- Updating knowledge through the Internet or television

- Keeping a file of your progress

Other

- Public service
- Voluntary work
- Courses

(See **http://www.hpc-uk.org/registrants/cpd/activities/**)

As you can see, any activity that involves learning, and as a result developing your practice, constitutes CPD. Therefore it is not possible to produce an exhaustive list of CPD learning opportunities. If the learning undertaken was a formal learning experience such as a course, conference, or study session, again it could be expedient to include in a personal professional profile the printed details of the event from the education provider. While CPD is not solely or required to be about undertaking formal learning events and acquiring certificates, retaining such information is useful.

Outcome of the learning activity (how did the learning relate to your work?)

Give a personal view of how the learning informed and influenced your work. What effect has this learning had on the way in which you work, or intend to work in the future? Do you have any ideas or plans for any follow-up learning?

'The way in which this learning has influenced my work . . .'

This last part of the document provides an opportunity to evaluate the learning experience in more detail. The NMC (2008c) specifies that this section is about what was learned from the CPD activity rather than just describing the learning event itself. The NMC (2008c) recommends that you should record how the learning related to your work and the effect that it has had on the way in which you work or intend to work. Particularly, this evaluation of learning needs to identify the type and content of future learning which might also link to action planning, your appraisal with your employer, or your personal/professional development plan linked to your role. A systematic approach to this process could be assisted by the use of a model for reflection, such as Gibbs (1998) or Johns (2004). As far as the NMC (2008c) is concerned, the key reflection necessary is the way in which this learning has influenced your work. Rolfe et al.'s (2001) model of reflection springs to mind as being useful because it prompts the reflector, in terms of a CPD learning activity, to consider the following.

- **What** (about the learning activity)?
- **So what** (about the learning activity in terms of my practice)?
- **Now what** (in terms of my future learning and practice needs)?

As discussed above, undertaking and recording CPD can be linked both to the appraisal process and to personal development planning. However, another recommendation in terms

---

Box 9.1 (continued)

of career planning is to link your individual CPD to the **NHS KSF** (DH, 2004b), particularly for those employed where this tool is utilized. The KSF is designed to:

- **identify the knowledge and skills that individuals need to apply in their post;**
- **help to guide the development of individuals;**
- **provide a fair and objective framework on which to base review and development for all staff;**
- **provide the basis of pay progression in the service.**

Use of the KSF in terms of planning, undertaking, and recording CPD will also be helpful because the DH White Paper (2007a) indicates that the NHS KSF will be used to provide the basis for revalidation. Revalidation is discussed later in this chapter.

The NMC (2008c) *Prep Handbook* provides a number of case studies as examples of how CPD learning activities can be both undertaken and documented using the structure it suggests. The NMC has included both structured and unstructured learning activities, divided into categories so that you can refer to the example most applicable to your practice situation. The case studies have been drawn from:

- acute care;
- midwifery;
- community/primary care;
- education and research;
- management;
- practising in other areas to cover those:
  - ○ not working, but using structured or formal learning;
  - ○ working, but not in professional practice, using unstructured or informal learning;
  - ○ working, but not in health care, using structured or formal learning.

CPD and compliance with the Prep CPD standard

The NMC has a number of statutory duties placed on it by legislation. One such duty is to ensure that the standards it sets for registrants are upheld. The Prep CPD standard is no exception. Therefore the NMC has devised a two-part system to ensure that registrants comply with the Prep standards.

The first part of the system affects everyone registered by the NMC. Each time a nurse re-registers, a **notification of practice (NOP) form** must be completed to declare compliance with the Prep CPD and Prep practice standard.

The second part of the system is the **Prep audit** whereby the NMC audits compliance with the Prep CPD standard. Nurses on a randomly selected basis might be asked to provide the NMC with brief evidence of their learning activities since their last re-registration point. This brief evidence should be provided on the **NMC CPD summary form**. At this point, the NMC does not want to view an individual registrant's personal professional portfolio, but if there is any doubt about an individual's Prep (CPD) summary form, the NMC will write to seek further clarification.

CPD and its place in professional regulation, accountability, and clinical governance

CPD and the current NMC Code (2008b)

The current Code (NMC, 2008b) stipulates that a registered nurse must:

> Provide a high standard of practice and care at all times.
>
> NMC (2008B: 4)

To ensure that this is provided, the NMC further requires of each nurse that they (2008b: 4):
- 'Use the best available evidence':
  - you must deliver care based on the best available evidence or best practice;
  - you must ensure that any advice you give is evidence-based if you are suggesting healthcare products or services;
  - you must ensure that the use of complementary or alternative therapies is safe and in the best interests of those in your care.
- 'Keep your skills and knowledge up to date':
  - you must have the knowledge and skills for safe and effective practice when working without direct supervision;
  - you must recognize and work within the limits of your competence;
  - you must keep your knowledge and skills up to date throughout your working life;
  - you must take part in appropriate learning and practice activities that maintain and develop your competence and performance.

It is interesting to note that this section of the NMC (2008b) Code does not include the term 'continuing professional development', nor indeed does it include this term in its entirety. However, for the nurse to fulfil the professional and statutory requirements laid down in the Code, CPD is an essential means of complying with it.

Other aspects of the Code clearly raise ongoing CPD implications. These implications may arise as a result of changes in healthcare treatments, the evidence base, and healthcare policy and legislation.

CPD and the NMC (2008b) Code: an example

A current example of how CPD can assist nurses to develop their practice and comply with the Code is provided here in relation to **patient consent**. The Code requires all nurses to 'ensure you gain consent' before any examination, treatment or care processes are undertaken (NMC, 2008b: 2). In addition to that statement, the NMC stipulates that nurses:

> must be aware of the legislation regarding mental capacity, ensuring that people who lack capacity remain at the centre of decision making and are fully safeguarded.
>
> NMC (2008B: 2)

Recent legal developments in the field of mental capacity for adults will mean that many nurses have CPD requirements to fulfil in relation to this aspect of their practice. In terms of safeguarding adults, a key piece of legislation is the **Mental Capacity Act 2005**. This legislation has been in force since April 2005 and came into effect in 2007. This Act created statutory provision for the protection of vulnerable adults, their carers, and the professionals who look after them. It clarifies, for instance, who can take decisions in terms of consent in identified situations and how these decisions should be determined and recorded. A key tenet of this Act is the fundamental point that a person has capacity unless determined otherwise and that all practical steps must be taken to help the person to provide consent. Therefore, since 2005, nurses working with adults have needed to understand the implications of this Act to their practice. A further amendment to the Mental Capacity Act 2005, entitled the Deprivation of Liberty Safeguards (formerly known as the **Bournewood Safeguards**), were introduced into the 2005 Act through the **Mental Health Act 2007** (DH, 2007b). The Mental Capacity Act Deprivation of Liberty Safeguards (MCADOLS) cover adults who lack mental capacity and for whom deprivation of liberty, within the meaning of section 5 of the **Human Rights Act 1998**, is considered after an independent assessment has deemed it necessary in their best interests to protect them from harm. The MCADOLS apply to all such adults in hospital, community setting, or registered care homes. Therefore nurses in these settings working with such patients need to be fully familiar with these safeguards. The means of achieving knowledge and understanding in relation to both the Mental Capacity Act and the Deprivation of Liberty Safeguards is by undertaking and providing evidence of relevant CPD. Recording evidence of CPD undertaken is important for many reasons. A key point to consider is that if decisions taken by a nurse in relation to mental capacity and/or deprivation of liberty were called into the question, so too might be the competence of that nurse. Therefore being able to provide a record of related CPD could assist in demonstrating that the nurse had taken reasonable steps to ensure that their knowledge and competence in this legislative area was kept up to date. We will provide an illustration on the means of undertaking CPD as well as other reasons for recording such activity later in the chapter.

CPD and revalidation

CPD is envisaged to become a key element of revalidation. Revalidation was first formalized by the Department of Health (2007a). The Department noted that previous and traditional systems of professional regulation saw individual health professionals, such as nurses, being deemed fit to practise for life following their initial professional qualification. Such individuals were registered with a professional or statutory body and remained on that register without having to demonstrate ongoing **fitness to practise** through CPD. Their place on the register was held on trust by society throughout their careers. This trust largely had its origins in social deference from the public and patients towards professionals and authority. However, the Department (2007a) also notes that, since the Second World War, a much greater informed and assertive public now increasingly rejects passive acceptance of authority and unquestioning obedience to establishments such as hospitals and professions such as medicine and nursing.

One of the reasons that the public is likely to challenge authority in health care is greater access to information that was once in the sole domain of healthcare professionals through the media and, within the past decade, the Internet. High-profile cases, particularly nationally within the last couple of decades, have challenged beliefs about the future of professional regulation for both the public and professions concerned. Such high-profile cases include those centred on the professional behaviour and conduct of enrolled nurse Beverley Allitt and Drs Harold Shipman, Richard Neale, Clifford Ayling, William Kerr, and Michael Haslam.

The Bristol Royal Infirmary and Alder Hey inquiries, as well as more recently the headlines from Maidstone and Tunbridge Wells Hospitals and the Mid Staffordshire Hospitals, revealed that many patients died due to both individual and organizational failings. In a more deferent age, such individual and collective failings might have escaped both public and media scrutiny. However, today, no such 'hiding place' exists, and the public has demanded that their politicians act.

The White Paper *Trust, Assurance and Safety: The Regulation of Health Professionals in the 21st Century*, presented before Parliament in 2007, seeks to implement new arrangements for professional regulation. Where individual healthcare professionals are concerned, professional regulation will introduce revalidation across all disciplines. Revalidation will require that individuals demonstrate periodically their continuous fitness to practise. In turn, a key requisite of revalidation will be CPD. However, ironically, surveys of public opinion indicate their belief that health professionals are already undergoing CPD and revalidation of their professional registration at least annually. More recently, the Department of Health (2008c) has set out principles for non-medical revalidation. CPD is included as principle 5. Here, the Department stipulates that CPD is:

> the process by which individual registrants keep themselves up to date with healthcare developments in order to maintain the highest standards of

professional practice. It should be seen as an integral part of revalidation and may provide supporting evidence that a practitioner submits to the regulatory body for consideration at the time of revalidation judgement. CPD needs to be relevant to the practitioner's scope of practise, where such scope has been defined.

DH (2008C: 12)

The NMC and other healthcare regulators, in response to the DH non-medical revalidation principles (DH, 2008c), began their response to the government White Paper (DH, 2007a), of which the first part was to set up a project in 2009 examining revalidation in nursing, taking into account:

- new areas of practice;
- specialist practice;
- advanced practice;
- non-medical prescribing;
- new ways of working.

This project also considered:

- introducing mandatory preceptorship;
- building an evidence base for a model of revalidation;
- undertaking an interim review of the Prep Standards.

The initial revalidation project identified five stage one findings. These include, in relation to revalidation:

- risk;
- appraisal;
- preceptorship;
- remediation;
- evidence.

To conclude this discussion on revalidation, while the NMC (2010a) undertakes stage two of its revalidation project as well as concludes its review of pre-registration nursing education (NMC, 2010b), issues of mentorship, preceptorship, and CPD remain dynamic. Therefore the nurse needs to keep aware of changes made to these important processes, which relate to their practice.

⊖ Theory into action

Visit **http://www.nmc-uk.org**, and navigate to and read the pages on revalidation and the pre-registration nursing education standards. Discuss with other nurses in your team what this will mean in terms of mentorship, preceptorship, and CPD.

CPD and clinical governance

According to Scally and Donaldson (1998), CPD is a vital component of clinical governance. The Royal College of Nursing (2009) agrees by asserting that integral to clinical governance is an initially trained and educated workforce, which is further developed through learning derived from CPD. The Department of Health (2007a) indicates that CPD is likely to be managed through the appraisal process, which again is a core component of clinical governance.

 Theory into action

> Examine the clinical governance policy in your employing organization and determine
> what it requires in terms of your CPD and whether it will be managed by your appraisal.

CPD and the interdisciplinary context

Other healthcare professional groups are now required to undertake CPD as a means of demonstrating fitness for re-registration. Allied health professionals have been required to meet the Health Professions Council (HPC, 2006) CPD standards. More recently, pharmacists are also required to meet such standards (Royal Pharmaceutical Society of Great Britain, 2009). Undertaking CPD with other professional groups is extremely valuable. As patient/client care involves an interdisciplinary approach, then it follows that CPD should involve joint learning to further develop the practice provided by all team members to their patient/client group. Equally, sharing resources from professional, statutory, and regulatory bodies related to CPD will be very useful to any healthcare professional and assist in maximizing resources. Joint CPD is indeed a learning activity itself if the outcome is a greater understanding of roles in the teams by the different disciplines.

 Theory into action

> Consider how you could undertake CPD with other professional groups in your practice
> area. Highlight the advantages and disadvantages.

CPD and *Modernising Nursing Careers*

The Department of Health (2010), through **MNC**, has provided a tool to assist the nurse in their career planning using the NHS Careers Framework. This tool is in the form of a segmented wheel diagram and recognizes that nurses no longer work mainly in hospitals. Indeed, their work may be beyond the NHS in the private, voluntary, and charitable sector, as well as social care.

A career in nursing could take a nurse into many different practice settings, such as:

- people's homes;
- community clinics;
- workplaces;
- schools;
- prisons;
- nursing homes;
- rehabilitation centres.

The tool also asserts that the nurse could provide care in many different identified pathway areas comprising:

- family and public health;
- acute and critical care;
- supporting long-term care;
- mental health and psychosocial care;
- first contact, access and urgent care.

The tool illustrates that, for each of these pathway areas, the nurse's career may be within the following contexts:

- research;
- education;
- management;
- clinical.

Finally, MNC indicates how nurses may use this tool to visualize not only their career pathways, but also their academic development. This leads us into reviewing how CPD can link to academic development.

CPD and academic accreditation

Your pre-registration nursing qualification is likely to have been academically accredited. This means that, in addition to qualifying as a nurse, you have achieved an academic qualification from a higher education institution (HEI) or university. This qualification is usually a diploma in higher education or a degree with or without honours. As discussed earlier, CPD can be undertaken in many forms and does not have to be associated with an academically accredited learning activity. This is, as we have already seen, is particularly underlined by the NMC (2008c) Prep CPD standard.

However, if some of your CPD is undertaken as an academically accredited learning activity, you may wish to consider whether you can or wish to use any of the academic credit gained towards a higher academic qualification relevant to your practice. Indeed, as pre-registration nursing education moves to become a graduate profession, the Department of Health (2006) recognizes that existing non-graduate nurses may wish to 'top up' their existing pre-registration nursing qualification from a diploma to a degree.

To manage your academic development, it is important to have some understanding of the higher education qualification and credit infrastructure. The **Quality Assurance Agency** for Higher Education (the QAA) has a national framework for higher education qualifications (QAA, 2008). This qualifications framework with academic levels is summarized in Table 9.1. There are three undergraduate levels (levels 4–6) and two postgraduate levels (levels 7–8). Levels 1–3 are within the preceding National Qualifications Framework and the Qualifications and Credit Framework (NQF/QCF).

The crucial point to bear in mind with the National Qualifications Framework is that the QAA (2008) sets out descriptors for the achievement of qualifications at each of its levels. These descriptors are usually written as learning outcomes for each overall qualification. HEIs that deliver these qualifications may use credit points to organize the delivery of their qualifications, but the QAA (2008) does not insist on such a system. If credit points are used, then they are usually attached to modules, which

Table 9.1 The QAA (2008) National Framework for higher education qualifications

Typical higher education qualification	Level
Doctoral, e.g. PhD	8
Master's, e.g. MSc or MA Postgraduate diplomas Postgraduate certificates	7
Bachelor's degrees with honours, e.g. BA/BSc (Hons) Bachelor's degrees qualifications Graduate diplomas Graduate certificates	6
Foundation degrees e.g. FdA, FdSc Diplomas of higher education (DipHE) Higher national diplomas (HND)	5
Higher national certificates (HNC) Certificates of higher education (CertHE)	4

then in turn form the overall academic qualification. Therefore, formal CPD learning activities that you undertake could provide, on successful completion, academic credits at a determined level. It may be useful to consider prior to undertaking such a learning activity whether the level of the credit enables you to complete a higher academic qualification.

Example

Referring to Table 9.1, if you already have a diploma in higher education (level 5), following the completion of your pre-registration nurse education, you may only choose to study academically accredited courses at the minimum of level 6 in order to progress towards an higher academic qualification.

In terms of accumulating academic credits, you then may wish to consider how you could transfer these credits towards a higher academic qualification. This requires using the **Credit Accumulation Transfer Scheme** (**CATS**). Therefore, you need to bear in mind how many credits you are accumulating and how many credits an academic award comprises in total. Another consideration is how the modules studied match the learning outcomes of a specific qualification towards which you may wish to transfer credit. The means of claiming credit using the CAT scheme is by the **accreditation of prior learning** (**APL**). This allows relevant formal and experiential learning to be claimed.

In order to successfully manage your academic development, it is best to seek advice from appropriate academic staff. It may also be useful to plan your academic development within your appraisal. Finally, it may be useful to identify whether the formal learning activities that you undertake are related to the KSF.

Personal and professional development planning and coaching

So far in this chapter, we have explored formal requirements and mechanisms that you may face as a newly qualified nurse. It is now appropriate to look at more informal, yet nonetheless worthwhile, strategies for your own development. The following section helps you to identify your needs and set goals, so that, as you embark on your career as a qualified nurse, you have some idea of a pathway for your future. This might mean identifying how to survive this initial period or to make longer-term plans and identify the steps needed to get there. These will be useful as a basis for your discussions with your preceptor or superiors in your workplace. It may also be helpful as a basis for the time when you might be the preceptor or coach for another newly qualified nurse.

Coaching

Henwood and Lister (2009) suggest that, in the modern world of health care, change is a constant and initial training, plus CPD is not always enough to deal with this. Staff need to be able to care for themselves. Coaching helps an individual to prepare for other aspects related to healthcare professional development such as preceptorship, mentoring, CPD, clinical supervision, and appraisal. Your preceptor may be able to assist you by using coaching techniques, which are increasingly used in professional careers. Coaching is not about giving advice; it is more about facilitating and pointing the individual in the direction in which they desire to go.

Machon (2010) suggests that coaching is about assisting individuals in relation to self-awareness, clarification of goals, expanding awareness around the goal, and focusing on how the goal can be met. Buckingham and Clifton (2005) suggest that strengths are an important factor in personal development, which relates to the awareness aspects suggested by Machon (2010). By recognizing your strengths, you can identify the patterns that you employ within them and make use of them by transferring them to other areas. In other words, by tying your strengths into your goals, you are able to shift the focus and perceptions of any problem and develop solutions or areas that you can develop more easily.

Self-awareness and goal-setting

Having another person act as a coach is very beneficial. However, as most of the approaches are facilitative, there are some of the aspects that you can initiate yourself. The most simple premise related to goal-setting is to state the goal in the positive— that is, to state what you actually want as opposed to what you don't want. Quite often, when problems occur, they are issues we don't want and individuals often think that the goal is to 'not have the problem anymore'; however, the real approach is to state what we actually want instead. When searching on a website, we often quickly get to the pages we want by stating the aspect we are searching for in clear terms. The more refined and specific our terms are, the more successful the search is. O'Connor (1998) suggests that we should ask the following questions.

- What is important to us? (Values)
- What do we want to accomplish? (Purpose)
- How do we want to accomplish it? (Goals, capabilities, resources, and strategy)

These aspects are similar to the concept of **logical levels** highlighted within the field of personal development known as **neuro-linguistic programming** (**NLP**—Roberts, 2006). Logical levels refer to the concept that individuals psychologically operate on a number of levels. In a similar way to Maslow's hierarchy of needs, the lower levels give

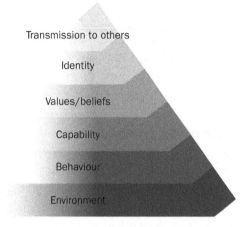

Figure 9.1 Logical levels

rise to the higher levels. Goals can be set in relation to the level at which the development is needed. The logical levels are shown in Figure 9.1.

The logical levels are **environment**, **behaviours**, **capabilities**, **beliefs/values**, and **identity** (Dilts & Epstein, 1995). Each level feeds into the one above, so in relation to setting goals for your development, you can ask further questions such as the following.

- In what environment do I want/need to work?
- What behaviours do I need to develop?
- What capabilities would I need?
- What are my values?
- What would that say about me?
- What kind of a person/nurse do I want to be?

These questions could alternatively be considered as follows.

- Where do I want to be?
- What do I want to do?
- How do I want to do it?
- Why do I want to do it?
- Who will I become?

Your situation can be analysed at each level to identify goals that would impact upon them. Bavister and Vickers (2005) suggest that this can be like a ripple effect and that changes at one level can have changes at a number of levels. For example, if an environment becomes contaminated, behaviour has to change as a result and so on. Therefore there is a need to understand what is happening at each level. Roberts (2006) suggests that these levels define understanding, which influences our thoughts and solutions in the world around us. In order to develop pertinent personal development questions as nurses, then, we can simply frame them in relation to the levels.

From these questions, we can set goals. This could be something as simple as: 'I want to work in intensive care environments.'

 Thinking about

Identify a list of issues with which you feel you would like preceptorship. Which of the logical levels do they fit in with: environment, behaviour, capability, values or identity?
Now set a positively stated goal (what you would actually want to achieve) for each one.

It is useful to note that if you get 'stuck' at one level, then you can look at the one below in order to set goals that will lead you to the higher level. For example, if it is a **capability** or skill that you feel you need to develop, then you might need to break the goal down into **behavioural** steps that build up the skill in order to master it.

According to Egan (2002), the basic premise of personal development planning or individual change goes through a process of understanding where you are now (**present state**) to where you want to be, or your goal (**desired state**), and how you intend to get there (**resources**). The goals that you set should be analysed and broken down into the various steps or stages that will take you through to the final process of achieving them. For example, if your desire is to become a nurse manager, then a smaller step might be to attend a management course. To get on a management course, your goal might be to seek out information on relevant management courses.

The discussion above has introduced the concept of setting outcomes that are relevant to your personal and professional development. By being able to create outcomes and identify resources, you can go into preceptorship, mentorship, clinical supervision, or appraisal armed with clear goals to discuss with your superiors, or in some cases your peers, and in doing so identify your CPD requirements. Being forearmed in such a way sends a clear message that you have well-formed ideas about your career development.

Personal and professional development planning will be an important part of your career. It will be something that occurs constantly and can be useful to you in your career as a nurse.

Summary

This chapter has focused on the aspects that you will need to consider in relation to your own development once you have become a qualified nurse. We have looked at issues related to what you can expect from a period of preceptorship and how to be involved in, and manage, this for yourself.

We discussed the CPD and the NMC requirements that you need to meet in order to continue to maintain your registration as a nurse with the NMC. The discussion has outlined some strategies and considerations that should assist you to do this. Remember, becoming a qualified nurse is not the end of your educational journey throughout your nursing career. You could liken it to having completed your driving test. You have met the required standard and are considered safe to drive. However, once functioning in the real world as a practitioner in your own right, you continue to learn how to operate and get used to everyday or unusual circumstances, just as you have to learn how to get used to driving without someone else providing you with instruction and supervision. So, really, it is just the beginning of a new phase. This means that you make lots of decisions. The difference from the driving analogy, however, as highlighted in this chapter, is that you can expect some guidance and supervision from a preceptor on qualifying. There should always be someone to whom you can turn for advice in these early transitional stages.

The need for continuing professional development is a requirement to demonstrate that you are up to date with current practices and that you continue to be safe to practise, and therefore deserve the right to continue being a registered nurse. The arenas in which nurses work are constantly changing, and you need to be able to change with the environments and approaches that are used in providing such a valuable public service.

Lastly, it is important to remember that this is your career. Therefore personal development planning is important in that it assists you to align your CPD to the plans that you might make as your career develops. You may need to be able to set short-term goals to identify how you can develop in relation to the area in which you may work, or longer-term goals to assist you to move in a desired career direction of your choice.

- **Preceptorship** is important in your transition to working as a qualified nurse.
- It is required to ensure the provision of safe and effective care whilst you are in this transition.
- It helps you to apply and develop your skills, knowledge, and confidence in your given field of practice.
- **CPD** is important in ensuring that you keep up to date with developing practice.
- It is a requirement to maintain your registration.
- **Personal development planning** assists in clarifying needs and goals.
- It helps to clarify your career direction and aspirations.

In this chapter, we have looked at:

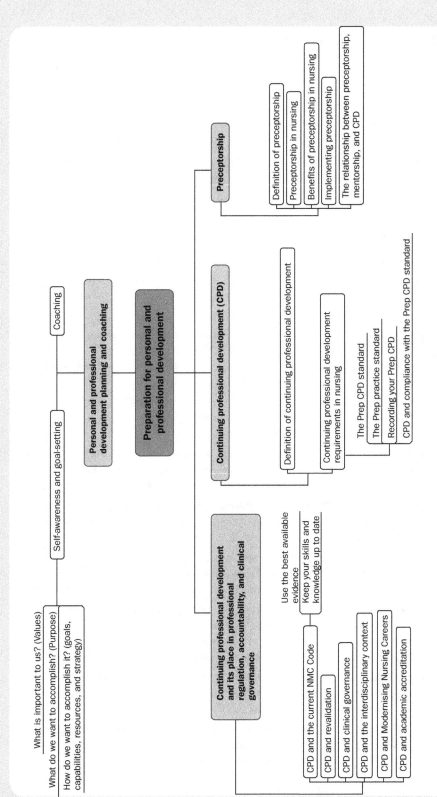

Figure 9.2

Online Resource Centre

 This textbook is accompanied by an Online Resource Centre that provides interactive learning resources and tools to help you to prepare for the transition from student to fully qualified member of staff. After you have completed each chapter and whenever you see this icon, please go to the ORC at your earliest convenience. If you have not done so already, save the ORC web address into your favourites: http://www.oxfordtextbooks.co.uk/orc/burton

References

Bavister S & Vickers A (2005) *Teach Yourself NLP*. Hodder Education, London.

Buckingham M & Clifton DO (2005) *Now, Discover your Strengths: How to Develop Your Talents and Those of the People You Manage*. Pocket Books, London.

Department of Health (2003) *Allied Health Professions Project: Demonstrating Competence Through Continuing Professional Development [CPD]—Final Report*. DH, London. Available at: http://www.dh.gov.uk/prod_consum_dh/groups/dh_digitalassets/@dh/@en/documents/digitalasset/dh_4067120.pdf

Department of Health (2004a) *Agenda for Change: Final Agreement*. DH, London. Available at: http://www.dh.gov.uk/en/Publicationsandstatistics/Publications/PublicationsPolicyAndGuidance/DH_4095943

Department of Health (2004b) *The NHS Knowledge and Skills Framework (NHS KSF) and the Development Review Process*. DH, London. Available at: http://www.dh.gov.uk/en/Publicationsandstatistics/Publications/PublicationsPolicyAndGuidance/DH_4090843

Department of Health (2006) *Modernising Nursing Careers: Setting the Direction*. DH, London. Available at: http://www.dh.gov.uk/prod_consum_dh/groups/dh_digitalassets/@dh/@en/documents/digitalasset/dh_4138757.pdf

Department of Health (2007a) *Trust, Assurance and Safety: The Regulation of Health Professionals in the 21st Century*. DH, London. Available at: http://www.dh.gov.uk/en/Publicationsandstatistics/Publications/PublicationsPolicyAndGuidance/DH_065946

Department of Health (2007b) *The Mental Capacity Act Deprivation of Liberty Safeguards*. DH, London. Available at: http://webarchive.nationalarchives.gov.uk/+/www.dh.gov.uk/en/SocialCare/Deliveringadultsocialcare/MentalCapacity/MentalCapacityActDeprivationofLibertySafeguards/index.htm

Department of Health (2008a) *A High Quality Workforce: NHS Next Stage Review*. DH, London. Available at: http://www.dh.gov.uk/en/Publicationsandstatistics/Publications/PublicationsPolicyAndGuidance/DH_085840

Department of Health (2008b) *Confidence in Caring: A Framework for Best Practice*. DH, London. Available at: http://www.dh.gov.uk/prod_consum_dh/groups/dh_digitalassets/@dh/@en/documents/digitalasset/dh_086388.pdf

Department of Health (2008c) *Principles for Revalidation: Report of the Working Group for Non-medical Revalidation.* DH, London. Available at: **http://www.dh.gov.uk/en/ Publicationsandstatistics/Publications/PublicationsPolicyAndGuidance/DH_091111** (accessed 20 June 2010).

Department of Health (2009) *Preceptorship Framework for Nursing.* DH, London. Available at: **http://www.dh.gov.uk/prod_consum_dh/groups/dh_digitalassets/@dh/@en/@ abous/documents/digitalasset/dh_109794.pdf**

Department of Health (2010) *Modernising Nursing Careers: Care for Your Future in Nursing.* DH, London. Available at: **http://www.dh.gov.uk/prod_consum_dh/groups/dh_ digitalassets/documents/digitalasset/dh_108369.pdf**

Dilts R & Epstein T (1995) *Dynamic Learning.* Meta Publications, Capitola, CA.

Egan G (2002) *The Skilled Helper: A Problem-management and Opportunity-development Approach to Helping,* 7th edn. Brooks Cole, Pacific Grove, CA.

Gibbs J (1998) *Realising Clinical Effectiveness and Clinical Governance Through Clinical Supervision Practitioner, Book 1.* Radcliffe Medical Press, RCN Institute, Oxford.

Health Professions Council (2006) *Continuing Professional Development and Your Registration.* Health Professions Council, London.

Henwood S & Lister J (2009) *NLP and Coaching for Healthcare Professionals.* John Wiley & Sons, Chichester.

Johns C (2004) *Becoming a Reflective Practitioner: A Reflective and Holistic Approach to Clinical Nursing, Practice Development, and Clinical Supervision,* 2nd edn. Blackwell Publishing, Oxford.

Machon A (2010) *The Coaching Secret: How to be an Exceptional Coach.* Pearson Education, Harlow.

Nursing and Midwifery Council (2006) *Preceptorship Guidelines,* NMC Circular 21/2006. NMC, London. Available at: **http://www.nmc-uk.org/Documents/Circulars/2006%20 circulars/NMC%20circular%2021_2006.pdf**

Nursing and Midwifery Council (2008a) *Standards to Support Learning and Assessment in Practice.* NMC, London. Available at: **http://www.nmc-uk.org/Documents/Standards/ nmcStandardsToSupportLearningAndAssessmentInPractice.pdf**

Nursing and Midwifery Council (2008b) *The Code: Standards of Conduct, Performance and Ethics for Nurses and Midwives.* NMC, London. Available at: **http://www.nmc-uk.org/ Nurses-and-midwives/The-code/**

Nursing and Midwifery Council (2008c) *The PREP Handbook.* NMC, London. Available at: **http://www.nmc-uk.org/Educators/Standards-for-education/The-Prep-handbook/**

Nursing and Midwifery Council (2010a) *Revalidation.* NMC, London. Available at: **http:// www.nmc-uk.org/About-us/Policy-and-public-affairs/Politics-and-parliament/Policy- areas/Revalidation/**

Nursing and Midwifery Council (2010b) *Review of Pre-registration Nursing Education (Phase 2).* NMC, London. Available at: **http://www.nmc-uk.org/Get-involved/Consultations/ Past-consultations/By-year/Review-of-pre-registration-nursing-education/**

O'Connor J (1998) *Leading with NLP.* Thorsons, London.

Quality Assurance Agency for Higher Education (2008) *The Framework for Higher Education Qualifications for England, Wales and Northern Ireland.* QAA, Gloucester. Available at: **http://www.qaa.ac.uk/academicinfrastructure/FHEQ/EWNI08/FHEQ08.pdf**

Roberts M (2006) *Change Management Excellence: Putting NLP to Work*, revised edition. Crown House Publishing, Wales.

Rolfe G, Freshwater D & Jasper M (2001) *Critical Reflection for Nursing and the Helping Professions.* Palgrave, Basingstoke.

Royal College of Nursing (2009) *Clinical Governance.* RCN, London. Available at: **http://www.rcn.org.uk/development/practice/clinical_governance**

Royal Pharmaceutical Society of Great Britain (2009) *Professional Standards and Guidance for Continuing Professional Development.* Royal Pharmaceutical Society of Great Britain, London. Available at: **http://www.rpsgb.org/pdfs/coepsgcpd.pdf**

Scally G & Donaldson LJ (1998) Clinical governance and the drive for quality improvement in the new NHS in England. *British Medical Journal,* **317**: 61–5.

Preparing for qualification: putting it all together

Rob Burton and Graham Ormrod

The aims of this chapter are to:

➲ consolidate the topics discussed in Chapters 1–9 in order to enhance your understanding of the roles and responsibilities of a newly qualified nurse;

➲ draw together the underpinning theories and explore how they are connected and related to each other by applying them to practice;

➲ explore the common challenges experienced by the newly qualified nurse and give you guidance on how to manage them.

Introduction

As highlighted in the preceding chapters of this book, while the role of a newly qualified nurse is complex and challenging, it is also rewarding and fulfilling. Hopefully, you are now ready to start this new period of your career, in which the benefits of your hard work, and your hopes, plans, and aspirations, will come to fruition. You are now, finally, about to become a registered nurse.

The preceding chapters will have helped you to clarify and confirm the roles and responsibilities of a registered nurse, such as:

- maintaining standards in the workplace;
- making decisions (accountable, ethical, and legal);
- teamworking;
- teaching and **mentoring** others;
- being in charge.

You should have gained insight and awareness into your current preparedness, and been able to recognize areas requiring further development. You will have also recognized where you might choose to invest your efforts and prioritize your time to ensure that you get the job that your commitment and hard work so richly deserves. There has also been scope to investigate the nature of your continuing personal and professional development.

This final chapter is an occasion to revisit some of the key learning opportunities that have been previously highlighted. We will look at how all of the complex and occasionally confusing aspects of professional practice can be brought together to ensure that you are appropriately confident and ready to take on the role of a qualified nurse. This should help to guarantee that you are fit for purpose as a nurse ready for registration. The aspects of a nurse's roles listed above may have been addressed as separate issues, however, in the real-world setting, everyday situations are not compartmentalized in such a way. You are not able to think 'I'll do the decision-making bit', then 'Now I'll do the teamworking bit', followed by 'Now I'll think about the leadership aspects'. All of these are inherent in each and every situation that you will face as a registered nurse. Therefore it is essential to recognize the interplay and interconnected nature of the concepts involved in your nursing practice.

First of all, it is important to be aware that some nervousness and anxiety are inevitable at this point. Consideration of what the future might hold and your preparedness for this are understandable and to be expected. Anyone about to embark on their new career who says that they have no hint of uneasiness is either being a little untruthful or profoundly lacking in self-awareness. Such overconfidence should also probably worry any future employer, as the potential employee will be implying that they have little or nothing left to learn. It is almost a truism to say that no one applies for a position or role for which they are already totally competent, and in the ever-changing professional context, reflection, self-awareness, and the grasping of the ethos of lifelong learning should be encouraged. This understandable nervousness is hopefully also coupled with a genuine enthusiasm and excitement at the career step that you are about to take.

What it means to be a front-line member of staff

According to the terms of reference for the *Front Line Care* report (Commission for Nursing and Midwifery, or CNM, 2010: 2), it was the report's aim:

> to identify the competencies, skills and support that front line nurses and midwives need to take a central role in the design and delivery of 21st century services for those that are sick, and to promote health and wellbeing.

This report highlights the need for nurses to ensure delivery of high-quality care in changing situations and environments, and places an emphasis on the development and leadership aspects of nursing. There is an importance placed on measuring outcomes and making sure that standards are met, as well as the innovation and promotion of nursing itself. The previous chapters in this book covered such aspects to raise your awareness of the complexities of each of these activities. Now, we will show you how these are brought together in everyday practice as we revisit some of the scenarios from earlier chapters and analyse them in relation to all of these activities.

Common issues faced by newly qualified nurses

As mentioned previously in Chapter 1, Mooney (2007) pointed out that the duties faced by most newly qualified nurses did not necessarily involve service user contact. Indeed, at this time, you may find yourself with more duties that relate to contacting and dealing with other professionals and services. Others may now expect you to provide the advice, guidance, and answers in some very complex situations. We have already emphasized that you should have a **preceptor** on qualifying to aid you through these transitions; however, the literature suggests there are still likely to be difficulties in this transition process and that, on occasions, you may have to face and take responsibility for some of these challenging issues (DH, 2009). As Gerrish (2000) points out, individual accountability, managerial responsibilities, delegating duties, and managing clinical situations such as death and dying may be some of the things with which qualifying nurses have to deal.

Let us revisit the thoughts of a newly qualified learning disability nurse from Chapter 1:

> When I qualified I went to work in a group home (registered nursing) for seven adults with learning disabilities and complex needs. Once there, I was often the shift leader and found that most of the challenging issues that I faced were related to managing the shift team. As the only qualified nurse on shift, delegation of duties was to unqualified staff; many of whom had worked within the home and/or company for several years. I had to overcome a significant age difference in conjunction with my newly qualified status—'proving my worth' was my most difficult task.

This nurse identifies some of the leadership and management skills required of a nurse when they take charge as a shift leader. These skills, as suggested by Gerrish (2000), include managing the team and delegating duties. Managing the care of seven individuals in any setting requires appropriate teamwork in order to make sure that all standards of care are met. There is a need to be aware of the relevant standards and

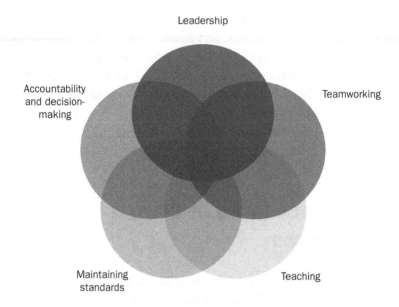

Figure 10.1 The overlapping concepts that newly qualified nurses face

be accountable for their implementation. This requires decision-making based on the knowledge of legal, ethical, and professional principles. Delegation needs firm leadership awareness, while also recognizing that the accountability still rests with those delegating. There may also be some practices or skills that need to be taught to the junior staff, as discussed in detail in the preceding chapters. Now, it is important to gain an overview of how all of these aspects contribute to successfully managing different situations. There is no line where leadership stops and management starts, or where accountability stops and maintaining standards start, or where teamwork stops and teaching starts. These concepts overlap. Awareness of this in such situations gives you scope to draw on your knowledge and skills and find alternatives that can help you to develop the best solutions available to you, as seen in Figure 10.1.

Scenario 10.1: responding to a medication error

Scenario 10.1 demonstrates an alarming and worrying, but all too common, occurrence that can happen in differing kinds of healthcare service (Brady et al., 2009).

As we have discussed, the leadership issues in Scenario 10.1 can be related to the leadership *styles* required in dealing with the situation (Marquis & Huston, 2009). Some authoritarian steps may need to be taken in dealing with the immediate issue of ensuring that the patient is safe. There are transactional leadership or transformational

Scenario 10.1

On arriving on duty, you find that you are the shift leader. On inspection, you find that the nurse (who has just completed a consecutive run of five night shifts) has made a medication error. This, fortunately, has not resulted in any harm to a patient.

From the brief information that you have in the above scenario, what do you consider to be the leadership priorities? What issues are there in relation to accountability? What elements might be considered important for teamworking? What actions do you need to take in relation to maintaining standards?

leadership considerations (Judge & Bono, 2000) to be made in how to approach the member of staff. Should you use sanctions or suggestions? Although you will not be directly involved in the human resource aspects of the care environment, you will still need to alert your senior colleagues to the situation, identifying any human resource factors that may have contributed to it. It is likely that you will be closest to the patient, and this will ensure that both junior and senior colleagues will view you as the prime information-holder (Phillips, 2005).

Clearly, there are also significant aspects of quality and clinical governance. As highlighted in Chapter 2, the complex aspects of risk management are the responsibility of all involved in the care of the patient (Healy & Spencer, 2007). This relates to your responsibilities in the processes of maintaining standards, including passing on and recording information accurately, and the subsequent steps taken. Lewis and Henderson (2000) emphasize that teams need collaboration, coordination, and communication with regards to issues of skill mix and accountability. A nurse having completed five nights might not be a good reflection of a positive team approach. The solving of this problem may need a team meeting of all staff to resolve it, as there may be fundamental issues that are beyond the scope of one qualified nurse to change on their own. The nurse in question and even the rest of the team may need to be involved in further training or instruction on the safe ways of medicine management in the workplace. Here, your skills of teaching may be put to the test, along with your understanding of learning styles and teaching approaches that are best suited to the learners, the topic, and the environment (Quinn & Hughes, 2007).

Scenario 10.2: delivering an evidence-based nursing teaching session

To continue on the notion of teaching and learning, once you are qualified, there will be an expectation that you not only contribute to the teaching of patients and their families, but also the development of junior nurses and the supervision and associate mentoring or full mentoring of student nurses. Clearly, you will be expected to utilize **evidence-based practice** in such instances. Providing instruction, demonstrations, and education is a recognized part of your role (NMC, 2010). Although most of this will take place informally, there may be occasions on which you are asked to do this in a more formal setting.

Scenario 10.2

Your charge nurse has set up a series of lunchtime seminars for the multidisciplinary team in your care area and you have been asked to fill one of the slots in two weeks' time as someone has backed out. You are given freedom to choose whatever relevant topic you want. How would you approach this to make it relevant and beneficial for the whole interprofessional team?

The most important factor involved in this is the need to plan thoroughly (Quinn & Hughes, 2007). This may include canvassing the staff team to find out what relevant topics they might be interested in. Getting to know what is on the rest of the programme is also important to avoid duplication or repetition. It would be good practice to attend similar seminars if possible to get a 'feel' for the environment, the topics, and the approaches taken. Muijs and Reynolds (2005) suggest that understanding the 'climate' of a learning environment is important. This relates to the general relationship dynamics in the setting. For example, how formal would it be? Is it likely to be a didactic session in which you are required to 'lecture' and provide information, or is it more likely to be an interactive environment in which you can act as a facilitator and create discussion? It is also essential to confirm what resources will be available, and as Race (2001) suggests, carefully check that all equipment needed is present, available, and in working order.

In the session itself, you will need to present up-to-date, evidence-based information. Maben and Griffiths (2008) highlight that part of the essential contribution you make to good nursing care is to ensure that you are knowledgeable and skilled and possess up-to-date knowledge. This ensures that standards for good practice can be identified and met. It also confirms your accountability to the NMC (2008b) that you must deliver care based on the best and current available evidence and practice. Such sessions can help to develop collaborative teamworking approaches to care. Handy (1999) suggests that they can help to develop motivation and joint working towards an organization's goals, and that being provided with such opportunities lends itself to more positive group cohesion, raised staff morale, and improved working relationships.

Scenario 10.3: professional behaviour

The maintenance of professional behaviour in the workplace is something with which you may have to deal on a regular basis. In order to qualify as a nurse, there is a requirement to have a statement of good character provided at the end of your course. The NMC (2009) suggests that good character is based on a person's conduct, behaviour, and attitude. Treating people as individuals with respect and integrity, and upholding the reputation of your profession is paramount. Obviously, more extreme examples, such as violence, criminal activity, and dishonesty, may be more easily identified, and may be managed in a relatively straightforward way due to clearly defined policies and laws. Similarly, there are sometimes situations in which professional behaviours are absent or demonstrated in behaviours such as rudeness to clients, colleagues, or others with persistent inappropriate attitudes or behaviour, such as poor communication skills and failure to accept and follow advice. However, it is also important to realize that, as a qualified nurse, you have a responsibility to manage situations and behaviours that are not always as explicit and with aspects that can be difficult to define or demonstrate.

Scenario 10.3

You are working with a third-year student while visiting a group of clients in a community nursing caseload. While conducting an assessment of a client, you notice that the student is distracted and disengaged. You note that she is using her mobile phone to send texts.

What professional issues are raised in this scenario? How would you deal with this situation?

Scenario 10.3 is clearly an example of inappropriate behaviour in which you may need to employ several strategies in order to fully address it. For example, it would appear to be appropriate to quietly and politely advise the student to put away the phone and to refocus on the client. In doing so, the student should be reminded that the client is their first concern, demonstrating dignity and respect. This would again be an example of adopting an authoritarian leadership style. It would also be important to remind the student that the NMC (2009) emphasizes that all students conduct themselves professionally at all times in order to justify the trust that the public places in the nursing profession. Such discussions should take place away from the immediate care environment to ensure confidentiality and fairness. This also relates to both your and their accountability.

You might conduct a tutorial with the student at a specified time during which you facilitate their understanding of the NMC (2009) guidance on conduct for student nurses and the NMC Code of Conduct (NMC, 2008b). Setting objectives, with an action plan related to the standards of **proficiency** in their portfolio, could be undertaken as a formative assessment. This particularly relates to the ethical and professional practice domain. The incident would also need to be reported to their mentor, including the actions taken and the student's response to the situation. Passing on information in such a circumstance helps to promote teamwork as it ensures that all involved are apprised of the situation (Doyle, 2008). However, working in community services might mean taking on more of a lone role, in which case, you need to communicate with the student's mentor and teachers if further action is needed.

Scenario 10.4: writing a staff rota

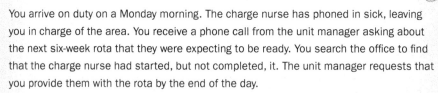

Scenario 10.4

You arrive on duty on a Monday morning. The charge nurse has phoned in sick, leaving you in charge of the area. You receive a phone call from the unit manager asking about the next six-week rota that they were expecting to be ready. You search the office to find that the charge nurse had started, but not completed, it. The unit manager requests that you provide them with the rota by the end of the day.

What do you need to do now that the responsibility to complete this task has fallen on you?

Although this scenario is very likely to raise anxiety and might be described as fundamentally unfair, it does indicate the need for all staff to recognize how the various aspects of an organization link together and how the management of an individual unit inevitably impacts in some way on the wider needs of the organization. This highlights the complexity and variety of the teams within which nurses work and confirms that healthcare systems require significant and varied resources to ensure that patients receive appropriate services and high-quality care. Similarly, it highlights the need for robust managerial leadership and clear recognition and understanding of accountability in relation to quality, patient safety, and risk management.

Clinical governance is fundamentally concerned with the *culture* of an organization and it would be legitimate to investigate whether such a situation had occurred previously. While the formulation of duty rotas might well be an appropriate development opportunity in the context of lifelong learning and professional development for a junior member of staff, it requires appropriate planning and supportive facilitation rather than simply having to deliver in such a pressured and acute situation.

Such a situation will give you opportunity to recognize the skills and insights that you have gained from your experience on the unit. As always, the safety of patients is paramount and it would be appropriate to negotiate time to complete this task if necessary. However, you will have gained awareness of the needs and requirements of those for whom you are caring and you may be very well placed to complete the rota recognizing both the client dependency and the requisite skill mix. This will also offer you the opportunity to call on the support and experience of colleagues, both to ensure the safe running of the unit and to contribute ideas and thoughts to complete the rota.

A note on the scenarios

The scenarios above provide a glimpse into some of the complex situations that you may face as a qualified nurse. The underpinning theories discussed throughout this book apply to them all. By raising your awareness of the theories, concepts, models, strategies, and approaches, you should be able to gain further understanding of the various aspects of nursing practice that you need to consider in solving such problems.

The above examples have not been field-specific, as they relate to principles that nurses in all settings and disciplines will recognize as familiar. Neither have we attempted to investigate all of the situations that you may face, or provided answers to such. Rather, we have given you a flavour of the kinds of situation in which you may find yourself and with which you may have to deal as a qualified nurse. Do remember that once you are a qualified nurse, you will gain experience in such situations; you will have someone to turn to for help, or at least you will be able to find some reference within this book or others that may provide you with insight into solving problems you may encounter.

Conclusion: putting it all together

We have covered with differing approaches the professional skills of maintaining standards of care, making ethical and legal decisions, being accountable, teamworking, teaching others, and being in charge. All of these are aspects of the role that you will undertake as a qualified nurse. It is necessary to reiterate for a final time that there is a certain amount of overlap in these concepts and you may be taking decisions and actions in day-to-day practice that are influenced by the concepts discussed.

This book has explored the 'quality agenda', the expectations of the public, and the changing responsibilities and expectations of nurses in maintaining standards and ensuring quality of care. Health care is seen as a partnership between health professionals and patients, and nurses, already accountable, will be scrutinized more closely in relation to various clinical outcomes—nurses may well be judged against such measures as nursing metrics. We have emphasized that nurses have a key role as **advocates** for patients and in their lead role within the multidisciplinary team. This may mean being involved in certain ethical dilemmas from time to time.

The use of an ethical framework can assist you in engaging in 'principled discussion' and subsequent actions; being aware of the principles of **autonomy, beneficence, non-maleficence,** and justice may help you to formulate solutions and inform your decision-making in relation to such challenging dilemmas. As discussed in scenarios within this chapter and elsewhere in this book, respect for individuals is the underpinning moral and ethical principle that informs current healthcare practice and the law. The essential concept of **informed consent** and **capacity** are reinforced throughout the book—once you qualify, it is imperative that you stay up to date with developments in relevant laws and their implications for your practice. We have discussed the differences in the accountability of students and registered nurses in practice—and don't forget, soon you will be the nurse and students will ask you: 'Can I do this?'

The importance of teamwork in health care has been highlighted, including what teamwork is and what the ingredients of an effective team are. We have emphasized that, during their career, nurses can work in a huge range of different types of team, so they will always need teamworking skills as well as the skills required to overcome the potential problems of teamworking!

The concepts of teaching and mentoring will be an important aspect of your role as a qualified nurse and we have explored the NMC standards (NMC, 2008a) about the nature of teaching, learning, and assessment in practice. Recognizing the individual learning needs and styles of students and junior staff provides a basis to develop appropriate strategies to meet their educational needs, including assessing and giving feedback.

You may soon find yourself in charge after qualifying. The major leadership theories, such as trait, style, situational, transactional, and transformational, have been discussed earlier in the book. In addition, some of the scenarios in this chapter have highlighted the fact that you need to be aware of these so that you can be flexible in your response to workplace situations in which you find yourself. Leadership is related to your people skills and your ability to observe the situation, identify problems, and create solutions. You need to be seen to be taking action, leading by example, evidence, and commitment, being involved and participating in the tasks that you would expect others to do. The concept of being a manager may seem to be some distance away for you in your career when you first become a qualified nurse. However, we have emphasized that awareness of theories of management can assist you by describing how organizational goals are aligned and your part in the strategies that are put in place to realize them. Management is about formal mechanisms in the day-to-day running of services, and following the policies and procedures set in place by your employing organization and profession. You may find yourself formally dealing with colleagues at all levels of an organization and have responsibility for reporting situations from the ground or 'coalface' level of service provision.

Within the book, we have also provided some advice for you to consider once qualified, so don't give this book away just yet! Chapter 6 includes ways in which to develop an effective CV and strategies for performing well in interview to get the jobs that you want, for the career that you want. Over the coming years, continuing professional development will be very important to you, and we have provided some advice on how you can meet these requirements.

A final note

Although there are many overlapping complexities in the theories and scenarios presented in this book and in the various issues that you may face as a qualified nurse, essentially nursing is an engaging and fulfilling profession. You may reflect on your reasons for entering the nursing profession and remember what made you take those first steps. It may have been a necessity that led you to nursing or a vocational drive. Whatever the reason, you can be assured that although a career in nursing is challenging, and at times stressful, you will find that it is a wonderful privilege to care for people in a variety of dynamic and exciting environments, in a professional field that is constantly changing and developing, yet highly publicly valued. We know that you will be glad of the efforts you put in when you attain your goals. We wish you the very best for your future as a qualified nurse.

Rob and Graham

Summary

The transition to qualified nurse:

- is challenging yet rewarding;
- is complex, yet principle-based;
- incorporates the application of all of the concepts previously discussed in earlier chapters;
- requires support and input across the whole interdisciplinary team;
- takes place in dynamic environments;
- is worth the journey.

In this chapter, we have looked at:

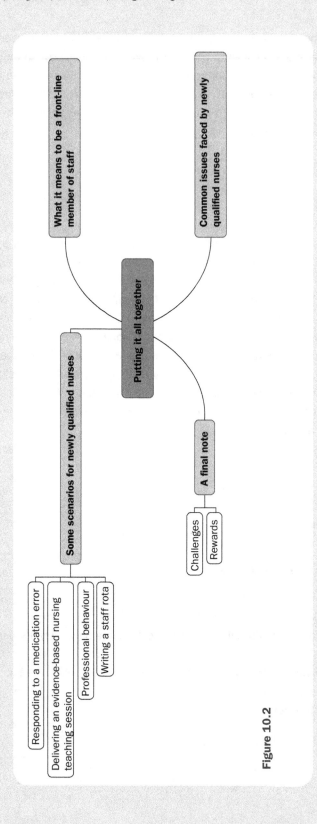

Figure 10.2

Online Resource Centre

 This textbook is accompanied by an Online Resource Centre that provides interactive learning resources and tools to help you to prepare for the transition from student to fully qualified member of staff. After you have completed each chapter and whenever you see this icon, please go to the ORC at your earliest convenience. If you have not done so already, save the ORC web address into your favourites: **http://www.oxfordtextbooks.co.uk/orc/burton**

References

Brady AM, Malone AM & Fleming S (2009) A literature review of the individual and systems factors that contribute to medication errors in nursing practice. *Journal of Nursing Management,* **17**(6): 679–97.

Commission for Nursing and Midwifery (2010) *Front Line Care: Report by the Prime Minister's Commission on the Future of Nursing and Midwifery in England.* COI, London.

Department of Health (2009) *Preceptorship Framework for Nursing.* DH, London.

Doyle J (2008) Barriers and facilitators of multidisciplinary team working: a review. *Paediatric Nursing,* **20**(2): 26–9.

Gerrish K (2000) Still fumbling along? A comparative study of the newly qualified nurse's perception of the transition from student to qualified nurse. *Journal of Advanced Nursing,* **32**(2): 473–80.

Handy C (1999) *Understanding Organisations,* 4th edn. Penguin, London.

Healy J & Spencer M (2007) *Surviving Your Placement in Health and Social Care: A Student Handbook.* McGraw-Hill, London.

Judge TA & Bono JE (2000) Five-factor model of personality and transformational leadership. *Journal of Applied Psychology,* **85**(5): 751–65.

Lewis P & Henderson E (2000) *Managing in Health and Social Care, Module 2: Managing People; Book 2: Managing Performance.* Open University Press, Milton Keynes.

Maben J & Griffiths P (2008) *Nurses in Society: Starting the Debate.* National Nursing Research Unit Kings College, London.

Marquis BL & Huston CJ (2009) *Leadership Roles and Management Functions in Nursing,* 6th edn. Wolters Kluwer & Lippincott, Williams & Wilkins, Philadelphia, PA.

Mooney M (2007) Professional socialization: the key to survival as a newly qualified nurse. *International Journal of Nursing Practice,* **13**: 75–80.

Muijs D & Reynolds D (2005) *Effective Teaching: Evidence and Practice,* 2nd edn. Sage, London.

Nursing and Midwifery Council (2008a) *Standards to Support Learning and Assessment in Practice,* 2nd edn. NMC, London.

Nursing and Midwifery Council (2008b) *The Code: Standards of Conduct, Performance and Ethics for Nurses and Midwives.* NMC, London.

Nursing and Midwifery Council (2009) *Guidance on Professional Conduct for Nursing and Midwifery Students.* NMC, London.

Nursing and Midwifery Council (2010) *Standards for Proficiency for Pre-registration Nursing Education.* NMC, London.

Phillips J (2005) Knowledge is power: using information management and leadership interventions to improve services to patients, clients and users. *Journal of Nursing Management,* **13**: 524–36.

Quinn FM & Hughes S (2007) *Quinn's Principles and Practice of Nurse Education*, 5th edn. Stanley Thornes Publishers, Cheltenham.

Race P (2001) *The Lecturer's Toolkit: A Practical Guide to Learning, Teaching and Assessment*, 2nd edn. Kogan Page, London.

Glossary of terms

A

Advanced directives Also known as advanced decisions, advanced medical decisions, or living wills, these indicate decisions made by a person, who has capacity, related to medical or surgical interventions that would be unacceptable to them in the future when they are no longer able to make decisions for themselves. The person must be at least 18 years old and the directive can only relate to *refusal* of treatment and cannot force a healthcare professional to offer specified treatment. The directive must be in writing if it relates to the refusal of life-sustaining treatment.

Advanced organizers This is information provided to a student with which to familiarize themselves before a learning event.

Advocate Somebody who acts or intercedes on behalf of another; somebody who supports or speaks in favour of someone. This is seen as a significant responsibility for nurses in their caring relationship with service users.

Autonomy The ability to think and act freely and independently or without interference. It relates to the idea of freedom and liberty, but does not mean that a person can simply act in any way they want, as the actions are also controlled by reason.

B

Beneficence The moral injunction to always do good. In health care, this means that the health professional should always do what is in the best interests of the patient.

C

Capacity A person's ability to make decisions with sufficient understanding and memory to comprehend in a general way the situation in which they find themselves and the possible consequences of the decision.

Clinical audit An evidence-gathering and quality-improvement process that seeks to improve patient care and outcomes through systematic review of care against explicit criteria. The key component of clinical audit is that performance is reviewed to ensure that what should be done is being done, and that, if not, a framework is being provided to enable improvements to be made.

Coaching A method of facilitation used to assist others in identifying goals, strategies, and resources in meeting their developmental or professional goals.

Consequentialism Ethical theories that claim that the rightness or wrongness of an act is based on the real or predicted consequences of the action.

Consumerism Consumerism in health care is based on the idea that individuals should have greater control over decisions affecting their health care. This includes empowering individuals with information and encouraging and supporting healthy behaviours.

D

Deontology An ethical framework that views *duty* as the basis of moral decision-making. The rightness or wrongness of an action is based on the action's adherence to a rule or set of rules. Compare with **consequentialism** and **utilitarianism**.

E

Emotional intelligence (EI) This is having the awareness and a set of skills recognizing that intelligence is not only about knowledge, but is also about the personal sensitivities that a person holds and having an ability to deal with others in relation to this.

Essential Skills Clusters (ESCs) Developed to help pre-registration nurses to achieve the Nursing and Midwifery Council (NMC) outcomes and proficiencies by promoting safe and effective practice, and maintaining public safety, trust, and confidence. Essential Skills Clusters have been developed for: care, compassion, and communication; organizational aspects of care; infection prevention and control; nutrition and fluid management; and medicines management.

Evidence-based practice The application of current best evidence in making decisions concerning patient care and nursing practice. It involves identifying valid, relevant, and research-based information, integrating it with clinical expertise and experience, and then implementing it in nursing practice to improve the quality of patient care. In order to practise evidence-based nursing, practitioners must understand how to accurately evaluate research.

F

Fidelity Devotion to duty or to obligations; loyalty; faithfulness.

Field of practice The discipline of nursing that an individual undertakes and becomes registered within by the Nursing and Midwifery Council (NMC). A discipline is sometimes referred to as a 'branch' of nursing. The various disciplines or branches are: adult; mental health; children's; and learning disability.

Fit to practise Defined as a person's ability to practise their profession in a way that meets appropriate standards, which means that they have the skills, knowledge, attitudes, character, and health to perform necessary functions safely and effectively.

Informed consent Legal requirement to ensure that a person knows all of the risks

and costs involved in any treatment. This includes informing them of the nature of the treatment, possible alternative treatments, and the potential risks and benefits. Informed consent can only be obtained from a person with capacity to understand the implications.

Integrated care pathway (ICP) A multi-disciplinary plan of anticipated care to help a patient with a specific condition to move progressively to positive outcomes.

Interprofessional teamworking The joint working approaches used by staff from different professions contributing to the care of individuals in the health or social care setting.

M

Mentor A registered nurse who supervises and assesses student nurses, following attendance and qualification on a recognized mentorship course.

N

Neuro-linguistic programming (NLP) The study of subjective experience. It is a set of techniques and approaches used in the fields of personal development, health, and education.

Non-maleficence Doing no harm to others. If a nurse cannot actually do good for others (beneficence), then at least they should do no harm.

Nursing and Midwifery Council (NMC) The regulatory body that sets standards for nursing and midwifery careers; the NMC holds the register onto which nurses enter on qualifying.

P

Paternalistic The practice of treating people in a fatherly manner, especially by providing for their needs, but without giving them rights or responsibilities.

Preceptor/preceptorship A qualified nurse who supervises and supports newly qualified nurses for a period of time following their registration and entry into the workforce.

Proficiency Demonstration of an ability or skill. This is used in relation to the standards set by the Nursing and Midwifery Council (NMC).

Q

Quality Assurance Agency (QAA) The organization responsible for ensuring standards of qualifications and education delivery across the higher education sector.

R

Revalidation The process by which nurses maintain their registration by demonstrating continuous practice and continuing professional development.

S

STAR approach Situation – Task – Action – Result. A technique used by interviewers to gather information about a person's capabilities and thereby their suitability for the job. It attempts to predict future performance based on the past.

SWOT analysis A strategic planning method used to evaluate the strengths, weaknesses, opportunities, and threats involved in any situation.

U

Utilitarianism Put simply, this philosophical concept promotes assessment of the rightness or wrongness of an action on its resultant 'greatest good for the greatest number'.

V

Veracity Adherence to the truth; truth-telling.

Index